IN VITRO EPITHELIA AND BIRTH DEFECTS

BOOKS PUBLISHED BY ALAN R. LISS, INC.
FOR MARCH OF DIMES BIRTH DEFECTS FOUNDATION

Birth Defects Compendium, Second Edition, Daniel Bergsma, *Editor*

BIRTH DEFECTS: ORIGINAL ARTICLE SERIES

1980 – Volume XVI

No. 1 **Enzyme Therapy in Genetic Diseases: 2,** Robert J. Desnick, *Editor*

No. 2 **In Vitro Epithelia and Birth Defects,** B. Shannon Danes, *Editor*

No. 3 **Diet in Pregnancy: A Randomized Controlled Trial of Nutritional Supplements,** by David Rush, Zena Stein, and Mervyn Susser

See pages 373–374 for other volumes in this series published by Alan R. Liss, Inc.

March of Dimes Birth Defects Foundation
Birth Defects: Original Article Series, Volume XVI, Number 2, 1980

IN VITRO EPITHELIA AND BIRTH DEFECTS

Proceedings of the workshop "Study of Human Birth Defects Using Cultured Epithelium" held at The Johns Hopkins Turner Auditorium in Baltimore, Maryland

Sponsored by the March of Dimes Birth Defects Foundation

Editor: **B. Shannon Danes, MD, PhD,** Associate Professor of Medicine, Cornell University Medical College, New York, New York

Associate Editors: *Part I*
William H. J. Douglas, PhD, Associate Professor of Anatomy, Tufts University School of Medicine, Boston, Massachusetts

Part II
Rody P. Cox, MD, Department of Medicine, Case Western Reserve University, Cleveland, Ohio

Assistant Editor: **Sue Conde Greene,** March of Dimes Birth Defects Foundation

ALAN R. LISS, INC., NEW YORK

To enhance medical communication in the birth defects field, the March of Dimes Birth Defects Foundation publishes the *Birth Defects Compendium (Second Edition)*, an *Original Article Series, Syndrome Identification,* a *Reprint Series,* and provides a series of films and related brochures.

Further information can be obtained from:

March of Dimes Birth Defects Foundation
Medical Education Division
1275 Mamaroneck Avenue
White Plains, New York 10605

Published by:

Alan R. Liss, Inc.
150 Fifth Avenue
New York, New York 10011

Views expressed in articles published are the author's, and are not to be attributed to the March of Dimes Birth Defects Foundation or its editors unless expressly so stated.

Library of Congress Cataloging in Publication Data

Main entry under title:

In vitro epithelia and birth defects.

(Birth defects original article series; v. 16, no. 2)
At head of title: March of Dimes Birth Defects Foundation
Includes bibliographical references and index.
1. Abnormalities, Human – Diagnosis – Congresses.
2. Epithelium – Congresses. 3. Epithelium – Diseases – Congresses. 4. Tissue culture – Congresses.
I. Danes, Betty Shannon, 1926– II. March of Dimes Birth Defects Foundation. III. Series: [DNLM: 1. Abnormalities – Etiology – Congresses. 2. Epithelium – Cytology – Congresses. 3. Cells, Cultured – Congresses. W1 BI96 v. 16 no. 2 QS675 I35]
RG626.B63 vol. 16, no. 2 [QM691] 616'.043s 80-7693
ISBN 0-8451-1036-5 [616'.043]

The **MARCH OF DIMES BIRTH DEFECTS FOUNDATION** is dedicated to the goal of preventing birth defects and ameliorating their consequences for patients, families, and society.

As part of our efforts to achieve these goals, we sponsor, or participate in, a variety of scientific meetings and symposia where all questions relating to birth defects are freely discussed. Through our professional educational program we speed the dissemination of information by publishing the proceedings of these meetings and symposia. From time to time, we also reprint pertinent journal articles to help achieve our goal. Now and then, in the course of these articles or discussions, individual viewpoints may be expressed which go beyond the purely scientific and into controversial matters. It should be noted, therefore, that personal viewpoints about such matters will not be censored but this does not constitute an endorsement of them by the March of Dimes Birth Defects Foundation.

Dedication

The research reported and the speculations/hopes for future research are dedicated to the families who through their participation have made and will continue to make such research possible.

The measure of this volume will be its ultimate influence on the lives of those with birth defects expressed in epithelium and of their families.

B. Shannon Danes, MD, PhD

Contents

Contributors

Howard P. Baden, Professor, Department of Dermatology, Massachusetts General Hospital, Boston, MA 02114 **[175]**

Alexander G. Bearn, Department of Medicine, Cornell University Medical College, New York, NY 10021. Present Address: Senior Vice President for Medical and Scientific Affairs, Merck, Sharp and Dohme, International, Rahway, NJ 07065 **[283]**

Paul J. Benke, Director of Clinical Genetics, Mailman Center and Department of Pediatrics, University of Miami School of Medicine, Miami, FL 33101 **[155]**

Michel Bergeron, Professor, Department of Physiology, Faculty of Medicine, University of Montreal, Montreal, Quebec, Canada H3C 3T8 **[305]**

D. Montgomery Bissell, Assistant Professor of Medicine, San Francisco General Hospital, San Francisco, CA 94110 **[283]**

Pablo Bringas, Jr., Research Senior Technician, Laboratory for Developmental Biology, University of Southern California, Los Angeles, CA 90007 **[211]**

Sharen L. Carey, Investigator, ALS Foundation, La Jolla, CA 92037 **[35]**

Graham Carpenter, Research Assistant Professor, Departments of Medicine and Biochemistry, Division of Dermatology, Vanderbilt University School of Medicine, Nashville, TN 37232 **[61]**

Rody P. Cox, Department of Medicine, New York University Medical Center, New York, NY 10016. Present Address: Department of Medicine, Case Western Reserve University, V.A. Medical Center, Cleveland, OH 44106 **[129, 361]**

B. Shannon Danes, Associate Professor of Medicine, Cornell University Medical College, New York, NY 10021 **[109, 275, 365]**

Monte A. Del Monte, Fellow in Ophthalmic Genetics, The Wilmer Institute, The Johns Hopkins Hospital, Baltimore, MD 21205 **[315, 327]**

Thomas I. Doran, Postdoctoral Fellow, Department of Dermatology, The Johns Hopkins Medical School, Baltimore, MD 21205 **[183]**

William H.J. Douglas, Associate Professor, Department of Anatomy, Tufts University School of Medicine, Boston, MA 02111 **[73, 161]**.

The number in brackets following each contributor's name is the opening page number of that author's paper.

Robert J. Fallon, Fellow, Medical Scientist Training Program, Department of Pharmacology, New York University Medical Center, New York, NY 10016 **[129]**

Diane K. Fast, Postdoctoral Fellow, De Belle Laboratory for Biochemical Genetics, McGill University-Montreal Children's Hospital Research Institute, Montreal, Quebec, Canada H3H 1P3 **[305]**

Jeanette S. Felix, Assistant Professor of Pediatrics, The Johns Hopkins Hospital, Baltimore, MD 21205 **[231]**

Ronald D. Fletcher, Professor and Associate Head, Department of Microbiology, University of Pittsburgh, School of Medicine, Pittsburgh, PA 15261 **[121]**

Aaron E. Freeman, Scientist, La Jolla Cancer Research Foundation, La Jolla, CA 92037 **[35, 169]**

Nimai K. Ghosh, Research Associate Professor, Department of Medicine, New York University Medical Center, New York, NY 10016 **[129]**

Robert J. Gorlin, Regents' Professor and Chairman, Department of Oral Pathology and Genetics, University of Minnesota School of Dentistry, Minneapolis, MN 55455 **[345]**

Martin Grodin, Research Technician, Laboratory for Developmental Biology, University of Southern California, Los Angeles, CA 90007 **[211]**

Fritz Herz, Associate Professor of Pathology, Montefiore Hospital and Medical Center, Bronx, NY 10467 **[85]**

Elvin A. Kabat, Professor, Department of Microbiology, College of Physicians and and Surgeons, Columbia University, New York, NY 10032 **[339]**

Winston W.-Y. Kao, Assistant Professor, Ophthalmology Research, Eye and Ear Hospital of Pittsburgh, Pittsburgh, PA 15213 **[53]**

Randall H. Kottel, Cell Biologist, La Jolla Cancer Research Foundation, La Jolla, CA 92037 **[35]**

Anne J. Krush, Assistant Professor of Medicine, Division of Medical Genetics, Johns Hopkins University School of Medicine, Baltimore, MD 21205 **[353]**

Joseph Kubilus, Research Associate, Department of Dermatology, Massachusetts General Hospital, Boston, MA 02114 **[175]**

MaryAnn C. Labant, Research Assistant, Department of Microbiology, University of Pittsburgh, School of Medicine, Pittsburgh, PA 15261 **[121]**

John W. Littlefield, Professor and Chairman, Department of Pediatrics, The Children's Medical and Surgical Center, The Johns Hopkins Hospital, Baltimore, MD 21205 **[231]**

Irene H. Maumenee, Assistant Professor of Ophthalmology and Medicine, The Wilmer Institute, The Johns Hopkins Hospital, Baltimore, MD 21205 **[315, 327]**

James A. McAteer, Department of Anatomy, Tufts University School of Medicine, Boston, MA 02111. Present Address: Assistant Professor of Anatomy, University of Virginia, School of Medicine, Charlottesville, VA 22909 **[73]**

Victor A. McKusick, Chairman, Department of Medicine, The Johns Hopkins Hospital, Baltimore, MD 21205 [**1**]

Barbara R. Migeon, Professor of Pediatrics, The Johns Hopkins University, School of Medicine, Baltimore, MD 21205 [**239**]

Orlando J. Miller, Professor, Department of Human Genetics and Development, College of Physicians and Surgeons, Columbia University, New York, NY 10032 [**339**]

Edmond A. Murphy, Professor of Medicine, The Moore Clinic, The Johns Hopkins Hospital, Baltimore, MD 21205 [**355**]

Marian R. Neutra, Assistant Professor of Anatomy, Harvard Medical School, Boston, MA 02115 [**261**]

Harold M. Nitowsky, Professor of Pediatrics and Genetics, Albert Einstein College of Medicine, Yeshiva University, Bronx, NY 10461 [**293**]

Stephanie Phillips, Research Associate, Department of Human Genetics and Development, College of Physicians and Surgeons, Columbia University, New York, NY 10032 [**339**]

Theresa P. Pretlow, Research Assistant Professor, Department of Pathology, The University of Alabama in Birmingham, University Station, Birmingham, AL 35294 [**95**]

Thomas G. Pretlow II, Professor, Department of Pathology, University of Alabama in Birmingham, University Station, Birmingham, AL 35294 [**95**]

Darwin J. Prockop, Chairman, Department of Biochemistry, College of Medicine and Dentistry of New Jersey, Rutgers Medical School, Piscataway, NJ 08854 [**53**]

Keen A. Rafferty, Jr., Professor, Department of Anatomy, College of Medicine, The University of Illinois at the Medical Center, Chicago, IL 60612 [**5**]

Charles R. Scriver, Professor of Biology and Pediatrics, De Belle Laboratory for Biochemical Genetics, McGill University-Montreal Children's Hospital Research Institute, Montreal, Quebec, Canada H3H 1P3 [**305**]

Seung-il Shin, Associate Professor, Department of Genetics, Albert Einstein College of Medicine, Bronx, NY 10461 [**145**]

Olli Simell, Department of Pediatrics, Helsinki University, Central Hospital, Helsinki, Finland [**305**]

Harold C. Slavkin, Professor of Biochemistry, Laboratory for Developmental Biology, University of Southern California, Los Angeles, CA 90007 [**211**]

Barry T. Smith, Assistant Professor of Paediatrics, Obstetrics and Gynaecology and Physiology, Queen's University, Kingston, Ontario, Canada K7L 3N6 [**249**]

Tung-Tien Sun, Department of Dermatology, The Johns Hopkins Medical School, Baltimore, MD 21205 [**183**]

A. Keith Tanswell, Assistant Professor of Paediatrics, Queen's University, Kingston, Ontario, Canada K7L 3N6 [**249**]

Louis Terracio, Research Associate, Department of Anatomy, Tufts University School of Medicine, Boston, MA 02111 **[161]**

Alda Vidrich, Postdoctoral Fellow, Department of Dermatology, The Johns Hopkins Medical School, Baltimore, MD 21205 **[183]**

Carl J. Witkop, Jr., Professor and Chairman, Division of Human and Oral Genetics, University of Minnesota, School of Dentistry, Minneapolis, MN 55455 **[197]**

Marie Yamada, Postdoctoral Fellow, Laboratory for Developmental Biology, University of Southern California, Los Angeles, CA 90007 **[211]**

Yutaka Yoshida, Pathologist, La Jolla Cancer Research Foundation, La Jolla, CA 92037 **[35]**

Foreword

I am personally delighted that Baltimore and Hopkins were picked as the site for this workshop. Hopkins is an appropriate place for this workshop because much of cell culture had its beginnings here – with Ross Harrison, Warren Lewis, George Gey, and others [1]. This is also the birthplace of the HeLa cell, derived just across the street in 1951 from Henrietta Lacks [2, 3].

The success of fibroblast cultures from skin biopsies in metabolic research is now well known. It is an important chapter in human biochemical genetics. David Harnden [4] has recently told the background of his 1960 paper [5] describing fibroblast culture for chromosome studies -- first on a piece of skin from his own arm. Certainly having logistic advantages over bone marrow material, it was shortly superseded, in the area of chromosome studies, by Hungerford's blood lymphocyte culture method. Nonetheless, a pleasant surprise was the discovery of the wide enzymatic repertory of cultured skin fibroblasts. In relation to homocystinuria, for example, normal skin on direct assay showed little activity of the relevant enzyme, and liver biopsy was considered necessary for enzymatic characterization of the disorder. Fortunately, Uhlendorf and Mudd [6] found that fibroblasts cultured from the same skin do show appreciable enzyme activity and that this activity is missing in homocystinuric fibroblasts.

It would be rewarding to repeat this success story with cultured epithelial cells. It is not necessary for anyone to speak long on the potential usefulness of that in the study of a large body of birth defects. The task clearly is a more difficult one, but in the process much may be learned about differentiation of epithelial tissues.

Victor A. McKusick, MD

Birth Defects: Original Article Series, Volume XVI, Number 2, pages 1–2

REFERENCES

1. Harvey AM: Johns Hopkins – The birthplace of tissue culture: The story of Ross G. Harrison, Warren H. Lewis and George O. Gey. Johns Hopkins Med J 136:142-149, 1975.
2. Jones HW Jr, McKusick VA, Harper PS, Wuu KD: The HeLa cell and a reappraisal of its origin. Obstet Gynecol 38:945-949, 1971.
3. Hsu SH, Schacter BZ, Delaney NL, Miller TB, McKusick VA, Kennett RH, Bodmer JG, Young D, Bodmer WF: Genetic characteristics of the HeLa cell. Science 191:392-394, 1976.
4. Harnden DG: Citation classics. (Letter) Current Contents (Life Sciences) 21(50):9, 1978.
5. Harnden DG: A human skin culture technique used for cytological examinations. Br J Exp Pathol 41:31-37, 1960.
6. Uhlendorf BW, Mudd SH: Cystathionine synthase in tissue culture derived from human skin: Enzyme defect in homocystinuria. Science 160:1007-1009, 1968.

PART I:
Proposed Systems for Study of Human Birth Defects Expressed in Epithelium

Methods in Hand: Classic Tissue Culture*

Keen A. Rafferty, Jr., PhD

I. INTRODUCTION

Review articles usually begin with exculpatory disclaimers, and the present is no exception. First, the scope of this review is not limited to epithelial cells, as the title of this volume implies that it should be, but instead deals broadly with organ parenchymal cells, comparing these with stromal cells of tissues and organs. This inevitably points up the contrast between the spectacular successes in fibroblast culture and the occasional triumph in the culture of most other cell types. For example, on the one hand, the catalog of the American Type Culture Collection [1] lists 171 currently available strains of fibroblasts derived from patients with congenital disease syndromes. On the other hand, no diploid epithelial strains of human origin are listed, and virtually all of the permanent, aneuploid, human epithelial lines have been identified as HeLa cell contaminants [2, 3]. To top this, no human genetic or developmental disorder has yet been detected through the examination of epithelial cells, in spite of the obvious fact that many such disorders involve the maldevelopment or malfunction of epithelial and other parenchymal cells. The argument for dealing with parenchymal cells as a group stems from the need to learn as much as we can about such cell types, in the hope that transfer of knowledge will be helpful.

The second disclaimer has to do with the matter of completeness concerning methodology, since organ culture methods are omitted entirely. The omission seems to be required by several factors, notably the immensity of the literature on both organ and cell and tissue culture, the rather fundamental differences in approach and objectives for the 2 techniques, and the fact that organ culture

*Supported in part by grant CA-13494 from the US National Cancer Institute.

Birth Defects: Original Article Series, Volume XVI, Number 2, pages 5–34

systems will be dealt with by others in this volume. This review will be limited, therefore, to parenchymal cell systems in which the goal is the propagation and study of cells in "pure" systems, in which cells are attached to solid substrates.

Although these methods have not been useful to date in practical clinical application, the message at the outset is that hardly any approach bears more promise for the future: there are numerous examples of the successful long-term cultivation of many parenchymal cell types (including epithelial cells in the strictest sense), and the prospects for the study of birth defects and genetic disease by these methods seem bright indeed. A principal conclusion of this paper will be that successes have generally involved close attention to methodology, often tailoring the technique to the characteristics of the particular cell type under study. Although many workers (for example, Wigley [4]) feel that the differentiated functions of parenchymal cells are usually lost in culture, we shall see that exceptions to the rule are so numerous as to indict the rule itself.

With these observations, specific discussion can begin on a very optimistic note.

II. PROBLEM SOLVING STRATEGIES

A. "Pure" Tissue Sources

An obvious way to eliminate fibroblast contamination of culture systems is to select tissues which lack them. Ideally, these consist of a single cell type, or at least of only one type that grows under the culture conditions.

1. Lymphocytes

It has been known for many years [5] that whole blood can produce lymphocyte cultures, but success has been spotty until the past decade. Moore and McLimans have had routine success [6] for years, while efforts in many other laboratories failed. Finally, it was realized that the key to development of permanent lines of lymphocytes lies in care in handling and in patience [7] : often 2 months are required to initiate lymphocyte lines, and during this period it is important to avoid shock from medium changes and from handling procedures. With this understanding, it seems to be the consensus of most workers in the field that a permanent line can be initiated from peripheral blood of almost any human individual. It is also believed that all such lines are infected by Epstein-Barr virus [8] , although not all liberate infectious virus into the medium. Nevertheless, since this agent is oncogenic, appropriate procedures must be used in handling such cultures [9] .

2. Mesothelial Cells

Normal and malignant cell strains have been initiated from aspirated pericardial effusions obtained from cancer patients or from those with inflammatory conditions [10] . Apparently normal as well as neoplastic cultures grew well under routine conditions but unfortunately were not followed for long term.

3. *Amnion*

Amnion culture has been one of the most frustrating of all approaches to the culture of epithelial cells, since this rich source has not produced any permanent lines in spite of repeated attempts (all claimed lines of human origin have been indicted as HeLa cell contaminants [3]). Some workers have achieved as many as 25 population doublings from such cultures, but this follows stationary phases of many months and intervals of slow growth [11, 12]. Since division potential has been demonstrated, and is about the equivalent of diploid fibroblasts isolated from human newborns, it would seem evident that this is an ideal system for the development of a specific medium which might also be useful in the long-term culture of other kinds of epithelial cells (see Media, p 000).

4. *Body Fluids*

a. Milk: Somewhat surprisingly, breast fluids expressed from human and primate subjects are rather rich in epithelial cells which grow fairly vigorously, without any very special precautions, at least for short periods [13, 14]. Rie and co-workers [15] initiated epithelial cell cultures from breast fluids of baboons aged 10–12 years. Using subcultures at the ratio of 1:2 they propagated the strain for only 7 passages but were able to accumulate 5×10^7 cells thereby.

b. Urine: This source also produces rather vigorously growing cells in short-term culture when human newborns are the donors [16–18]. Although the cells are epithelial, their origin is unknown: a urothelial source would seem obvious, except that what is known of the growth of other epithelia in situ would make it appear unlikely that cells with mitotic potential would be released into the urine from this source. One difficulty with such cultures is that adults are poor donors, as are some individual infants. Hence, the method cannot be used dependably to establish cell lines, but success in development of short-term cultures is frequent. Microbial contamination is a problem in cultures initiated from female donors.

c. Peritoneal Exudate: Induced in animals by the injection of thioglycolate medium, the exudate contains mononuclear cells that do not usually appear to be present in the peritoneal cavity [19]. Moreover, they are capable of growing in soft agar if conditioned medium is used, suggesting that they may be hemopoietic elements. Later work, in which cell growth was augmented by use of medium conditioned by mouse L cells, indicated that the cells were in fact macrophages, since they readily engulfed erythrocytes [20].

B. Exclusion of Cell Types by Dissection

Perhaps next best to the use of uncontaminated cell sources is the use of tissues which can be rather easily dissected to remove unwanted cells. It should be remembered in this respect that complete elimination of fibroblasts is often not necessary, since kinetic considerations mean that fibroblasts present in small numbers may exhaust their division potential without being able to repopulate the cell strain.

1. Retinal Pigment Cells

Originally cultured from chick embryos, these can be peeled off the sclera from the inside of the orb after the retina is first removed, and yield cell populations with little or no contamination with other cell types [21]. These grow vigorously, although they are limited in their in vitro life-span. An interesting feature of such cell strains is their continued production of melanin in culture, an obviously useful factor in characterization and identification. It also illustrates the point that cell strains often retain functional characteristics in culture, contrary to some theories and expectations.

The method has also been applied successfully to human retinal pigment cell culture. Mannagh et al [22], using human donor eyes found unsuitable for corneal transplant, removed the anterior portion (including the vitreous) and peeled the retina from the pigment cell layer with a scalpel. The posterior segment was then filled with pronase in saline free of divalent cations, and the pigment cells were pipetted off after an incubation period. Primary cultures were heavily pigmented, but pigment tended to diminish in subcultured strains. A remarkable observation is that 7 such strains eventually gave rise to heteroploid (presumably permanent) cell lines, some of which occasionally produced pigment. The anterior pigmented region (the uveal tract) of human eyes was used by Giovanella et al [23]. Minces of the tract were trypsinized, and most fibroblasts were preferentially removed by transferring suspensions to new vessels early in primary culture, taking advantage of the fact that fibroblasts attach more rapidly. Fibroblast colonies that did develop in later primary cultures were differentially removed. This method gave some melanin-producing strains which were serially propagated.

2. Endothelium

These cells are obtained from the endothelial lining of aortic arches or umbilical veins of fetal calves, by rubbing them off the surface with a cotton swab [24–26]. Growth is vigorous in the presence of fibroblast growth factor, and secondary cultures can readily be cloned by the cylinder method. Strains initiated in this manner can be continuously subcultured for months, possibly becoming aneuploid in later passages. This method was first applied by Lewis et al [27] to endothelial cells derived from human umbilical veins. These were scraped off, trypsinized, and cultured in an enriched medium (but one lacking growth factors in addition to those present in the serum supplement). The doubling time was 40 hours, and subcultures were made at split ratios of 1:6 for at least 5 serial passages, a minimum of 13 population doublings. The cells were characterized by demonstrating the presence of ABO blood group antigens and of thrombosthenin.

3. Smooth Muscle

Smooth muscle cells are obtained from the same material that yields endothelial cells, by continuing the erosion of the vessel wall after the endothelial cells have been removed [24]. In this case, a surgical scalpel is used to scrape away the tunica intima (which is essentially acellular) and to dissect off fragments of smooth muscle. These may then be cultured as fragments from which smooth muscle cells migrate, or dissociated by digestion with collagenase. As in the case of endothelial cells, secondary cultures may be cloned and continuously subcultured for a number of generations. Both epidermal and fibroblastic growth factors are effective in promoting growth [25].

4. Chondroblasts

Dissociation of chick embryo cartilage after dissecting away the perichondrium gives cultures of uncontaminated chondroblasts which can be plated at clonal density in primary culture with the addition of embryo extract to the medium [28]. Colonies of these cells produce sulfated mucopolysaccharides (detected by staining with metachromatic dyes), but only after an interval following culture or subculture, and only at the center of the colonies. Hence, this differentiated feature is expressed only in crowded, presumably contact-inhibited, cells, and not in sparse, rapidly growing, cultures. A factor in clonal growth of chick embryo cells which may need to be taken into account is the fact that the doubling potential is only about 25. Since about 21 doublings are required for a single cell to populate a small tissue culture flask (2×10^6 cells), most of the doubling potential is exhausted by cloning itself. Hence, cloned cultures cannot be used to establish cell strains.

5. Colon

Of particular interest is the success reported by Lycette and Whyte [29] in developing primary cultures of vigorously growing epithelial cells derived from adult bovine colon obtained at slaughter. Surprisingly, repeated washing with sterile saline reduced the bacterial count to the point where the medium antibiotics were apparently able to control microbial contamination. The mucosa was scraped off, minced, and trypsinized with a mucolytic agent, after which washed pellets of cells were seeded in culture flasks. Unfortunately, the cells were subcultured only once and no attempt was made to follow them for long periods. They were characterized by the production of periodic acid: Schiff-positive mucin. The method was applied successfully to human colon as well.

It remains to be seen whether microbial contamination can be controlled in long-term cultures from such sources. In any case, it would certainly seem advisable to test for the presence of mycoplasma contamination in apparently clean cultures, and possibly to use antibiotics (such as kanamycin and gentamycin) which are helpful in controlling such growth.

6. Neuroglia

A number of reports have established that human and animal normal neuroglia and glioma cells (the former obtained from wound debridement or surgery for hematoma or aneurysm) grow well with no special precautions. Experience with long-term cultures of human origin [30] demonstrated a limited doubling potential on the order of that observed with human diploid fibroblasts taken from adults. Cultures initiated from brain tissue might be expected to have some fibroblasts, since these are present in the medium-sized and smaller blood vessels. In fact, however, it appears to be comparatively easy to identify and dissect out such sources of contaminating cells, and fibroblast overgrowth has not been reported as a problem [31].

Glial cell cultures can also be initiated from chick embryo neural plate and brain [32]. Postmitotic neural cells are eliminated on subculture. Cultures from embryos of 36 hours or less contain proliferating neural precursor cells which terminally differentiate in the presence of glial cells, and are thus eliminated [32]. In cultures on plastic surfaces, oligodendrocytes also tend to degenerate eventually, but the identification of the remaining cells is sometimes in question. Extracts of brain [33] or mesenchymal tissue, and medium conditioned on other glial cell cultures, stimulate some differentiation in glial cultures, but this stops short of the formation of myelin [32]. Epidermal growth factor effectively stimulates proliferation in glial cell cultures [34]. A number of lines and strains from human and rodent sources are available [35].

7. Neuronal Cells

Cell lines thought to be of neuronal origin were intitated from brain tissue of mouse embryos, using thimerosal (see Heavy Metal Compounds, p 16) to discourage growth of fibroblasts and certain glial cell populations [36]. It is not clear how thoroughly these were characterized, or whether they terminally differentiated in culture.

8. Urothelium

The cells of transitional epithelium of bladder and kidney have shown good growth ability in vitro. Using human surgical tissue, Peterson et al [37] dissected the mucosa from the lamina propria. The epithelium was minced and fragments affixed to the culture vessel surface by compression beneath coverslips, after which sheets of cells migrated over the surface. Fibroblasts are presumed to be present in such tissue, but migration of the epithelial cell sheet tends to enclose the fragment and prevent the migration of fibroblasts (see Encapsulation of Fibroblasts, p 14. Stone et al [38] used a similar technique with epithelia from both bladder and kidney, but reported extensive success in subculturing: kidney epithelium was carried for 45 serial passages, and bladder epithelium for 70 subcultures, presumably representing at least that many population doublings. Roszell et al [39] everted rat urinary bladders on syringe needles, inflated them, and incubated them at 4°C for 4 hours, after which they were shaken at 37°C for 5–7 minutes. This technique of partial digestion released epithelial cells that were readily cultured and carried through at least 5 subcultivations. A factor in this system was the requirement of the polyamines, putrescine, spermine, and spermidine, for maximum growth.

9. Lens Epithelium

Epithelial cells are easily dissected from the lens and have proven readily able to grow in culture. Using calf lenses from eyes collected on ice at the time of slaughter, van Venrooij and co-workers [40] incubated them in collagenase and dispersed the lens cells by stirring. Since lens fibers are postmitotic, there is no opportunity for contamination by other cells once the lens is removed from the eye. Another method used was to dissect the inert capsule and lens epithelial sheet from the lens and to dissociate it by squirting through a syringe needle. Capsule fragments were subsequently removed when media were changed. Explants of undissociated epithelial sheets were also found effective. These strains were serially subcultivated at 1:3 split ratios about 50 times, or approximately 79 population doublings (personal communication, van Venrooij). The cells were shown to synthesize crystallins throughout their culture history, so presumably some cells were continually undergoing terminal differentiation, possibly being lost at subcultivation. These workers [41] also showed that the synthetic glucocorticoid, dexamethasone, caused cells in long-term culture to elongate and orient parallel to each other, somewhat as they do during lens fiber formation, without altering the synthesis of crystallins. Taylor-Papadimitriou et al [42] repeated this work, using epithelial sheets stripped off the lens. They observed much lower division potential [5–8] which was increased by the use of mitomycin C-killed 3T6 feeder layers. Using dissociated epithelium from chick lenses, Eguchi et al [43] observed the development of lentoid bodies. Hence, lens cells show pronounced retention of their ability to differentiate in culture, as well as good growth potential.

10. Myoepithelial Cells

Hackett and colleagues [44] developed cell lines from neoplastic human breast tissue. One cell line, initiated from tissue adjacent to the tumor masses, proved to be diploid and had the characteristics of myoepithelial cells. This line, derived from a 74-year-old donor, went through at least 30 population doublings.

C. Clonal Analysis

Cloning from primary culture is an elegant technique for obtaining strains of cells from mixed tissues and for eliminating fibroblasts or other cells that tend to overgrow the cultures. This method suffers from the fact that the doubling potential of the cells is more-or-less exhausted in the production of a single flask of cells from typical sources (ie chick or adult human), or else selects heavily for aneuploid cells in the case of species that transform spontaneously. It is also a method that requires meticulous attention to medium composition and culture conditions, both of which must usually be worked out through repeated experimental trials in which these factors are tailored to the particular cell type and species. Frequently, special additives, such as embryo extract, are required, but sometimes they are found to be deleterious. In each case, special lots of fetal calf serum are selected by testing them in clonal density cultures with the cells to be studied. Careful attention must be paid to such factors as water quality and pH, and many workers advocate preparation of media in the laboratory from the basic chemicals. Aside from possibly giving more reliable results, this approach permits varying the composition of the media. Surprisingly, most clonal analysis to date from primary cultures has not involved the direct addition of hormones or growth factors, but these may be presumed to be present in the sera and other additives, especially embryo extract.

1. Liver

Coon [45] developed a number of epithelial cell lines from rat liver by clonal density techniques and applied the method to a variety of other cell types, ie salivary gland, thyroid, pancreas, spleen, kidney, cardiac muscle, and skeletal muscle. The liver cell lines were aneuploid but nevertheless were shown to produce and liberate into the medium a number of proteins which corresponded electrophoretically to some serum albumins from the same species. Although this is not absolute proof that the proteins are identical, these cell lines can grow quite well in the complete absence of serum and support the growth of other cells as well, constituting the best evidence that they are indeed hepatocytes and capable of producing critical serum constituents. The products of these lines were treated as growth factors by Smith and Temin [46], who referred to their action as "multiplication-stimulating activity" (MSA) (see p 18). Kaighn and Prince [47] and Kaighn [48] developed strains of cells from human liver, using similar methods. Although these produced proteins which matched some of the electrophoretic bands from human serum, the cultures resembled those of fibroblasts or at least consisted of elongated cells. The method involved tissue dispersal in a mixture of chicken serum, trypsin, and crude collagenase.

2. Prostatic Epithelium

This approach was used by Kaighn and Babcock [49] to develop strains of epithelial cells from normal and hyperplastic human prostatic tissue. A strain of similar morphology derived from benign hyperplasia was shown to be positive for tartrate-inhibited acid phosphatase. Although this suggests origin from the glandular components, it is not conclusive.

3. Type II Pneumocytes

Using basically the same methods, with gentle dissociation by rocking the lung tissue fragments in the enzyme mixture, followed by pipetting to liberate cells, Douglas and Kaighn [50] established epithelial strains by cloning from primary cultures. The occurrence of specific cellular organelles (multilamellar bodies) in these strains strongly suggested their identity as the producers of pulmonary surfactant, or as type II pneumocytes (great alveolar cells or granular pneumocytes). Kniazeff et al [51] produced similar cultures from cat fetuses near term, cloning in conditioned medium by the cylinder method. These underwent 55 subcultures before being lost.

4. Pancreas

Wilson [52], using newly weaned rabbits, obtained epithelial cell cultures of pancreas with no particular attention to the elimination of fibroblasts except for careful dissection. Mass cultures produced lipase, amylase, insulin, and glucagon activities, although these functions dwindled rapidly and had disappeared in 4 days. However, when primary digests were aggregated in a gyratory shaker, they preserved these functions for 28 days, the longest interval tested. By means of aggregation, function could be recovered from mass monolayer cultures, but only up to the ninth day. Cells could be cloned from low density cultures, but it was not possible to show hormonal or enzymatic activity, presumably because of the rapid disappearance of function. It would be interesting to initiate such cultures in media conditioned by fibroblasts, or containing certain growth factors or hormones.

5. Skeletal Muscle

Chick embryo myoblasts were cultured at low density by Konigsberg [53]. These divided well in culture but fused to become postmitotic myotubes as the cell density increased. Fibroblast-like cells present in the cultures did not participate in this fusion, indicating that the myoblasts were embryologically determined by the developmental stage used.

6. Glial and Neuroblastoma Cells

Glial cells of human and rodent origin may be cloned directly in primary culture [54], and a number of such lines exist (see Pfeiffer et al [35] for review). Many of these have distinguishing characteristics, although it is not always certain from which cell type they are derived. Neurons from normal tissue do not survive in "pure" culture [32], but rodent and human neuroblastoma cells lend themselves somewhat readily to cloning, and a number of strains and permanent lines are available which show various combinations of differentiated properties [55]. Fedoroff [54] identifies 6 different colony morphologies in primary cultures seeded at clonal density with cells derived from mouse cerebral hemisphere dissociated by forcing the tissue through Nitex.

Postmitotic neurons from normal tissue may be studied in primary cultures but ordinarily become overgrown by glial elements. Fluorodeoxyuridine has been used to prevent or retard such overgrowth [56].

D. Selective Removal of Fibroblasts in Primary or Secondary Culture

1. Encapsulation of Fibroblasts

This method depends for its success on the imprisonment of fibroblasts in the center of a tissue fragment through the migration and extension of the epithelial sheet to enclose the fibroblasts in the center, with the sheet then continuing to migrate on the culture surface. Fibroblasts can then be removed completely by removing the original explant. We have seen that this method was successful with urothelium [37, 38]. At an earlier date, Flaxman et al [57] developed epithelial cultures from human skin and buccal mucosa but were unable to subculture them successfully. Subsequent studies [58, 59] have indicated that epidermal cell subculture requires conditioning factors or possibly culture surfaces with dermis-like physical features.

Epithelial cell cultures were obtained by partial encapsulation in explants of mouse mandibular salivary gland, with migration enhanced by addition of insulin and hydrocortisone [60]. Subculture of the epithelial cells was unsuccessful, however, with the culture vessels being rapidly overgrown by "mesenchymal" cells.

2. Differential Trypsinization

Rheinwald and Green [58] cultured human keratinocytes by enzymatic dissociation of skin after the removal of as much dermis as possible, through preliminary dissection. Cells from dissociated tissues were mixed with irradiated 3T3 mouse fibroblasts and hydrocortisone, and seeded in culture vessels. The epidermal cells form colonies directly on the vessel surface, with the fibroblasts (both irradiated 3T3 and contaminating human) forming sheets around them. Fibroblasts are then removed, since they detach more rapidly than epithelial cells, by pipetting with a trypsin-EDTA mixture, then removing the epidermal cells with a second application of enzyme. In later experiments [61] contaminating fibroblasts were completely removed by 2 successive differential trypsinizations. The later experiments also indicated that growth is improved by the addition of epidermal growth factor, and that feeder layers could be dispensed with by using conditioned medium.

The cultures were shown to produce keratins and were diploid. Keratinocytes from newborn donors underwent 25–51 population doublings before the cultures deteriorated, and those from individuals aged 3–34 years terminated after 20–27 doublings. As noted, melanocytes [23] can also be isolated in culture by selective removal of fibroblast colonies.

In a series of experiments, remarkable results were obtained with this method, by Owens [14] and Owens et al [62], using a variety of normal and neoplastic epithelial tissues of human and murine origin, ie skin, kidney, bladder, and fetal intestine. In general, these were dissociated by incubating fragments in collagenase overnight and then pipetting. Cell clumps, which consisted largely of epithelial cells, were removed with some selectivity by allowing them to settle out rapidly.

Fibroblasts that persisted in subsequent cultures were removed by the trypsin-EDTA method. Depending upon the source, the cultures then survived for 7–35 subcultivations as epithelial cells.

3. Differential Adhesion

Although fibroblasts are among the first cells to detach from culture surfaces, they are also the first to attach. Kasten [63] exploited this property by culturing digests of rat cardiac tissue in Rose chambers, which are enclosed by 2 apposed coverslips. In this case, the problem was the separation of endothelial cells from myoblasts. When the chambers were incubated in one position for 90 minutes, and then turned over for a longer incubation period, it was found that endothelial cells attached first on the surface, originally in the down position. The chambers could then be dismantled and the slips cultured separately, but overgrowth of myoblasts by endothelial cells eventually occurred. It is also possible to seed culture vessels serially with cell suspensions for predetermined intervals, transferring the remaining unattached cells to new vessels.

As noted earlier, selective removal and differential adhesion seldom accomplish the removal of all fibroblasts (or other offending cells) but succeed by reason of the fact that such cells cannot dominate cultures if they are initially reduced to a small number, since they often lack an adequate population doubling potential: in fact, many fibroblast clones have rather low doubling potentials [64].

4. Progressive Digestion

Gaffney et al [65] obtained cultures enriched in epithelial cells by progressive digestion of normal human mammary tissue obtained through reduction mammoplasty or even through autopsy. Minces were digested in collagenase, but only for a limited time, with the finding that stromal cells were liberated more slowly. Predominantly epithelial primary cultures were kept for as long as 2 months, but were contaminated by fibroblasts and could not be subcultured successfully. A similar method was used by Raul et al [66] to provide cultures of villus and crypt cells from rat intestine. Segments of intestine of young rats were removed, everted, and incubated in a mixture of versene and dithiothreitol. These were then incubated, with shaking on a gyratory shaker. Serial harvests were made at 10-minute intervals, each being used to initiate a single culture. With time, the relative proportion of villus to crypt cells decreased. This was shown by means of tritiated thymidine incorporation, since cells of the villi are postmitotic. It is not clear whether fibroblast contamination was a problem in these experiments. As noted earlier, a similar method gave epithelial cultures from urinary bladders [39].

5. Mechanical Disaggregation After Enzymatic Digestion.

Some workers feel that epithelial cells are vulnerable to proteolytic enzymes, particularly while tissue fragments are being digested: presumably, this is the result of the disruption of tight junctions and desmosomes. At any rate, some tissues, especially embryonic ones, seem to yield more and healthier epithelial cells by mincing alone or in combination with collagenase digestion. Lasfargues and Ozzello [67] seem to have been the first to use this method, which they referred to as the "spilling" technique. Using human surgical material from carcinoma, gastrointestinal and urinary epithelia, Owens et al [14, 62] minced them with scalpels into 2-mm fragments and incubated them in purified collagenase at 37° C for 18–24 hours. The suspensions were then pipetted to break up the fragments as much as possible. This resulted in the liberation of clumps of epithelial cells and more-or-less completely dispersed fibroblast elements. After allowing a short interval for the clumps to settle, about 90% of the medium (and most of the fibroblasts) could be removed by careful aspiration. This method yielded epithelial islands (interspersed with fibroblasts) about 40% of the time. Fibroblasts were then selectively detached with a trypsinversene mixture, which was also used for subcultivation of the epithelial cell cultures. All proved to consist of rather slowly growing cells, however. The method was applied successfully to various tissues from fetal to adult mice (skin, ovary, liver, mammary gland), although these cultures rapidly became aneuploid.

E. Biochemical Selection

1. Heavy Metal Compounds

Braaten and co-workers [68] pioneered the use of several organic compounds containing heavy metals (notably mercury and gold) as cytotoxic elements with some differential action on fibroblasts. These are usually regarded as toxic for epithelial cells as well, but less so. They seem to exert their effect through reversible inhibition of sulfhydryl enzymes, since the cytotoxic action of the mercury compounds is inhibited by glutathione. This group has applied the method to isolated islets of Langerhans, which yield epithelial cells cultures of endocrine cells virtually free of fibroblasts. An important consideration is to add the inhibitor as the culture is initiated, and then to remove it in a few days. Fibroblasts are reported to be killed, while epithelial cells are able to recover. The compound most frequently used was sodium ethylmercurithiosalicylate, known as thimerosal.

This method was used by Bulloch et al [36] to derive neuronal cell cultures from mouse embryonic brain, with the observation that thimerosal removed some glial cell populations as well as fibroblasts, if added in 2–3 day pulses: they reported, in fact, that neuronal cells actually seemed to be stimulated to grow by thimerosal.

The method does not, however, seem to work with all epithelial sources of tissue, and there is controversy concerning the general utility of thimerosal. An important factor seems to be the inclusion of thimerosal at the very beginning of culture rather than delaying its introduction until fibroblasts are established.

2. Growth Factors

This group constitutes a jungle of elements, some of which seem to be similar or identical to others. The following discussion does not pretend to be complete, but the subject was reviewed in 1976 by Gospodarowicz and Moran [69], to whom the reader is referred for further information. The most generally useful elements are epidermal growth factor (EGF) and fibroblast growth factor (FGF), which seem to be virtually required for growth of some cell types. These are now commercially available. In the ensuing discussion it should be borne in mind that most growth factors are supplied as constituents of the serum supplement, which may be the reason for the importance of using selected serum lots for the successful culture of some cell types. Many tissue culturists can ignore growth factors for this reason, but they become crucial considerations as the serum level is reduced. All of the growth factors discussed here are proteins or polypeptides.

a. Epidermal Growth Factor. First isolated in 1962 by Cohen [70], EGF was derived from mouse submaxillary gland (preferably male) and was at least as active in its effect on differentiation as in stimulating growth per se, since it accelerated incisor eruption and eyelid opening in newborn animals. It was subsequently found in varying amounts in other tissues, but submaxillary gland remains one of the best sources. In addition, EGF was shown to be effective in promoting growth of a variety of cell types, including fibroblasts [71]. It is effective in stimulating growth of human glial cells, for example, when these are grown in sparse populations where density-dependent growth inhibition normally occurs [34]. Rheinwald and Green [72] found that EGF increased the culture lifetime of human epidermal keratinocytes from 50–150 population doublings.

b. Fibroblast Growth Factor. FGF was purified from bovine pituitaries in 1975 by Gospodarowicz [73]. When assayed through stimulation of DNA synthesis in contact-inhibited 3T3 cells, it was effective in concentrations as low as 2×10^{-13}M, with saturation at 1×10^{-10}M. Used with dexamethasone, it can sustain multiple division cycles in serum-starved cells. It lacks cell and species specificity, and acts on fibroblasts, chondrocytes, an adrenal cell line, glial cells, and endometrial cells obtained from mouse, cattle, and human sources. It can also be isolated from mammalian brain [25]. Gospodarowicz et al [24] showed that FGF was effective in growth of both endothelial and smooth muscle cells, while EGF was effective in promoting the growth of smooth muscle, but not endothelial, cells. Many epithelial cells, such as cornea, adrenal cortex, and luteal cells, require FGF, not EGF [26].

c. Platelet Factor. This factor is liberated from platelets, is found in serum prepared from whole blood, but is not found in plasma (see Ross and Vogel [74], for review). Its action is fairly general and seems to be required by 3T3, glial, and fibroblast cells, among others. It rather strikingly resembles FGF, except that it is not very mitogenic for endothelium. The authors cited noted that whole blood serum is a pathologic fluid, and not a physiologic substance. It contains factors from platelet degradation and coagulation cascade, so that cells in vivo are exposed to serum constituents under conditions of injury and blood coagulation. On this basis, it is not surprising that injury response and fibroblast proliferation are promoted. Platelet factor is heat stable and has been partially purified.

d. Nonsuppressible Insulin-Like Activity (NSILA). NSILA activity is not suppressible by antibodies against insulin [75]. It is a component of human serum and, like insulin, has general growth-promoting properties.

e. Multiplication-Stimulating Activity (MSA). Smith and Temin [46] purified a growth substance from tissue culture medium that had been conditioned by a rat liver cell line. This source was used because such media support the growth of cells without any serum.

f. Conditioned Medium. Medium conditioned by a variety of cell types has, of course, been in use for many years, and no attempt will be made to discuss these efforts comprehensively. Aside from medium conditioned by rat liver cells, that conditioned by mouse cells (3T3 and L929) seems to be the most generally effective. Some investigators [61] feel that conditioning factors are useful for the support of epithelial cells in general. It has already been noted that the medium conditioned by mouse 3T3 cells can replace irradiated fibroblast feeder layers in promoting the growth of epidermal keratinocytes.

g. Nerve Growth Factor. Discovered in 1951 by Levi-Montalcini and Hamburger [76], nerve growth factor was originally isolated from a mouse sarcoma but later was also found in rodent salivary glands. It has the rather specific action indicated by the name, and also promotes the outgrowth of nerve fibers in post-mitotic cultures of neurons.

h. Colony-Stimulating Factor. As in the case of nerve growth factor and epidermal growth factor, colony-stimulating factor is derived from mouse submaxillary glands, but some is also found in lung, kidney, and spleen. It is very specific in its activity, however, stimulating the growth of macrophages and granulocytes in vitro [69].

i. Ovarian Growth Factor. Isolated from bovine pituitaries, as in the case of fibroblast growth factor [77], ovarian growth factor acts on a permanent cell line derived from rat ovary.

j. Mesenchymal Factor. Ronzio and Rutter [78] have partially purified a factor that substitutes for mesenchyme in stimulating the growth of pancreatic epithelial cells from chick embryos. Although these are dependent upon mesodermal cells for their differentiation, mesenchymal factor is regarded as a growth factor rather than one that stimulates differentiation. It is not clear whether this factor is similar or identical to factors described by others, or how general its action is.

3. Hormones

Hormones have been largely ignored in culture systems because most are reasonably thermostable and are presumed to be supplied by the serum supplement. Yet there are a number of instances in which the addition of particular hormones to serum supplemented media results in increased growth of various cell types. The most detailed studies of hormone requirements of cells in culture are those of Sato's group [79], which have been able to replace serum altogether by adding a mixture of hormones to cultures of a permanent rodent cell line. Although this work is of considerable interest, it usually does not impinge upon the activities of most tissue culturists, who use conventional serum supplements on the order of 10% and often deal with diploid cells. The following notes emphasize cases in which hormones seem to amplify growth when added to conventional media containing undefined supplements.

a. Hydrocortisone. A number of reports implicate hydroxycortisone as an agent important in the stimulation of growth. Two that deal with epithelial cells are those of Yuan and Chang [80] and Wigley and Franks [60]. The former showed that the addition of hydrocortisone prolonged the postmitotic life-span of human amnion cells. The latter showed that explants of tissue from mouse salivary glands gave epithelial outgrowths in which mitosis was intensified by the addition of hydrocortisone. In addition, Rheinwald and Green [58] found that hydrocortisone was important (in addition to feeder layers) for the growth of human keratinocytes.

b. Insulin. For most cell requirements, this hormone seems to be stable enough to persist at adequate levels in selected serum batches, as in the case of hydrocortisone. Insulin is not an effective mitogen but seems to act instead as a potentiating agent for other factors [69]. Wigley and Franks [60] found that both insulin and cortisone resulted in enhanced growth of their cultures of mouse salivary epithelium.

c. Somatomedins. These are insulin-like peptide growth factors, production of which is under the control of growth hormone [81,82]. They are present in serum, stimulate proteoglycan synthesis in cartilage, and act on skeletal tissue cells generally. Somatomedin A may be the same as MSA, and Somatomedin B may be the same as NSILA, but these identities have not been determined with certainty.

d. Estrogens and Androgens. It might be expected that sex hormones would act in vitro upon cells concerned with reproductive activities. On the other hand, 17β-estradiol is reported to stimulate growth of human diploid fibroblasts, as shown by Milo et al [83]. Brehmer et al [84] found that testosterone promoted growth of hyperplastic and neoplastic human prostatic epithelia, but normal human prostatic epithelium grows well without it [49].

Progesterone appears to inhibit the growth of most tissue culture systems in which it has any effect at all. As one specific example, it has been reported to interfere with the growth of human diploid fibroblasts [83].

e. Glucocorticoids. This group (represented by dexamethasone) stimulates partial differentiation in cultured lens epithelium [41]. A permanent rabbit kidney cell line was shown to have dexamethasone-inducible proline oxidase activity, and it has been suggested (see Proline, p 20) that it might be used to select for epithelial cell growth in proline-deficient media [85].

f. Erythropoietin. This highly specific hormone stimulates mitosis in cultured proerythroblasts [86].

4. Auxotrophic Methods

These are methods in which the attempt is made to select for growth of parenchymal cells in mixed cultures by taking advantage of special synthetic activities. They suffer from the disadvantage of "feeder" effects, in which fibroblasts, for example, receive the required substance from the cells that produce it. For this reason, perhaps, there is considerable disagreement about their effectiveness. Nevertheless, it seems likely that the producer cells would have some advantage, and some successes have been reported. Our experience is that feeder effects are minimized by culture at low cell density.

a. D-Valine. Gilbert and Migeon [87] reported that epithelial cells possess D-amino acid oxidase activity (lacking in fibroblasts), which converts D-valine to 2-ketoisovaleric acid, this in turn being converted to L-valine by a ubiquitous enzyme. Since L-valine is an essential amino acid, it follows that presence of activity of oxidase is essential for growth in deficient media. Success in selection in mixed culture has not always been observed, presumably because of feeder effects, but Gilbert and Migeon obtained success in cultures of fibroblasts mixed with epithelial cells from fetal human kidney, fetal lung, and umbilical cord. These workers feel that it is important for deficient media to be used from the very beginning of culture initiation. Benke and Dittmar [88] pointed out that lymphoid cells are also deficient in activity of the oxidase and cannot grow in valine-deficient media.

b. Proline. Downing and colleagues [85, 89] have reported that fibroblasts, unlike some epithelial cells, also lack proline oxidase activity. Since activity is inducible in a rabbit kidney cell line by dexamethasone, they have pointed out that this may be the basis of a selective system. Although proline is not an essential amino acid, even nonessential amino acids are important additives in culture media. It is not clear that this approach has as yet succeeded in practical situations.

c. Proline Analogues. Although not an "auxotrophic" method, this is grouped under the heading for convenience. It involves inhibition of fibroblast growth by substitution of *cis*-hydroxyproline for L-proline, which prevents collagen chains from folding into the triple helical conformation [90]. Deposition of this form on the culture surface seems to be required for growth of fibroblasts, since such growth can be enhanced by artificial coating of culture surfaces. Substitution of the analog has no effect on growth of a human epithelial cell line (KB) or on a neuroblastoma line (Type Culture Collection, CCL-131).

5. Vitamins

Inspection of the formulae of defined media effective in promoting growth in the absence of serum indicates that the water-soluble vitamins are required for cell growth, but not the fat-soluble vitamins, which are required for the intact organism only. With this as background, only 2 examples will be discussed, as they seem to involve special situations.

a. Vitamin A. DeLuca et al [91] have pointed out that bioassays in gut tissue show that vitamin A controls synthesis of the fucose-glycopeptide constitutent of goblet cell mucus. The practical effect on cultured gut epithelium is that lack of the vitamin results in squamous metaplasia, while its presence causes differentiation of goblet cells and mucous secretion by goblet cells. Hence, its level is important in characterization of many epithelial cells. In addition, the vitamin is said to inhibit development of epithelial tumors.

b. Vitamin E. The effect of relatively large doses of vitamin E (as DL-α-tocopherol) on the culture life-span of human diploid fibroblasts has been studied by Packer and Smith [92], and by Balin et al [93]. The first group augmented the level of the vitamin beginning at the 45th population doubling (near the end of the normal culture life-span) and showed an increase in doubling potential from 65–100, using a concentration of 100 μg/ml. This concentration does not enhance either growth rate or plating efficiency, however [94].

6. Essential Fatty Acids

These are usually considered to be oleic, linoleic, linolenic, and arachidonic acids, although some are derived from others. They make up constituents of membranes of diploid cells, although many permanent cell lines dispense with them by substituting other fatty acids in serum-free media. They are required only in very small amounts and are generally provided by serum, although they are not very stable. Jenkin and Anderson [95] were able to replace serum in growth of a monkey kidney cell line by the addition of oleic acid. A caution has to do with the essential fatty acid levels in commercial dry powder media, since desiccation is reported to destroy them in media in which they are constituents (Nutrient media F10, F12, MCDB 104, etc). If these media are used with low serum levels, or with unusually sensitive cells, the fatty acids should be added again.

7. Polyamines

There are sporadic claims in the literature that growth of particular cell types may be enhanced by polyamines. It was noted earlier [39] that rat urinary bladder cells were reported to require the addition of putrescine, spermine, and spermidine for maximum growth.

8. Phorbol Diesters

These compounds, which are tumor promoters, have been reported to be very effective in promoting the growth of chick embryo fibroblasts [96] and may be shown to have activity with other cell types.

F. Biologic Methods

1. Feeder Layers

The technique of using cultures of inviable cells to promote growth (usually at clonal density) is time-honored, and only a few recent applications will be mentioned here. The use of irradiated feeder layers of 3T3 mouse fibroblast cells to culture human epidermal keratinocytes has been mentioned [58]. These cells are especially useful for this purpose because, in addition to being better than most for conditioning, they are subject to contact inhibition and therefore produce neatly arranged monolayer pavements of cells before they are irradiated. In the case at hand, irradiation was necessary to prevent overgrowth by them during subcultivations.

Taylor-Papadimitriou et al [42] have recently used feeder layers of mouse 3T6 cells for the culture of calf lens epithelium, after the mouse cells were rendered inviable by mitomycin-C. They also found an increase in culture life-span with the use of such support, from 5–8 to 16–20 population doublings.

2. *Conditioning*

Conditioning factors have been discussed elsewhere, with respect to their study as growth components [46] and their ability to substitute for feeder layers [61]. As in the case of media used to support serumless growth of diploid chick fibroblasts conditioned by rat liver cell lines [46], Shodell [97] had reported earlier that conditioning factor produced by L-929 mouse fibroblasts can substitute for serum in growth of the permanent cell line BHK/21. The use of conditioning factors is certainly more convenient than feeder layers, and the literature seems to indicate that feeder layers can be replaced by conditioning factors in many cases. A common practice is to mix conditioned with unconditioned medium to replace components that may be inactivated during conditioning, but the rule is that these parameters must usually be worked out with the particular system in use.

3. *Aggregation*

As discussed in an earlier section (Pancreas, p 13) Wilson [52] found a rapid decline in functional activity of epithelial cells cultured as monolayers from rabbit pancreas. When primary cultures were initiated as aggregates (made from dissociated cells using a gyratory shaker), however, retention of functional activity was increased from 4–28 days, the longest period tested. Function was regained when cells of primary cultures were aggregated after as much as 7 days, but aggregation of older cultures indicated that functional capability was lost at that time. This points up the need to consider culture form in the characterization of cell types.

4. *Species' Differences*

A final biologic consideration in the culture of epithelial cell types is that there can be striking differences in the morphology of cells obtained in cultures initiated from various species but using the same methods. Comparing lung tissues of various primate species with those of the ferret and rat has shown that fibroblastic cells dominated after serial subculture of primate cells, while cells of clearly epithelial appearance resulted from cultures of the second 2 species. The last, moreover, gave rise to permanent cell lines, while the primate strains all degenerated spontaneously [98]. Hence it is quite possible that choice of species can be a major factor in the success of particular culture approaches.

G. Physical Methods in Cell Separation

For a variety of reasons, the use of physical methods in cell separation has enjoyed a resurgence in recent years. First, it can be shown from mathematic and physical considerations that it is theoretically possible to separate cells on the basis of quite small differences in a number of factors, such as size, density, and surface charge. Such methods have obvious potential in the development of characterized strains of organ parenchymal cells, which often differ from stromal cells in some or all of these factors. A second reason for renewed interest is that earlier methods tended to produce inviable cells, while more recent techniques are often succeeding in the separation of cells that can subsequently produce vigorous cultures. Some of these are briefly reviewed below.

1. Cell Density

a. Density Gradient Techniques. These have suffered in the past from the liability that most employed sucrose as the gradient material, or Ficoll (a sucrose polymer) that was contaminated with inorganic material. The result often was that the gradient osmolarity was too high for the separation of viable cells, or the viscosity was too high for practical separation. In addition, some density gradient methods, even with the use of preformed gradients, require rather high centrifugal forces, which can be deleterious for cell survival. When attention is paid to the method of preparing Ficoll, however, viable cells may be obtained [99]. To cite only one example from among a number, Fusenig [100] dissociated mouse skin with trypsin and separated epithelial cells by centrifuging them at 800 rpm on 3 discontinuous Ficoll gradients. In this system, epithelial cells separated out first (ie were the most dense) and were apparently free of fibroblasts. These were successfully cultured.

b. Isopycnic Separation. Munthe-Kaas and Seglen [101] have used metrizamide as a gradient medium in isopycnic separation of rat liver cells. Although this material does not have high viscosity at the required densities (1.05–1.16 gm/cm^3) it can be toxic, and batches must be tested beforehand for this property. A further problem is that centrifugation to equilibrium requires centrifugal speeds of 3,000–10,000 rpm. The method is extremely sensitive, giving cell separations by densities ranging from 1.10–1.12 gm/cm^3. Unfortunately, cells separated by this method were not cultured. They did, however, exclude trypan blue and convert fructose to glucose at the normal rate. It remains to be seen whether this method can produce fully viable separated cells.

c. Centrifugal Elutriation. Another sensitive density separation method is that of centrifugal elutriation, with an example from the work of Mitchell and Tupper [102], who were able to obtain synchronized cultures of 3T3 cells by separation on the basis of their position in the cell cycle. This method is based in turn upon the fact that cell size increases during the S period of the cell cycle (and density presumably decreases), permitting good separation of G_1 and G_2 cells, presumably with some contamination by cells at the very beginning and end of the S period. Cell volume is reported to double from G_1 to M [103].

2. Combination Methods: Cell Size and Cell Density.

Among those not trained in biophysics, there has been considerable confusion concerning some methods of cell separation, in determining whether multiple factors are involved in separation. Some of these interpretations are still debated from time to time.

a. Velocity Sedimentation at Unit Gravity. Good success has been obtained in separating cells by allowing them to fall through solutions of low viscosity and density, a method introduced by Mel [104]. A special advantage of this method is that the media used are mixtures such as serum, serum-culture medium, and bovine serum albumin-saline mixtures which can be fully compatible with viability. The process is relatively rapid as well, and cultures can often be constructed directly from the sedimentation system. In practice, gradients are usually made, to reduce turbulence and the mixing of layers during loading and unloading. A further point is that these techniques sometimes require fairly simple and inexpensive equipment. Finally, centrifugation is usually not required.

In recent years there has been rather vehement controversy among practitioners of the methods, regarding whether separation takes place on the basis of cell size alone [103, 105–107], or a combination of size and density, which is the more current and prevailing view [99, 108–110]. These conclusions are based upon reasonably complex mathematic theory and in some instances will matter little to the cell culturist who enjoys practical success in separating cell types of interest.

Miller and Phillips [103] and MacDonald and Miller [105] used gradients of fetal bovine serum and phosphate buffered saline (PBS) to separate mouse L cells into synchronized fractions. They used a gradient maker to construct a gradient of 3–30% serum in PBS, which has a density range of 1.004–1.009 compared with densities on the order of 1.06 gm/cm^3 and up for the cells themselves. A specially constructed chamber permits loading as many as 10^9 cells, which fall through the gradient at about 1.5 mm/hr in the cold. At this rate 4 hour runs are sufficient for separation. Volume separations of suspension-cultured mouse L cells are on the order of 1,400–2,000 nm^3. Viability remains high, yielding plating efficiencies of 40% and 60% for sedimented and unsedimented cells, respectively. Catsimpolas and Griffith [108] use a commercially available apparatus (Buchler PolyPrep 200) for their sedimentation chamber, and use cell aliquots containing as many as 5×10^7 human blood cell elements. Using a bovine serum albumin (BSA)-PBS gradient they are able to separate platelets, erythrocytes, mononuclear and polymorphonuclear cells. A problem pointed out by them, with this and other sedimentation methods, is that the concentration of cells in the starting zone is limited by sample and gradient-interface instability, so that a relatively wide starting zone is needed when a large number of cells are used. Hence, the bands widen as they fall. Despite these objections, the method is quite useful.

Shall [106, 107] used basically similar methods, but with sucrose gradients ranging to 10%, and therefore presumably hypertonic. Although synchronized populations of mouse fibroblasts were obtained by this method, long-term cell viability was not determined. Stephenson and Axelrad [111], using a BSA gradient, separated erythropoietin-sensitive cells from fetal mouse liver, and Davis and Schuetz [112] separated germinal cells of immature rat testis by a similar method. Unfortunately, there is a paucity of studies involving long-term culture of separated fractions, but Mitsui and Schneider [113] and Houghton [114] separated populations of human diploid fibroblasts (WI-38) into 2 size populations by a velocity sedimentation technique and propagated them to the end of their life-span, with the result that both grew for the same length of time, and for as long as control cultures, before culture deterioration occurred.

b. Isokinetic Gradients. Pretlow et al [99, 115] have developed isokinetic gradients (ones in which cells sediment at constant velocity) using Ficoll in tissue culture medium and a gradient maker. Further, they accelerated sedimentation by centrifuging at 55 g for 21 minutes. The method was applied to separation of cells from carcinomas and a variety of normal epithelial cells. Since a final isopycnic sedimentation was used, cell density was an important parameter in the separation process. The authors point out that the densest cells are those with the highest concentrations of cytoplasmic protein, eg mast cells, parotid and pancreatic acinar cells, and cardiac myocytes, all of which were separated successfully from fibroblasts. Long-term viability studies were not done.

3. Combination Methods: Surface Charge and Cell Density

Methods of density gradient electrophoresis have been developed which separate cells on the basis of surface charge and density combined and which can manage large numbers of cells (ie 10^8): this is the subject of a recent extensive review [108]. Electrophoresis is conducted in an iso-osmolar Ficoll-sucrose gradient and gives good separation of mixtures of rabbit and mouse erythrocytes.

4. Cell Membrane Properties: Two-Polymer Aqueous Phase System

Some very recent studies [116] have indicated that cells may be separated on the basis of complex interacting combinations of membrane-surface properties, related to such factors as charge, lipid content, specific receptors, etc. Separation is accomplished at boundaries of immiscible aqueous phases, in this case polyethylene glycol and dextran. It is too early to tell whether this technique will be useful in separating viable cells for tissue culture.

5. Cell Sorting for Various Properties

Viable cells can be separated through fluorescence-activated cell sorting, based upon a number of parameters for which the sorter can be programmed [117]. The method appears to be a practical one but as yet has had few applications to tissue culture, possibly because of the high cost of the equipment. In addition, sorters process fewer than 10^7 cells per hour, and viability is doubtful.

6. Special Substrates

As we have seen, epidermal cells do not thrive in the absence of conditioned medium or feeder cells, but these factors can also be replaced by autoclaved pigskin as a surface for the growth of epithelial cells from human foreskin [59]. Subcultivation can be done, and cultures can be maintained for as many as 48 population doublings. Moreover, cell division occurs throughout the culture, not only at the edge of cell colonies. The method will be discussed further in this volume. Other substrates, especially collagens, have been used and may be helpful in special cases.

7. Treated Substrates

Basic polymers are useful in altering surface charge to encourage attachment of cells in situations where very low serum levels are used. Poly-L-lysine is used by McKeehan and Ham [118] in clonal growth of fibroblasts in serum at levels down to 0.5%.

8. Centripetal Separation of Adipocytes.

Human adipose tissue derived from infants at laparotomy was disaggregated and adipocytes removed from the top of the tube after centrifuging [119]. These were plated in dishes containing small amounts of medium and were observed to lose their lipid inclusions after a time. Some division then occurred and subcultivation was possible. Mitotic potential was seen only in adipocytes taken from infants 20 months old or younger.

III. CULTURE CONDITIONS AND SPECIAL REQUIREMENTS

A. Media

Choice of medium for any particular purpose is often a matter of educated guesswork, but every experienced tissue culturist knows that it is very important – even though there is usually no rational basis for the selection. In his review of the history of medium development, Ham [120] pointed out that cell culture in general suffers from the fact that most of the commercially available media were developed using permanent, malignant, lines of fibroblasts or carcinoma cells (ie mouse L or HeLa) as the test cells. Ironically, these cells were chosen in the first place because they were the ones that grew best in the primitive early media and had, in fact, been selected for this property. Recent, sophisticated studies of cell nutrition by Ham and McKeehan [94] have shown that rational medium composition becomes crucial when serum level is reduced. The results of these studies, on several cell and species types, indicated that there is no reason why any cell that has growth potential in vivo cannot be propagated in vitro. In this regard, there is mounting (almost undeniable) evidence that the "stem" cells of some epithelia – such as intestinal crypts – have in vivo doubling potential limits that are very high, indeed, and very likely in the hundreds [121, 122].

Cell nutrition studies also indicate that the tailoring of media to cell type and species is extremely effective. Rational medium development, as practiced by Ham's group [120, 123] is an elaborate one, in which diploid cells are subcultured at clonal density and both plating efficiency and colony size are assayed in separate trials of each proposed medium ingredient, tested in a range of dilutions designed to reach the minimum effective at one extreme and the toxic level at the other. In this approach, an "ideal" concentration is arrived at as the logarithmic center of this range. When this task is performed for each of the scores of ingredients tested, the entire process must be repeated at least once more, since optimal concentrations of some ingredients affect those of some others. Moreover, the future addition of a new ingredient may require further retesting.

There is thus small wonder that most media have been developed largely by guesswork, usually as modifications of preexisting media that were also developed by guesswork. Typically, these are then applied to the culture of cell types and species origin for which they were not intended.

It is, of course, possible to argue that the use of serum at high level abrogates these difficulties (since diploid fibroblasts certainly will grow in most common media containing 10% fetal bovine serum from a selected lot), but these considerations do not seem to explain the multitude of failures experienced in propagating epithelial cells that should grow well in culture, on the basis of what we know of their behavior in vivo. What is important are the successes, because they indicate what is possible. There would seem to be great hope in the development of media for various species and epithelia. This preamble also sets the stage for the point that media which are made up 'from scratch' in the laboratory are said to be generally superior to commercially available media. They offer the added advantage that concentration of specific ingredients can be varied quite easily, since final medium batches are assembled from a number of stock ingredients, each usually containing only a few constituents. The original organization of the project requires some effort, but the compatible stocks, and solution and storage techniques, have been worked out [123], and the process is surprisingly painless.

B. Sera

The use of selected serum lots for the cultivation of fastidious cell types is so well recognized that supporting citations are unnecessary. Fetal bovine serum seems to give the best results in most systems, but some cell types (or variants) do seem to require other sera, or to be adapted to them. The usual method is to test sera against cells plated at clonal density (usually a few hundred cells per culture vessel), assessing plating efficiency and colony size. The cell type to be studied should be used for this testing. The effect of heat inactivation (usually 56°C for 30 minutes) should also be determined.

C. Carbon Dioxide and Oxygen Toxicity

Some evidence is accumulating that media saturated with atmospheric air at 37°C have oxygen concentrations that are somewhat toxic for fibroblasts and perhaps even more so for epithelial cells, a possible reflection of the fact that these are higher than tissue levels of dissolved oxygen in vivo. This may, in fact, be the basis for the efficacy of the 5% CO_2 usually added to the gassing atmosphere, in that it leads to a slight reduction in the partial pressure of oxygen. Taylor et al [124] showed that the growth of WI-38 human diploid fibroblasts and Vero cells (a permanent epithelial line) was enhanced by cultivation in an atmosphere of only 1% oxygen, a result confirmed by McKeehan et al [125] in clonal growth of WI-38 cells at low serum concentrations. Selenium, apparently by reducing oxygen availability, was found to be an essential trace element under these conditions. Balin et al [93] tested the effect of oxygen level on the replicative life-span (as distinguished from growth at clonal density) of WI-38 cells and found no effect when reduced levels were compared with normal atmospheric levels. Life-span was markedly shortened, however, when the oxygen level was elevated much above atmospheric levels. The effect of oxygen level on the propagation of epithelial cells early in their culture history does not appear to have been tested.

D. Water Quality

This is a crucial factor and requires careful attention by those who make their own media or salines, or who use media made up from 10-fold concentrated commercial stocks. Historically, the standard has been the use of triple distilled water prepared in a quartz glass still. Fortunately, this laborious process is no longer necessary with the availability of mixed bed resins, which typically are used to process tap water before the single distillation most culture laboratories now use. The still should have a "scrubber," or chamber (sometimes with a baffle) to deter heavy metal ions from entering the condenser, and a vent at the top of the condenser, with the condenser cooling rate arranged so that a continuous wisp of steam escapes, in order to remove volatile gasses such as chlorine. The distillate should have an electrical resistance in the megohm range, and is best stored in polyethylene bottles. Stills need not be made of quartz glass: tin-lined stills are also satisfactory. With the insertion of a micropore filter at the end of the system, sterile water can be delivered.

E. pH

Although many cell types tolerate a wide range in pH, growth stops very rapidly, as a rule, when the limits are exceeded, and cells can easily be injured or killed. Growth of almost all cells ceases below pH 6.8 but may persist to quite high levels (ie 7.8) in some cells. Unfortunately, this level is all too often exceeded in bicarbonate buffered systems when the culture medium is not equilibrated in the gassed environment. The use of HEPES buffer with or without bicarbonate [94] is a great improvement.

Some cell types (especially transformed ones) produce large amounts of acid and for that reason pH control problems can make it difficult to produce confluent monolayers. By setting initial pH levels high and using HEPES buffer, sometimes with daily adjustment of pH using iso-osmolar NaOH (0.14 N), this problem can usually be overcome. Like most other parameters, exact pH level tends to become more important at clonal density, if for no other reason than the cells are less able to regulate their own pH.

F. Osmolarity

Most cells tolerate fluctuations in osmolarity on the order of 10% about the norm for mammalian plasma (ie 300 ± 30 mOsm), but this factor should be tested in clonal density systems.

REFERENCES

1. "The Human Genetic Mutant Cell Repository." Camden: Institute for Medical Research, 1978.
2. Gartler S: Genetic markers as tracers in cell culture. Natl Cancer Inst Monogr 26:167–181, 1967.
3. Nelson-Rees WA, Flandermeyer RR, Hawthorne PK: Banded marker chromosomes as indicators of intraspecies cellular contamination. Science 184:1093–1096, 1974.
4. Wigley CB: Differentiated cells in vitro. Differentiation 4:25–55, 1975.
5. Paul J: Establishment of permanent cell strains from human adult peripheral blood. Nature 182:808, 1958.
6. Moore GE, McLimans WF: The life span of the cultured normal cell: Concepts derived from studies of human lymphoblasts. J Theor Biol 20:217–226, 1968.
7. Nilsson K: High-frequency establishment of human immunoglobulin-producing lymphoblastoid lines from normal and malignant lymphoid tissue and peripheral blood. Int J Cancer 8:432–442, 1971.
8. Miller G: Human lymphoblastoid cell lines and Epstein-Barr virus: A review of their interrelationships and their relevance to the etiology of leukoproliferative states in man. Yale J Biol Med 43:358–384, 1971.
9. "Biological Safety Manual for Research Involving Oncogenic Viruses." Bethesda: National Cancer Institute (Office of Research Safety), 1977.

10. Castor CW, Naylor B: Characteristics of normal and malignant human mesothelial cells studied in vitro. Lab Invest 20:437–443, 1969.
11. Chang RS: Observations on the growth phases of human amnion cell cultures. J Natl Cancer Inst 40:491–503, 1968.
12. Conover JH, Hirschhorn K: Establishment and genetic stability of human amnion cell lines. Lab Invest 24:38–40, 1971.
13. Buehring GC, Williams RR: Growth rates of normal and abnormal human mammary epithelia in cell culture. Cancer Res 36:3742–3747, 1976.
14. Owens RB: Selective cultivation of mammalian epithelial cells. Methods Cell Biol 14:341–355, 1976.
15. Rie EJ, Rie IP, Buehring GC: Short-term line of normal baboon mammary epithelial cells. J Natl Cancer Inst 57:607–611, 1976.
16. Sutherland GR, Bain AD: Culture of cells from the urine of newborn children. Nature 239:231, 1972.
17. Sutherland GR, Bain AD: "U"-cell culture – A new technique. Arch Dis Child 49:74, 1974.
18. Sutherland GR, Grace E, Bain AD: Metaphase chromosomes from neonatal urine. Humangenetik 17:273–275, 1973.
19. Lin H-S, Stewart CC: Peritoneal exudate cells. I. Growth requirement of cells capable of forming colonies in soft agar. J Cell Physiol 83:369–378, 1974.
20. Stewart CC, Lin H-S, Adles C: Proliferation and colony-forming ability of peritoneal exudate cells in liquid culture. J Exp Med 141:1114–1132, 1975.
21. Cahn RD, Cahn MB: Heritability of cellular differentiation: Clonal growth and expression of differentiation in retinal pigment cells in vitro. Proc Natl Acad Sci USA 55:106–114, 1966.
22. Mannagh J, Arya DV Irvine AR Jr: Tissue culture of human retinal pigment epithelium. Invest Ophthal 12:52–64, 1973.
23. Giovanella BC, Stehlin JS, Santamaria C, Yim SO, Morgan AC, Williams LJ Jr, Liebovitz A, Fialkow PJ, Mumford DM: Human neoplastic and normal cells in tissue culture. I. Cell lines derived from malignant melanomas and normal melanocytes. J Natl Cancer Inst 56:1131–1142, 1976.
24. Gospodarowicz D, Moran J, Braun D, Birdwell C: Clonal growth of bovine vascular endothelial cells in tissue culture: Fibroblast growth factor as a survival agent. Proc Natl Acad Sci USA 73:4120–4124, 1976.
25. Gospodarowicz D, Moran JS, Braun DL: Control of proliferation of bovine vascular endothelial cells. J Cell Physiol 91:377–386, 1977.
26. Gospodarowicz D, Greenburg G, Bialecki H, Zetter BR: Factors involved in the modulation of cell proliferation in vivo and in vitro: The role of fibroblast and epidermal growth factors in the proliferative response of mammalian cells. In Vitro 14:85–118, 1978.
27. Lewis LJ, Hoak JC, Maca RD, Fry GL: Replication of human endothelial cells in culture. Science 181:453–454, 1973.
28. Coon HG: Clonal stability and phenotypic expression of chick cartilage cells in vitro. Proc Natl Acad Sci USA 55:66–73, 1966.
29. Lycette RR, Whyte S: Monolayer culture of bovine colon epithelium. Res Vet Sci 14:121–122, 1973.
30. Pontén J, Macintyre EH: Long term culture of normal and neoplastic human glia. Acta Pathol Microbiol Scand 74:465–486, 1968.
31. Pontén J: Human glia cells. In Kruse PF Jr, Patterson MK Jr (eds): "Tissue Culture Methods and Applications." New York: Academic Press, 1973, pp 50–53.

32. Sensenbrenner M: Dissociated brain cells in primary cultures. In Fedoroff S, Hertz L (eds): "Cell, Tissue, and Organ Cultures in Neurobiology." New York: Academic Press, 1977, pp 189–213.
33. Lim R, Turriff DE, Troz SS, Koto T: Differentiation of glioblasts under the influence of glia maturation factor. Ibid, pp 223–235.
34. Westermark B: Density dependent proliferation of human glia cells stimulated by epidermal growth factor. Biochem Biophys Res Commun 69:304–310, 1976.
35. Pfeiffer SE, Betschart B, Cook J, Mancini P, Morris R: Glial cell lines. Supra #32, pp 287–346.
36. Bulloch D, Stallcup WB, Cohen M: A new method for the establishment of neuronal cell lines from the mouse brain. Life Sci (Submitted for publication).
37. Peterson LJ, Paulson DF, Bonar RA: Response of human urothelium to chemical carcinogens in vitro. J Urol 111:154–159, 1974.
38. Stone KR, Paulson DF, Bonar RA, Reich CF III: In vitro culture of epithelial cells derived from urogenital tissues. Urol Res 2:149–153, 1975.
39. Roszell JA, Douglas CJ, Irving CC: Polyamine-stimulated growth of cultured rat urinary bladder epithelial cells. Cancer Res 37:239–243, 1977.
40. van Venrooij WJ, Groeneveld AA, Bloemendal H, Benedetti EL: Cultured calf lens epithelium. I. Methods of cultivation and characteristics of the cultures. Exp Eye Res 18:517–526, 1974.
41. van Venrooij WJ, Groeneveld AA, Bloemendal H, Benedetti EL: Cultured calf lens epithelium. II. The effect of dexamethasone. Exp Eye Res 18:527–536, 1974.
42. Taylor-Papadimitriou J, Shearer M, Watling D: Growth requirements of calf lens epithelium in culture. J Cell Physiol 95:95–104, 1978.
43. Eguchi G, Clayton RM, Perry MM: Comparison of the growth and differentiation of epithelial cells from normal and hyperplastic lenses of the chick: Studies of in vitro cell cultures. Dev Growth Diff 17:395–413, 1975.
44. Hackett AJ, Smith HS, Springer EL, Owens RB, Nelson-Rees WA, Riggs JL, Gardner MB: Two syngeneic cell lines from human breast tissue: The aneuploid mammary epithelial (Hs578T) and the diploid myoepithelial (Hs578Bst) cell lines. J Natl Cancer Inst 58:1795–1806, 1977.
45. Coon HG: Clonal culture of differentiated rat liver cells. (Abstract) J Cell Biol 39:29a, 1968.
46. Smith GL, Temin HM: Purified multiplication-stimulating activity from rat liver cell conditioned medium: Comparison of biological activities with calf serum, insulin, and somatomedin. J Cell Physiol 84:181–192, 1974.
47. Kaighn ME, Prince AM: Production of albumin and other serum proteins by clonal cultures of normal human liver. Proc Natl Acad Sci USA 68:2396–2400, 1971.
48. Kaighn ME: Human liver cells. Supra #31, pp 54–58.
49. Kaighn ME, Babcock MS: Monolayer cultures of human prostatic cells. Cancer Chemother Rep 59:59–63, 1975.
50. Douglas WHJ, Kaighn ME: Clonal isolation of differentiated rat lung cells. In Vitro 10:230–237, 1974.
51. Kniazeff AJ, Stoner GD, Terry L, Wagner RM, Hoppenstand RD: Characteristics of epithelial cells cultured from feline lung. Lab Invest 34:495–500, 1976.
52. Wilson GL: Functional analysis of rabbit pancreatic cells in vitro. Thesis, University of Illinois at the Medical Center, 1976.
53. Konigsberg IR: Clonal analysis of myogenesis. Science 140:1273–1284, 1963.
54. Fedoroff S: Tracing glial cell lineages by colony formation in primary cultures. Supra #32, pp 215–221.

55. Nelson PG: Neuronal cell lines. Supra #32, pp 347–365.
56. Godfrey EW, Nelson PG, Schrier BK, Breuer AC, Ransom BR: Neurons from fetal rat brain in a new culture system: A multidisciplinary analysis. Brain Res 90:1–21, 1975.
57. Flaxman BA, Lutzner MA, Van Scott EJ: Cell maturation and tissue organization in epithelial outgrowths from skin and buccal mucosa in vitro. J Invest Dermatol 49:322–332, 1967.
58. Rheinwald JG, Green H: Serial cultivation of strains of human epidermal keratinocytes: The formation of keratinizing colonies from single cells. Cell 6:331–344, 1975.
59. Freeman AE, Igel HJ, Herrman BJ, Kleinfeld KL: Growth and characterization of human skin epithelial cell cultures. In Vitro 12:352–362, 1976.
60. Wigley CB, Franks LM: Salivary epithelial cells in primary culture: Characterization of their growth and functional properties. J Cell Sci 20:149–165, 1976.
61. Green H: Cell culture for the study of epithelial cells. Natl Cancer Inst Monogr 48:259–262, 1978.
62. Owens RB, Smith HS, Nelson-Rees WA, Springer EL: Epithelial cell cultures from normal and cancerous human tissues. J Natl Cancer Inst 56:843–849, 1976.
63. Kasten FH: Functional differentiated culture systems. In Vitro 8:115–116, 1972.
64. Smith JR, Hayflick L: Variation in the life-span of clones derived from human diploid cell strains. J Cell Biol 62:48–53, 1974.
65. Gaffney EV, Polanowski FP, Blackburn SE, Lambiase JT, Burke RE: Culture of normal human mammary cells. Cell Diff 5:69–81, 1976.
66. Raul F, Simon P, Kedinger M, Haffen K: Intestinal enzyme activities in isolated villus and crypt cells during postnatal development of the rat. Cell Tissue Res 176:167–178, 1977.
67. Lasfargues EY, Ozzello L: Culture of human breast carcinomas. J Natl Cancer Inst 21:1131–1148, 1958.
68. Braaten JT, Järlfors U, Smith DS, Mintz DH: Purification of monolayer cell cultures of the endocrine pancreas. Tissue Cell 7:747–762, 1975.
69. Gospodarowicz D, Moran JS: Growth factors in mammalian cell culture. Annu Rev Biochem 45:531–558, 1976.
70. Cohen S: Isolation of a mouse submaxillary gland protein accelerating incisor eruption and eyelid opening in the new-born animal. J Biol Chem 237:1555–1562, 1962.
71. Carpenter G, Cohen S: Human epidermal growth factor and the proliferation of human fibroblasts. J Cell Physiol 88:227–238, 1976.
72. Rheinwald JG, Green H: Epidermal growth factor and the multiplication of cultured human epidermal keratinocytes. Nature 265:421–424, 1977.
73. Gospodarowicz D: Purification of a fibroblast growth factor from bovine pituitary. J Biol Chem 250:2515–2520, 1975.
74. Ross R, Vogel A: The platelet-derived growth factor. Cell 14:203–210, 1978.
75. Bürgi H, Müller WA, Humbel RE, Labhart A, Froesch ER: Non-suppressible insulin-like activity of human serum. I. Physicochemical properties, extraction and partial purification. Biochim Biophys Acta 121:349–359, 1966.
76. Levi-Montalcini R, Hamburger V: Selective growth stimulating effects of mouse sarcoma on the sensory and sympathetic nervous system of the chick embryo. J Exp Zool 116:321–362, 1951.
77. Gospodarowicz D, Jones KL, Sato G: Purification of a growth factor for ovarian cells from bovine pituitary glands. Proc Natl Acad Sci USA 71:2295–2299, 1974.
78. Ronzio RA, Rutter WJ: Effects of a partially purified factor from chick embryos on macromolecular synthesis of embryonic pancreatic epithelia. Dev Biol 30:307–320, 1973.
79. Hayashi I, Larner J, Sato G: Hormonal growth control of cells in culture. In Vitro 14:23–30, 1978.

80. Yuan GC, Chang RS: Testing of compounds for capacity to prolong postmitotic life-span of cultured human amnion cells. Effect of steroids and Panax ginseng. J Gerontol 24:82–85, 1969.
81. Van Wyk JJ, Underwood LE, Hintz RL, Clemons DR, Voina SJ, Weaver RP: The somatomedins: A family of insulinlike hormones under growth hormone control. Recent Prog Horm Res 30:259–295, 1974.
82. Van Wyk JJ, Furlanetto RW, Plet AS, D'Ercole AJ, Underwood LE: The somatomedin group of peptide growth factors. Natl Cancer Inst Monogr 48:141–147, 1978.
83. Milo GE, Malarkey WB, Powell JE, Blakeslee JR, Yohn DS: Effects of steroid hormones in fetal bovine serum on plating and cloning of human cells in vitro. In Vitro 12:23–30, 1976.
84. Brehmer B, Marquardt H, Madsen PO: Growth and hormonal response of cells derived from carcinoma and hyperplasia of the prostate in monolayer culture. A possible in vitro model for clinical chemotherapy. J Urol 108:890–896, 1972.
85. Kowaloff EM, Phang JM, Granger AS, Downing SJ: Glucocorticoid induction of proline oxidase in LLC-RKl cells. J Cell Physiol 97:153–159, 1978.
86. Terada M, Cantor L, Metafora S, Rifkind RA, Bank A, Marks PA: Globin messenger RNA activity in erythroid precursor cells and the effect of erythropoietin. Proc Natl Acad Sci USA 69:3575–3579, 1972.
87. Gilbert SF, Migeon BR: D-valine as a selective agent for normal human and rodent epithelial cells in culture. Cell 5:11–17, 1975.
88. Benke PJ, Dittmar D: Human lymphocyte response to D-valine media. Biochim Biophys Acta 451:635–637, 1976.
89. Downing SJ, Phang JM, Kowaloff EM, Valle D, Smith RJ: Proline oxidase in cultured mammalian cells. J Cell Physiol 91:369–376, 1977.
90. Kao WW-Y, Prockop DJ: Proline analogue removes fibroblasts from cultured mixed cell populations. Nature 266:63–64, 1977.
91. DeLuca L, Maestri N, Bonanni F, Nelson D: Maintenance of epithelial cell differentiation: The mode of action of vitamin A. Cancer 30:1326–1331, 1972.
92. Packer L, Smith JR: Extension of the lifespan of cultured normal human diploid cells by vitamin E. Proc Natl Acad USA 71:4763–4767, 1974.
93. Balin AK, Goodman DBP, Rasmussen H, Cristofalo VJ: The effect of oxygen and vitamin E E on the lifespan of human diploid cells in vitro. J Cell Biol 74:58–67, 1977.
94. Ham RG, McKeehan WL: Development of improved media and culture conditions for clonal growth of normal diploid cells. In Vitro 14:11–22, 1978.
95. Jenkin HM, Anderson LE: The effect of oleic acid on the growth of monkey kidney cells (LLC-MK_2) Exp Cell Res 59:6–10, 1970.
96. Driedger PE, Blumberg PM: The effect of phorbol diesters on chicken embryo fibroblasts. Cancer Res 37:3257–3265, 1977.
97. Shodell M: Environmental stimuli in the progression of BHK/21 cells through the cell cycle. Proc Natl Acad Sci USA 69:1455–1459, 1972.
98. Rafferty KA Jr: Morphology and longevity of cells cultured from primate, carnivore and rodent tissues. Differentiation 1:363–372, 1973.
99. Pretlow TG II, Pretlow TP: Separation of viable cells by velocity sedimentation in an isokinetic gradient of Ficoll in tissue culture medium. In Catsimpoolas N (ed): "Methods of Cell Separation." New York: Plenum Press 1977, vol 1, pp 171–191.
100. Fusenig NE: Isolation and cultivation of epidermal cells from embryonic mouse skin. Naturwissenschaften 58:421, 1971.
101. Munthe-Kaas AC, Seglen PO: The use of metrizamide as a gradient medium for isopycnic separation of rat liver cells. FEBS Lett 43:252–256, 1974.
102. Mitchell BF, Tupper JT: Synchronization of mouse 3T3 and SV40 3T3 cells by way of centrifugal elutriation. Exp Cell Res 106:351–355, 1977.

103. Miller RG, Phillips RA: Separation of cells by velocity sedimentation. J Cell Physiol 73:191–202, 1969.
104. Mel HC: Sedimentation properties of nucleated and non-nucleated cells in normal rat bone marrow. Nature 200:423–425, 1963.
105. MacDonald HR, Miller RG: Synchronization of mouse L-cells by a velocity sedimentation technique. Biophys J 10:834–842, 1970.
106. Shall S: Cells at defined stages of the cell cycle. B. Sedimentation in sucrose and Ficoll gradients of cells grown in suspension culture. Supra #31, pp 198–204.
107. Shall S: Selection synchronization by velocity sedimentation. Separation of mouse fibroblast cells grown in suspension culture. Methods Cell Biol 7:269–285, 1973.
108. Catsimpoolas N, Griffith AL: Preparative density electrophoresis and velocity sedimentation at unit gravity of mammalian cells. Supra #99, pp 1–24.
109. Pretlow TG II, Weir EE, Zettergren JG: Problems connected with the separation of different kinds of cells. Int Rev Exp Pathol 14:91–204, 1975.
110. Pretlow TG II, Pretlow TP: Cell electrophoresis. Int Rev Cytol (In press).
111. Stephenson JR, Axelrad AA: Separation of erythropoietin-sensitive cells from hemopoietic spleen colony-forming stem cells of mouse fetal liver by unit gravity sedimentation. Blood 37:417–427, 1971.
112. Davis JC, Schuetz AW: Separation of germinal cells from immature rat testes by sedimentation at unit gravity. Exp Cell Res 91:79–86, 1975.
113. Mitsui Y, Schneider EL: Characterization of fractionated human diploid fibroblast cell populations. Exp Cell Res 103:23–30, 1976.
114. Houghton BA: Velocity sedimentation separation of human diploid fibroblast subpopulations. (Abstract) In Vitro 14:357, 1978.
115. Pretlow TG II, Scalise MM, Weir EE: Separation of hamster testicular cells in successive stages of differentiation by velocity sedimentation in an isokinetic gradient of Ficoll in tissue culture medium. Am J Pathol 74:83–94, 1974.
116. Walter H: Cell partitioning in two-polymer aqueous phase system. Trends Biochem Sci 3:97–100, 1978.
117. Herzenberg LA, Sweet RG, Herzenberg LA: Fluorescence-activated cell sorting. Sci Am 234:108–117, 1976.
118. McKeehan WL, Ham RG: Stimulation of clonal growth of normal fibroblasts with substrata coated with basic polymers. J Cell Biol 71:727–734, 1976.
119. Adebonojo FO: Monolayer cultures of disaggregated human adipocytes. In Vitro 11:50–54, 1975.
120. Ham RG: Nutritional requirements of primary cultures. A neglected problem of modern biology. In Vitro 10:119–129, 1974.
121. Leblond CP, Greulich RC, Pereira JPM: Relationship of cell formation and cell migration in the renewal of stratified squamous epithelia. In Montagna W, Billingham RE (eds): "Advances in Biology of Skin: Wound Healing." Oxford: Pergamon Press, 1964, vol 5 pp 39–67.
122. Cheng H, Leblond CP: Origin, differentiation and renewal of the four main epithelial cell types in the mouse small intestine. I. The columnar cell. Am J Anat 141:461–480, 1974.
123. Ham RG: Cloning of mammalian cells. In Prescott DM (ed): "Methods in Cell Physiology." New York: Academic Press, 1972, vol 5, pp 37–74.
124. Taylor WG, Richter A, Evans VJ, Sanford KK: Influence of oxygen and pH on plating efficiency and colony development of WI-38 and Vero cells. Exp Cell Res 86:152–156, 1974.
125. McKeehan WL, Hamilton WG, Ham RG: Selenium is an essential trace nutrient for growth of WI-38 diploid human fibroblasts. Proc Natl Acad Sci USA 73:2023–2027, 1976.

Growth and Characterization of Functional Epithelial Cells on Selective Substrates

Yutaka Yoshida, MD, PhD, Sharen L. Carey, BS, MT (ASCP), Randall H. Kottel, PhD, and Aaron E. Freeman, PhD

Studies of metabolic disorders in cell culture are hampered by three major difficulties in technique.

1) Most in vitro studies have been carried out with fibroblasts and not the functional cells characteristic of specific organs. Emphasis on the study of fibroblasts has been necessary, because they are the dominant cells under in vitro conditions and epithelial cells are very difficult to culture.
2) Cell cultures are usually established from mixed cell populations. The ancestry of the cells which grow is difficult or impossible to define.
3) Most normal cells grow only when attached to some kind of surface or substrate and then growth characteristically tends to be monolayered. The lack of cellular organization and properties of the substrate often interfere with histochemical analysis of the cells.

In this paper, we will briefly review certain culture techniques for growing selected functional cells on substrates made of glass, polystyrene, cellophane, gas-permeable membranes, histone coat, collagen coat, and stainless steel raft. Further, we will present new data on the use of pigskin as a collagen bed or keratin bed, respectively, for the culturing of organotypic lung or liver epithelial cells.

SELECTIVE CONDITIONS FOR CULTURING EPITHELIAL CELLS

Successful culturing of epithelial cells depends upon some sort of selective pressure to discourage fibroblast takeover. This paper will focus on the use of the pigskin substrate, which tends to select for epithelial cell growth. Within the methods discussed in this paper there are usually specific techniques which are designed to discourage growth of fibroblasts. As an example, the technique of

Birth Defects: Original Article Series, Volume XVI, Number 2, pages 35–52

Flaxman [1] for growing skin epithelial cells on glass depends on a differential rate of cell migration from explants. Keratinocytes rapidly mobilize within 2–3 days; dermal fibroblasts are not mobilized for up to 12 days. Removal of the original explant before fibroblast migration begins results in virtually pure cultures of epithelial cells [2]. For each method discussed in this paper, we will try to point out similar techniques which exert selective pressure for survival of epithelial cells. There are, however, two powerful methods – clonal isolation and selective trypsinization – which may be applicable with many substrates and which deserve special review.

Clonal Isolation

One method to prevent fibroblast overgrowth of epithelial cells is to separate the cell types by clonal isolation. The procedure for clonal isolation begins with selection of a relatively pure donor tissue. (Obviously, whole embryos are not good donors for lung epithelium.) The donor tissue is then broken down to cellular elements by enzymatic digestion, usually with trypsin and/or collagenase. Cells are seeded so that individual colonies can be isolated. In primary culture, epithelial cell colonies are readily distinguished from fibroblastic colonies [2]. Physical isolation and subsequent outgrowth of epithelial colonies result in cultures which have functional markers of their epithelial cell ancestry. Cell lines established by this method include rat alveolar cells [3] and rat hepatocytes [4]. In some cases continuous culturing of epithelial cells is further facilitated by establishing the clones on feeder layers of other cell types. As an example, the Rheinwald and Green [5] method for culturing human skin epithelial cells is dependent on the use of irradiated mouse fibroblasts as feeder cells.

Selective Trypsinization

A major advance in the culturing of continuous epithelial cell lines was the development of the selective trypsinization procedure. When fibroblasts and epithelial cells are growing together in the same glass or plastic dish, exposure to trypsin results in detachment of the fibroblasts first, often within minutes. Epithelial cell detachment by trypsin is usually comparatively slow. Repetitive weeding of the fibroblasts yields cultures more and more rich in epithelial cells. This method has been used to establish continuous strains of human colon, bladder, and kidney epithelial cells [6].

Substrates

The Tissue Culture Association (TCA) Manual is a very useful reference which includes detailed descriptions of procedures for growing specific functional cell types on a variety of substrates. Most of the following topics are abstracted from volumes 1–3 of the TCA Manual.

Substrate	Cell Type	Reference
glass	keratinocytes, human skin	[1]

Split-thickness pieces of human skin, 2–4 mm on a side, are held in place on glass coverslips by a chick plasma clot. After the clot dries, the cultures are fed 2 ml of Eagle's Minimum Essential Medium per 35-mm dish and incubated in 5% CO_2 at 37°C. Within 4–5 days, outgrowth of the epithelial keratinocytes can be seen around 95% of the explants. The cultures continue to proliferate for 3–4 months, but all attempts at subculture have failed. **Note that fat tissue inhibits growth of the epithelial cells!**

Substrate	Cell Type	Reference
glass or plastic	mammary epithelium	[7]

Normal mammary glands are carefully dissected from muscle fibers, connective tissue, accumulated collagen, blood vessels, and lymph nodes. The gland fragments are minced to a pulp and treated with collagenase for 1 hour or longer at 37°C. After a series of washes, the cell pellet is seeded into 25-cm^2 flasks.

Neoplastic mammary epithelium is excised into tumor chunks, free of muscles; the fibrous-limiting membranes; and necrotic tissue. Tumor fragments are minced by crosscutting action of two scalpels. The tumor mince is distributed into 25-cm^2 flasks.

The procedures yield fairly pure cultures of mammary epithelium. Selection of epithelial cells from fibroblasts is facilitated because fibroblasts attach first to the substrate; thus, replanting of cells remaining in suspension for 24 hours results in virtually pure cultures of epithelial cells.

Subcultures are made by classical trypsinization procedures. Cell lines are sometimes established.

Substrate	Cell Type	Reference
cellophane	central nervous system	[8]

The brains of 20- to 21-day rat embryos are dissected and 0.5 to 1.0-mm^3 tissue bits are planted on a 35 × 40-mm cellophane rectangle. The explants are anchored into place by a second cellophane sheet placed on top. The cellophane sandwich is fed just enough medium to cover the upper cellophane sheet. Incubation is in 5% CO_2 at 37°C.

Outgrowth from the explants proceeds with notable migration within 24 hours, appearance of neurites within 5 days, and development of myelinated axons within 2 weeks. The cultures remain viable for 3 months or longer.

Overgrowth of fibroblasts is held in check because fibroblasts migrate through the cellophane perforations to the floor of the vessel, while glial and nerve cells develop between the 2 layers of cellophane.

Substrate	Cell Type	Reference
histone-coated plastic	plasmacytoma	[9]

Mouse plasmacytoma cells are neoplastic cells which grow as floating clusters. When plastic is treated with histone, however, the cells adhere and form monolayers. This facilitates observation, counting, colony formation, and cloning.

Substrate	Cell Types	Reference
rafts, stainless steel	many	[10]

Tissue explants not larger than 8 mm^3 are placed on absorbent disks resting on a stainless steel wire mesh platform. Medium is introduced below the platform until the tissue comes into contact but is not submerged by the medium. Organ explants may be maintained up to 2 weeks.

Substrate	Cell Type	Reference
collagen-coated cellulose sponge	epithelial tumor cells	[11]

Collagen dispersed in 50% methyl alcohol is impregnated into slices of cellulose sponge. As the methanol evaporates, the collagen fibers coalesce and adhere to the sponge. Solid tumor explants 1 mm in diameter are placed on the surface of the sponge, which is contained in flat culture tubes. The explants lose their original shape and blend into the surrounding surface. Outgrowth of tissue is meager and continues for no more than 17 days; however, the growth obtained often has a three-dimensional architecture, typical of the organ of cell derivation.

THE PIGSKIN GRAFT METHOD

The procedures for growing cells, by a variety of techniques, on collagen-coated surfaces has been reported for chicken fibroblasts [12], human diploid malignant cells [13], muscle clones [14], and embryonic tissues [15]. Primarily related to our work are reports for growing rabbit and human skin epithelium on the dermal collagen surface of dead sterile pigskin [16–18]. The pigskin method of epithelial cell culture in vitro will be presented in detail elsewhere in this volume. Briefly reviewed, however, rabbit and human skin cultured on the pigskin dermis form maturating epithelium consisting of basal, squamous, granular, and keratin layers. The cultures can be carried for several months and, when grafted to a wound in the donor, provide rapid and excellent permanent epithelial coverage. This paper describes the use of pigskin as a substrate for culturing and characterizing other types of epithelial cells.

Dermis vs Epidermis as a Substrate

Mouse embryonic liver explanted on pigskin dermis degenerated and died after 1 week in culture (Fig. 1).

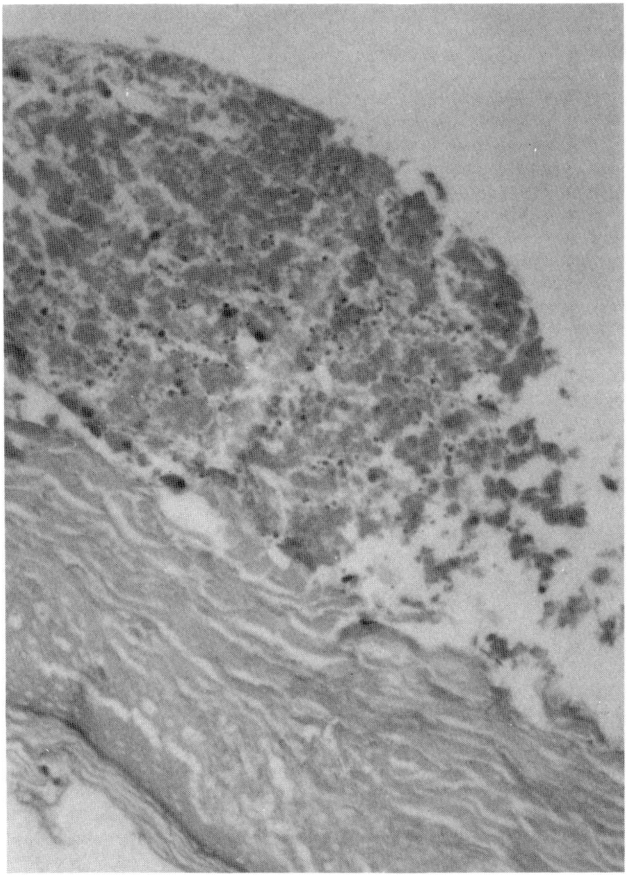

Fig. 1. Mouse embryonic liver on pigskin dermis, 1 week (H & E, X350).

When explanted on the epidermal surface, however, the embryonic liver cells not only survived for periods up to 5 weeks, but also proliferated by undermining and digesting the pigskin epithelium (Fig. 2).

In contrast, pregnant mouse mammary gland epithelium (Fig. 3), embryonic mouse pancreas (Fig. 4), embryonic mouse kidney, and adult rabbit and human skin all grew preferentially on or in the dermal pigskin surface.

Growth and Characterization of Embryonic Mouse Lung Cells on Pigskin Dermis

Histologic and histochemical evidence of organotypic structure and metabolic function in embryonic lung cultures. The original mouse embryo lung tissue, at the time of explanting, contained bronchial tubes and numerous alveolar sacs but no complete alveolar structures (Fig. 5).

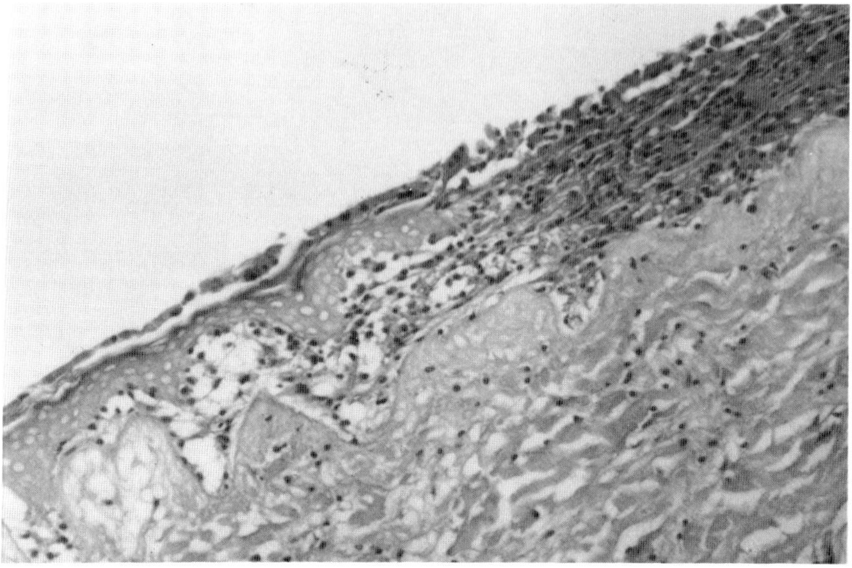

Fig. 2. Mouse embryonic liver on pigskin epidermis, 5 weeks. Note invasion of cells into the pigskin dermal collagen (H & E, X350).

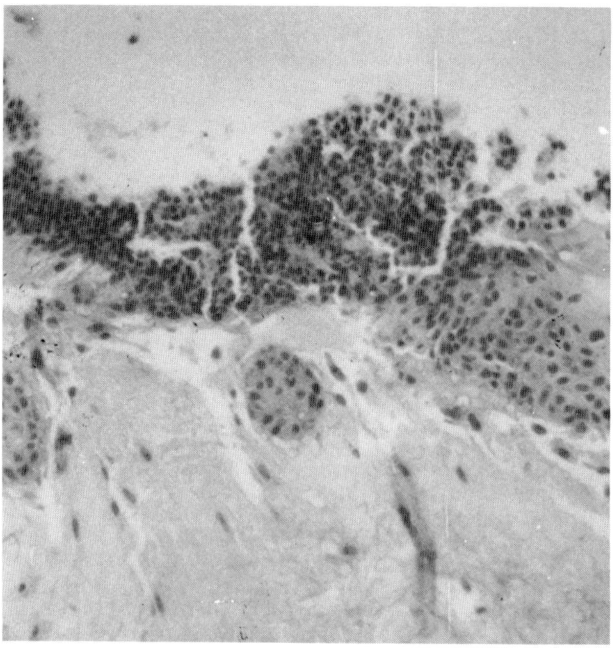

Fig. 3. Pregnant mouse mammary gland on pigskin dermis. Note epithelial cell invasion into the pigskin dermal collagen (H & E, X350).

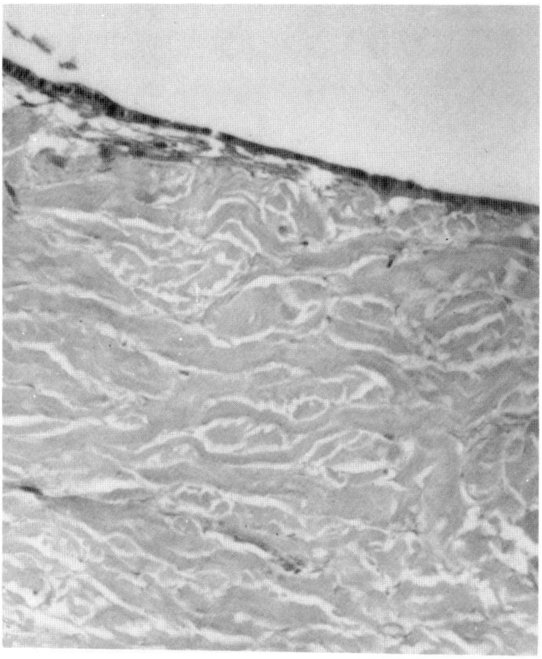

Fig. 4. Mouse embryonic pancreas on pigskin dermis. Note columnar cells (H & E, X350).

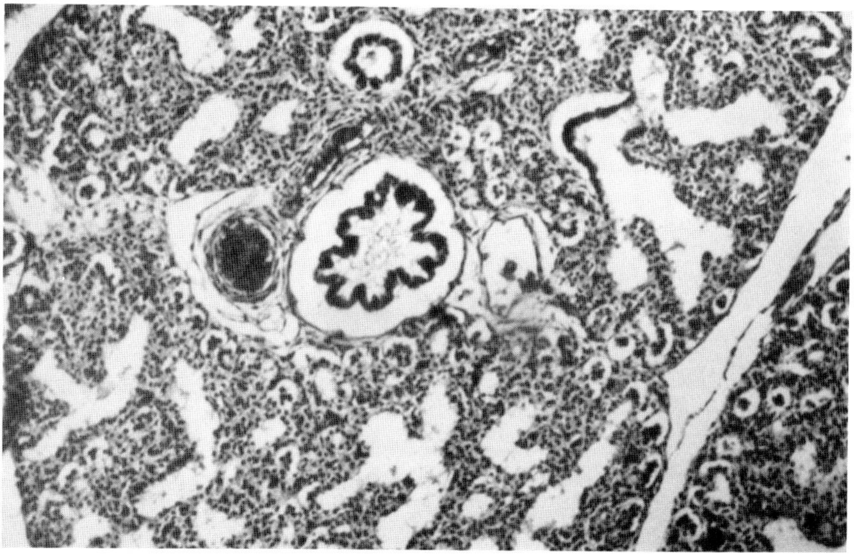

Fig. 5. Full-term mouse fetal lung (H & E, X320).

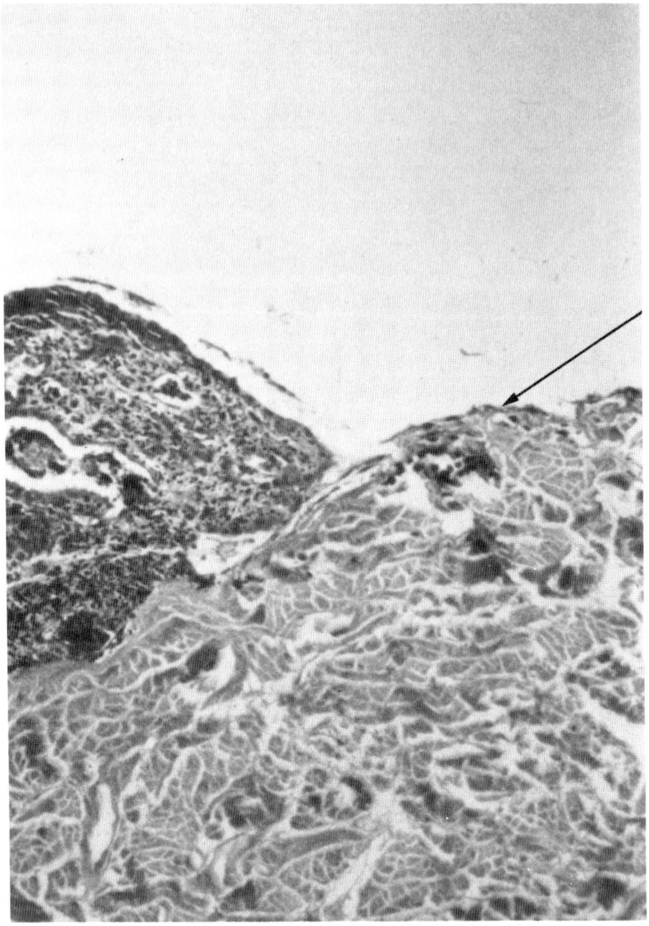

Fig. 6. Full-term fetal lung explanted on pigskin dermis, 1 week (H & E, X320).

After 1 week in culture, the tissue retained an organoid structure. It had an alveolus-like structure together with glandular structure composed of tall columnar cells. Among the epithelial cells were compactly arranged mononuclear cells. A cell population showing onionskin-like nuclear arrangement was noted. Certain areas within the explant showed degenerative changes and even cellular necrosis. Some cells began to spread onto and beneath the surface of the pigskin dermal collagen (Fig. 6).

Mitotic figures were detected within the explant (Fig. 7).

Histologic appearance of the explants remained stable after 3 weeks in culture. The explants were moderately cellular, contained well-developed gland-like struc-

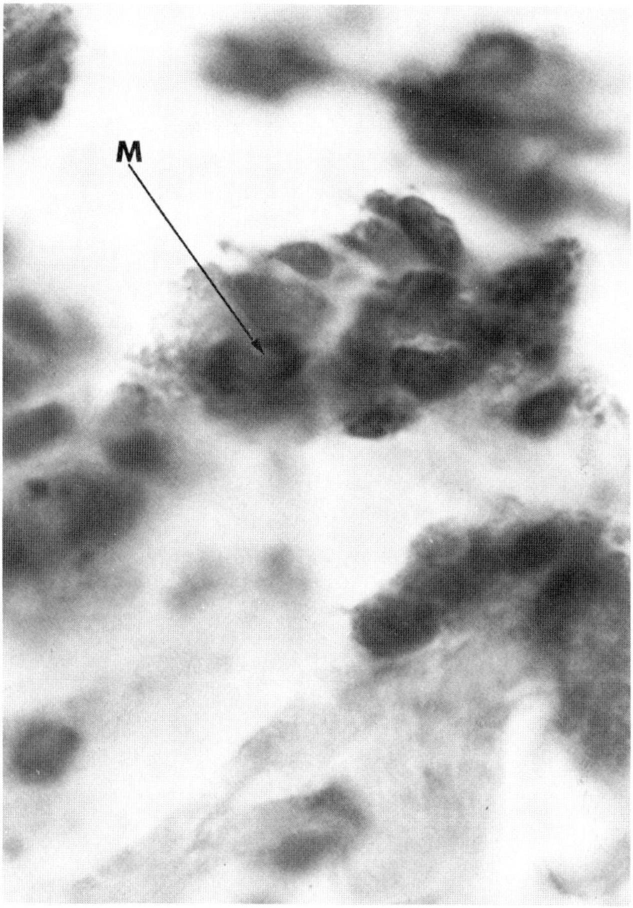

Fig. 7. Note mitotic figures (M) (H & E, X1,280).

tures, alveolus-like structures, and some degenerated cellular debris. However, between the explants, sheets of cells were widely spread on and under the dermal pigskin surface (Fig. 8).

After 3 weeks, highly differentiated ductular structures were found in the cell culture outgrowth, tightly adhering to pigskin collagen between explants. The epithelial cells in the cultures regularly had nuclei located at the base of the cytoplasm. Mitotic figures were detected randomly. Epithelial cells lining the ductular structure had cilia at the surface border (Fig. 9).

When epithelial cells lining the ductular structures were stained with PAS–Alcian blue, mucin was conspicuous on the free surface of the cells (Fig. 10).

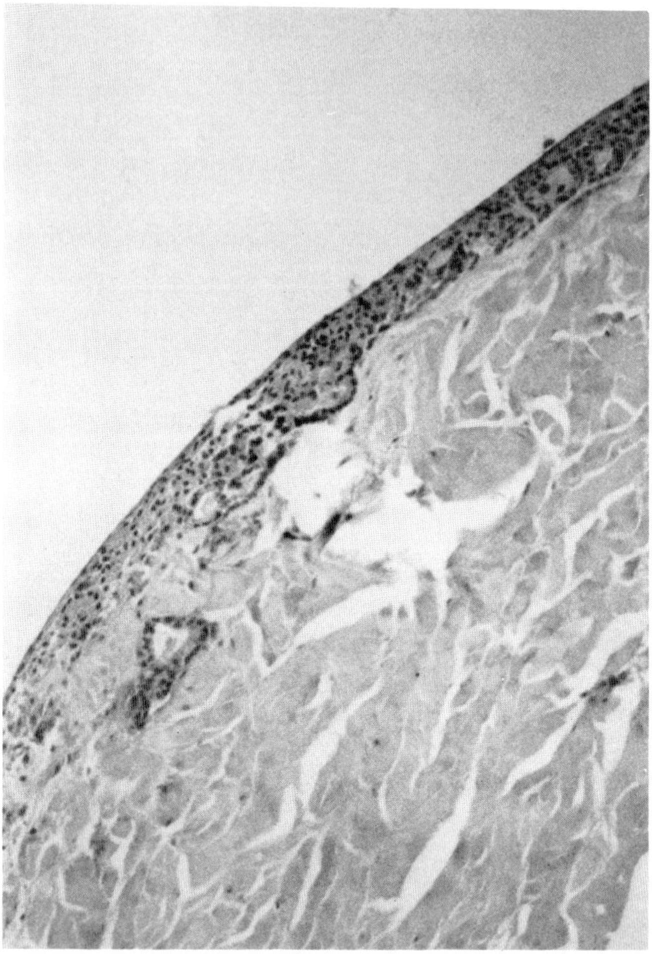

Fig. 8. Full-term fetal lung on pigskin dermis, 3 weeks (H & E, X320).

Based on the data presented we conclude that the mouse embryonic cultures growing on pigskin dermis are proliferating, ciliated, mucin-producing lung epithelial cells. However, it is our intention to further demonstrate the origin, function, and differentiation of the cultured cells by comparing in vitro activity of specific enzymes with the expression of the same gene products during normal ontogenetic development in vivo. Our preliminary studies have focused on alkaline phosphatase (ALP) and gamma-glutamyl transferase (GGT) as enzyme markers. The activity and distribution of ALP and GGT during the normal ontogenetic process of mouse lung are shown in Table 1.

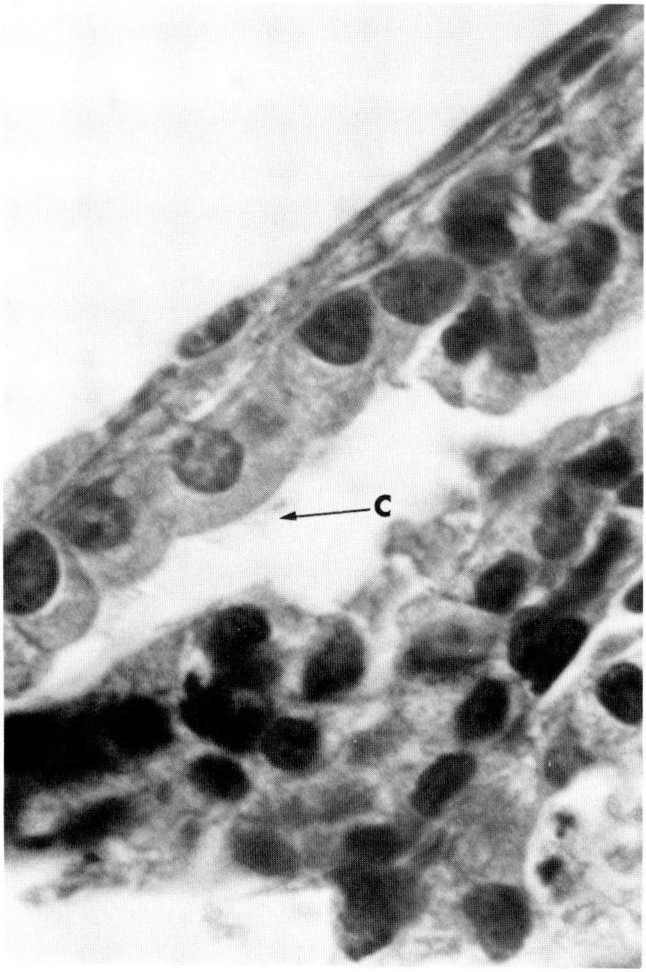

Fig. 9. Note cilia (C) at surface border (H & E, X1,280).

GGT activity was found only for a short period following birth and was confined to the respiratory bronchial epithelium. Thus, no GGT activity could be demonstrated in newborn mouse lung tissue at the time of explant. After 1 week in culture, however, some GGT activity was noted in the lung explant (Fig. 11). After 3 weeks in culture, GGT activity could no longer be observed in the explant. These findings seem to indicate some differentiation of the newborn mouse lung cells in culture.

ALP was found in the newborn mouse lung 3 days after birth and was maintained thereafter. We have not yet determined the cell type responsible for the

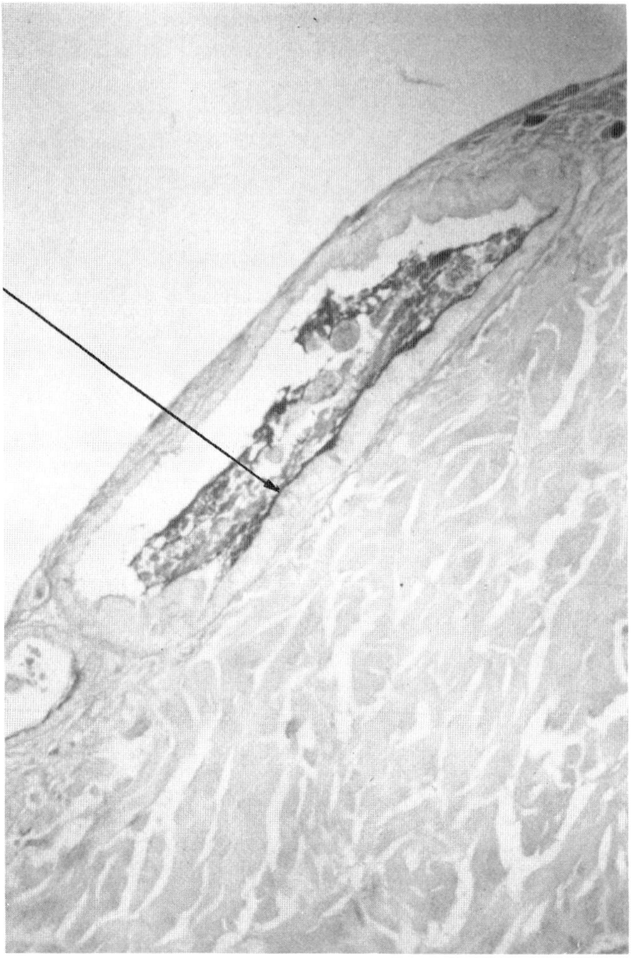

Fig. 10. Mucin production by epithelial lung cells within a ductular structure (PAS–Alcian blue, X320).

TABLE 1. Histochemical Activity of GGT and ALP During Normal Ontogenetic Process of Mouse Lung

	Early embryo	Full term	Newborn Day 1	Day 2	Day 3	Day 4	Day 7	Day 14	Adult
GGT	–	–	–	+	+	+	–	–	–
ALP	–	–	–	–	+	+	+	+	+

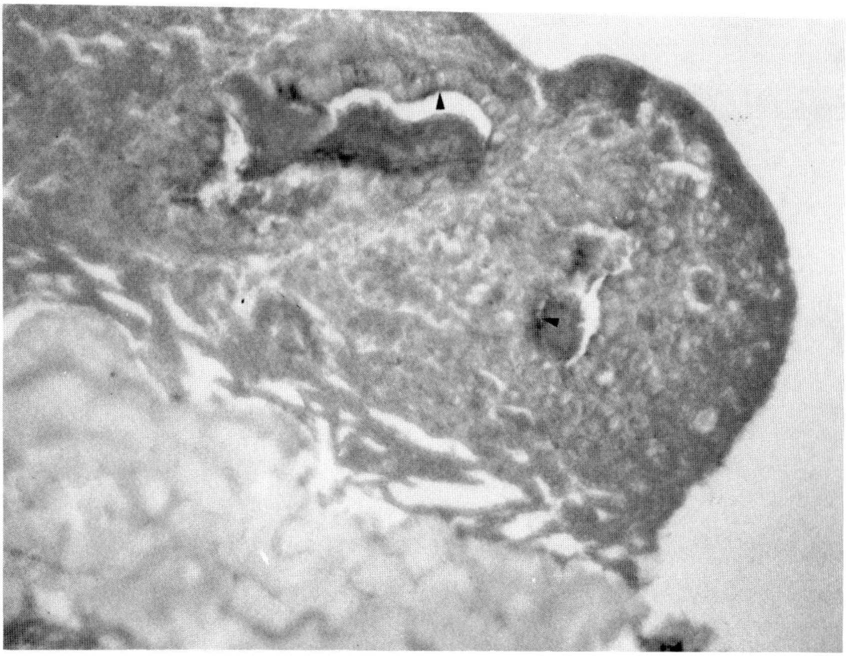

Fig. 11. GGT activity in lung explant, 1 week (GGT stain, X500).

ALP activity in the mouse; however, in the fetal rat ALP activity was limited to the epithelial cells lining the alveolar tubes (Fig. 12).

After 3 weeks in culture, ALP activity could be demonstrated in embryonic and newborn mouse cells spreading onto the surface of the pigskin (Fig. 13). This would tend to confirm that the spreading cells were derived from the epithelial cells lining the alveolar tubes, that cellular differentiation may occur, and that the cells remained functional after 3 weeks in culture.

Biochemical evidence of organotypic metabolic function in lung and liver cultures. Explants of embryonic and newborn mouse liver and newborn mouse lung were planted onto pigskin and cultivated for 5 weeks. At that time, the cultures were overlaid with 4 ml of fresh medium containing 2 μCi tritiated benzo(a)-pyrene (BaP)/ml, specific activity = 56 Ci/mmole. After 24 hours, the supernatants were removed and assayed for hexane–soluble and water–soluble counts by the Diamond assay. Virtually all of the radioactive material in the blank or pigskin control plates remained in the hexane fraction (Table 2), thus indicating little hydrocarbon metabolizing activity (HMA) activity. The reduction in hexane–soluble counts from 47,086 cpm/plate in the blank as compared to 23,423 cpm/plate in the pigskin control represents binding of BaP to the pigskin. The newborn

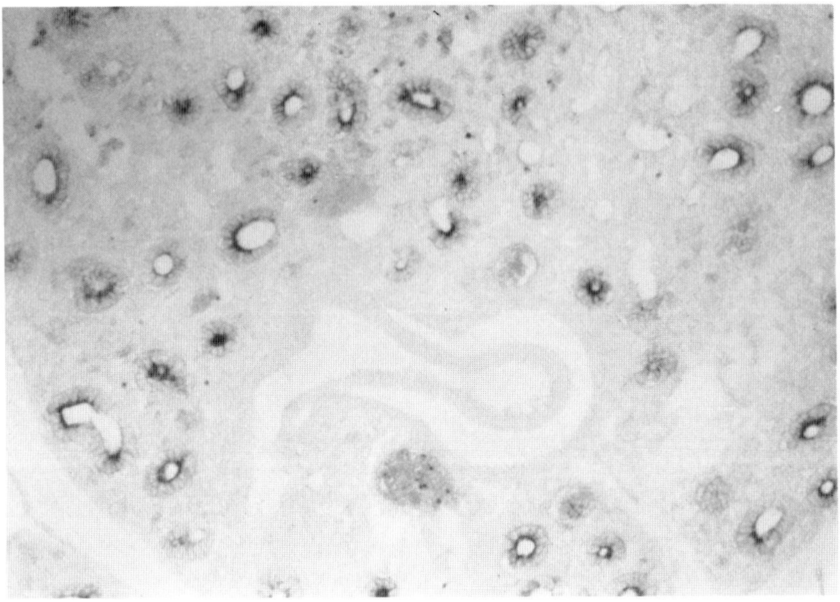

Fig. 12. Alkaline phosphatase activity in rat fetal lung (ALP stain, X320).

liver culture had no more HMA activity than the pigskin blank. Newborn lung, however, had 1,983 cpm/dish and embryonic liver had 5,020 cpm/dish, indicating that these two cultures had relatively high levels of hydrocarbon metabolizing activity.

We must point out that these are preliminary experiments carried out in single dishes, which may be subject to variance because of problems in the methodology. Nevertheless, these promising qualitative results indicate that liver and/or lung cultures remain metabolically functional under in vitro culture conditions.

TABLE 2. Hydrocarbon Metabolizing Activity of 5-Week-Old Mouse Lung and Liver Cultures on Pigskin

	cpm/dish	
Cells cultured	Hexane soluble	Acetone – H_2O soluble
Blank	47,086	277
Pigskin	23,423	791
Newborn lung	27,544	1,983
Newborn liver	26,103	440
Embryonic liver	16,737	5,020

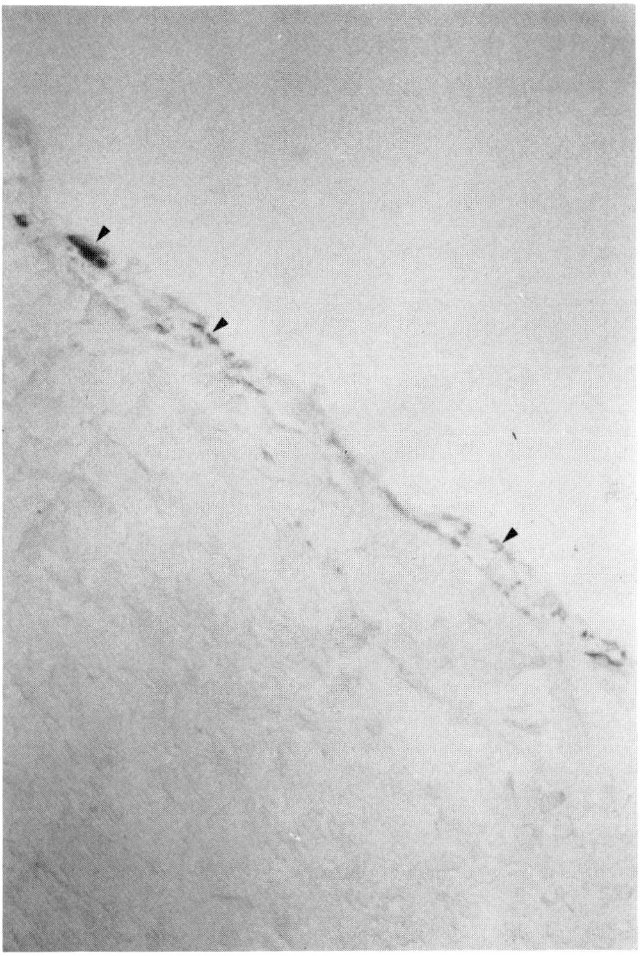

Fig. 13. Alkaline phosphatase activity in 3-week culture of mouse fetal lung on pigskin dermis (ALP stain, X320).

Biochemical analysis of liver explant. Finally, we were concerned with proving that the small organ explants contained enough enzymatic activity to allow for biochemical analysis. As yet, we have no preliminary data with lung explants, but offer the following data with liver explants to support our hypothesis.

The results of comparable analyses of adult and fetal liver explants are shown in Table 3. It can be seen that the ALP levels for both adult and fetal liver remained constant over the 1-week time period. Fetal ALP activity was found to be approximately 4 times greater than corresponding adult activity at each point.

TABLE 3. Comparative Enzymology of Mouse Adult and Fetal Tissues

Specimen	Source	Time in culture (days)	Enzyme specific activity ALP[a]	GGT[b]	LDH[c]	G6PD[d]
Liver	Adult	0	2.3	ND	492	2.3
		7	2.2	ND	1,021	13.0
	Fetal	0	10.0	9.0	1,514	4.3
		7	8.9	5.5	747	11.0

[a]Expressed as nmole p-nitrophenol/min/mg protein.
[b]Expressed as milliunits/mg protein.
[c]Expressed as Wacker units/mg protein.
[d]Expressed as milliunits/mg protein.

Of interest is the fact that GGT activity was found in fetal liver at Day 0 and this activity was observed to decrease (approximately 50%) in the 7-day explants. In contrast, fetal and adult G6PD activity increased markedly during the 7-day period of culture.

DISCUSSION

We conclude that a number of specific functional epithelial cell types can be cultured in vitro through the use of selective procedures which help control fibroblast takeover. The use of specific substrates not only facilitates epithelial cell outgrowth but also may enable the cells to form an organotypic three-dimensional structure. When epithelial cells are grown on pigskin, demonstration of organotypic structure can be made by sectioning and staining the samples by histochemical methods. Specific stains can then be used to demonstrate specific functions indicative of cell ancestry, function, and differentiation. Sufficient functional growth occurs so that biochemical analyses can also be made. Further application of these epithelial cell culture systems to human cell types and human metabolic diseases can lead to a better understanding of the nature of birth defects and improved methods of early diagnosis and treatment.

SUMMARY

In vitro culturing and characterization of functional epithelial cells can be facilitated by use of selective substrates. The substrates include glass, plastics, perforated cellophane, histone-coated plastic, collagen-coated cellulose sponge, and stainless steel rafts. A pigskin raft method has been used to produce primary proliferating organotypic cultures of human and rabbit skin, embryonic mouse liver, lung, kidney and pancreas, and pregnant mouse mammary gland. Most cell types grow preferentially on the pigskin dermis; however, mouse embryonic liver cells grow preferentially on pigskin epidermis. Cultures grown on pigskin can be sectioned, stained, and evaluated by classical histochemical procedures.

Embryonic mouse lung cells which proliferate on pigskin dermis form organotypic structures consisting of ciliated or mucin-producing cells. Alkaline phosphatase or gamma-glutamyl transferase activity can be demonstrated in the cultured cells or explants even though the starting donor material was negative for these enzymes. A comparison of enzyme activity in vitro with expression of these enzymes. A comparison of enzyme activity in vitro with expression of these same gene products during normal ontogenetic development indicates that the cultured lung cells are derived from cells which line the alveolar sacs. Further, differentiation of enzyme function continues during cultivation.

REFERENCES

1. Flaxman BA: Primary epithelial outgrowth cultures of keratinocytes from human skin. Procedure No 42621. Tissue Culture Association (TCA) Manual 1:21–22, 1975.
2. Lake RS, Freeman AE, Igel HJ, Pezzutti MR, Korpko ML: In vitro culture of diploid human skin epithelial cells for chemical transformation studies. In Saffiotti U, Autrup H (eds): "In Vitro Carcinogenesis. Guide to the Literature, Recent Advances and Laboratory Procedures." NCI Carcinogenesis Tech Rep Ser No 44. DHEW Publ No (NIH) 78-844, 1978, pp 283–291.
3. Douglas WHJ, Kaighn ME: Clonal isolation of differentiated rat lung cells. In Vitro 10: 230–237, 1974.
4. Williams GM, Stromberg K, Kroes R: Cytochemical and ultrastructural alterations associated with confluent growth in cell cultures of epithelial-like cells from rat liver. Lab Invest 29:293–303, 1973.
5. Rheinwald JG, Green H: Serial cultivation of strains of human epidermal keratinocytes: The formation of keratinizing colonies from single cells. Cell 6:331–344, 1975.
6. Owens RB, Smith HS, Nelson-Rees WA, Springer EL: Epithelial cell cultures from normal and cancerous human tissues. J Natl Cancer Inst 56(4):843–849, 1976.
7. Lasfargues EY: Primary explanation of normal and neoplastic mammary epithelium. Procedure No 46135. TCA Manual 2:269–271, 1976.
8. Cole R, De Vellis J: The cellophane sandwich explant system. Procedure No 41175. TCA Manual 2:261–263, 1976.
9. Keay L: A method for cloning plasmacytoma cells by attachment to histone-coated plastic surfaces. Procedure No 78199. TCA Manual 1:177–180, 1975.
10. Douglas WHJ, Kahn RH: Raft cultures. Procedure No 43122. TCA Manual 2:409–410, 1976.
11. Leighton J, Mark R, Justh G: Patterns of three-dimensional growth in vitro in collagen-coated cellulose sponge: Carcinomas and embryonic tissues. Cancer Res 28:286–296, 1968.
12. Gey GO, Svotelis M, Foard M, Bang FB: Long-term growth of chicken fibroblasts on a collagen substrate. Exp Cell Res 84:63–71, 1974.
13. Elsdale T, Bard J: Collagen substrata for studies on cell behavior. J Cell Biol 54:626–637, 1972.
14. Hauschka SD, Konigsberg IR: The influence of collagen on the development of muscle clones. Proc Natl Acad Sci USA 55:119–126, 1966.

15. Leighton J: Collagen-coated cellulose sponge. In Kruse P Jr, Patterson MK (eds): "Tissue Culture Methods and Applications." New York: Academic Press, 1973, pp 367–371.
16. Freeman AE, Igel HJ, Waldman NL, Losikoff AM: A new method for covering large surface area wounds with autografts. I. In vitro multiplication of rabbit-skin epithelial cells. Arch Surg 108:721–723, 1974.
17. Igel HJ, Freeman AE, Boeckman CR, Kleinfeld KL: A new method for covering large surface area wounds with autografts. II. Surgical application of tissue culture expanded rabbit-skin autografts. Arch Surg 108:724–729, 1974.
18. Freeman AE, Igel HJ, Herrman BJ, Kleinfeld KL: Growth and characterization of human skin epithelial cell cultures. In Vitro 12:352–362, 1976.

Can Proline Analogues Be Used to Prevent Fibroblasts From Overgrowing Cultures of Epithelial Cells?*

Winston W.-Y. Kao, PhD and Darwin J. Prockop, MD, PhD

One of the problems in culturing epithelial cells is that cultures of such cells are frequently overgrown by fibroblasts. We have recently made an observation which apparently provides a new technique for eliminating fibroblasts from cultures of mixed cell populations [1]. We have tested this technique with 2 different kinds of fibroblasts and with 2 nonfibroblastic cell lines. It has also been tested with a few additional cell lines by other investigators [2]. We have not, however, tested the procedure with epithelial cells and therefore we present the technique here only as a proposal which may be useful to investigators who are actively working with cultures of epithelial cells.

The technique has the appeal of simplicity. Also, the rationale for the technique has been fairly extensively investigated.

This technique consists of adding the proline analogue, *cis*-4-hydroxy-L-proline, to cell cultures. As indicated in Figure 1, the presence of 100 μg/ml *cis*-hydroxyproline markedly inhibited the growth of fibroblasts from chick embryo tendons, but it did not inhibit the growth of a cultured line of cells from a human epidermoid carcinoma. Also, it had no effect on the growth of a line of neuroblastoma cells. As indicated in Figure 2, the analogue in a concentration of 100–200 μg/ml also inhibited the growth of L-929 mouse fibroblasts. Higher concentrations of the analogue were required to inhibit L-929 fibroblasts than fibroblasts from chick embryos, an observation which may be related to the fact that the chick embryo fibroblasts employed here were about 5 times more active in synthesizing collagen than L-929 fibroblasts [1]. At much higher concentrations, the analogue also inhibited the growth of KB cells and neuroblastoma cells, but there appeared to be an adequate margin of safety between the effects on these cells and on the fibroblasts we have examined.

*Supported in part by NIH research grants AM-16, 516, and AM-16, 186.

Birth Defects: Original Article Series, Volume XVI, Number 2, pages 53–59

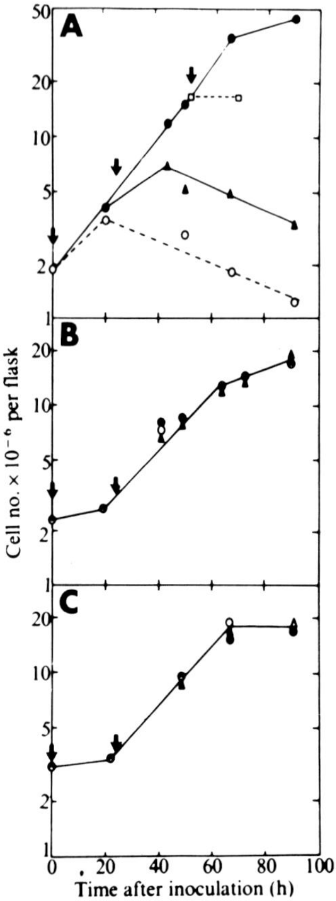

Fig. 1. The effects of *cis*-hydroxyproline on the growth of A) tendon fibroblasts from chick embryos, B) KB cells, and C) neuroblastoma cells. Tendon fibroblasts were obtained by limited enzymic digestion of tendons from 17-day-old chick embryos. KB cells (CCL-17) and neuroblastoma cells (CCL-131) were obtained from the American Type Culture Collection. The culture media were changed every other day after inoculation. *cis*-Hydroxyproline, at a concentration of 100 μg/ml, was added to the culture at the time indicated by the arrows. Cultures were grown under control conditions (●) or with *cis*-hydroxyproline added at the time of inoculation (0), 24 hours after inoculation (▲), or 54 hours after inoculation (□). (Figs. 1 and 2 from Kao WW-Y, Prockop DJ: Proline analogue removes fibroblasts from cultured mixed cell populations. Nature 266:63, 1977, with permission.)

More recently we have found that the analogue also inhibits the growth of chondrocytes from chick embryo cartilage (Fig. 3). The concentrations required to inhibit the growth of these cells is higher than the concentrations required to inhibit the L-929 fibroblasts or the chick embryo tendon fibroblasts. This observation may well be related to the fact that cartilage cells synthesize Type II procollagen and collagen, whereas the fibroblasts synthesize Type I procollagen and collagen. It also may be related to the fact that the cartilage cells bind to the surface of the culture dishes by a different mechanism than the fibroblasts (see below).

There are 2 aspects to the current rationale for the procedure presented here: The effects of proline analogues on collagen biosynthesis and the consequences of inhibiting collagen synthesis in cultures of fibroblasts.

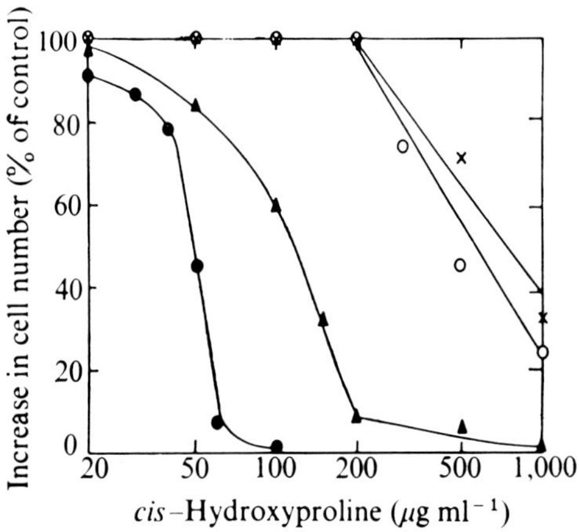

Fig. 2. Dose dependency of effect of *cis*-hydroxyproline on the growth of the cells. Various amounts of *cis*-hydroxyproline were added to the cultures at mid-log phase about 48 hours after inoculation. In each case the experiment was terminated after the cell number in control cultures had doubled. Cells used were tendon fibroblasts (•); L-929 fibroblasts (▲); KB cells (0); and neuroblastoma cells (X).

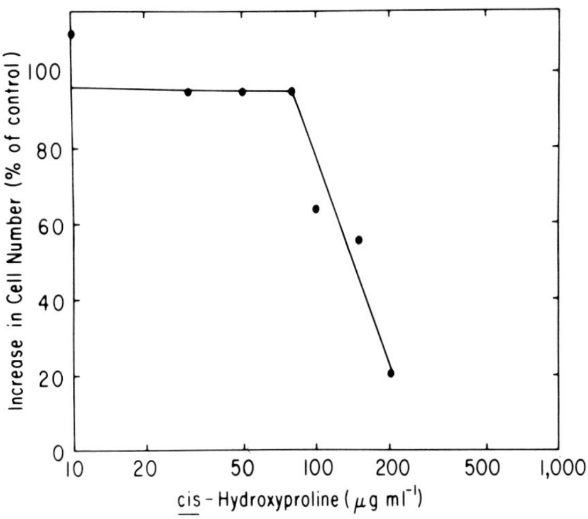

Fig. 3. Effect of *cis*-hydroxyproline on the growth of chondrocytes from chick embryo cartilage. The cells were prepared from sternal cartilages of 17-day-old chick embryos by enzymic digestion as described previously [8]. Primary cultures were then prepared with the same technique used previously for the preparation of tendon fibroblasts from chick embryos [1]. Other conditions were as in Fig. 2.

The effects of proline analogues on collagen biosynthesis involve 3 events: 1) proline analogues are incorporated into the polypeptide chains of the precursor of collagen known as procollagen; 2) the presence of the analogues in the pro-α chains of procollagen prevents these chains from folding into the native triple-helical conformation of the protein; 3) because the polypeptides do not fold into their native conformation, the protein remains biologically inactive and cannot form collagen fibers. The experimental data for these events have been reviewed elsewhere [1, 3–8]. The general effects of proline analogues on protein synthesis have been reviewed by Fowden et al [9] and their effects on inhibiting collagen synthesis have been examined in a number of different systems [10,11]. For the present purposes, suffice it to say that proline analogues differ from the analogues of most other amino acids in that they are readily incorporated into proteins. In the case of collagen biosynthesis it has been shown that 4 or 5 different proline analogues are readily incorporated into the precursor of collagen known as procollagen [4]. Incorporation of these analogues into the procollagen polypeptides has extensive consequences primarily because collagen is unusually rich in proline and in the closely related amino acid hydroxyproline. The general structure of the polypeptides of collagen is $(Gly\text{-}X\text{-}Y)_n$ in which the X- and Y- positions are frequently occupied by proline and hydroxyproline. The presence of proline and hydroxyproline in these X- and Y- positions is critical for the molecule to fold into its native conformation which consists of 3 polypeptide chains wrapped around each much like the strands of a rope. This triple-helical conformation of collagen is essential for the molecule to self-assemble into collagen fibers. Since the hydroxyproline in collagen is synthesized by the hydroxylation of peptidyl proline, incorporation of proline analogues alters both the X-positions occupied by proline and the Y-positions occupied by hydroxyproline in the molecule. One proline analogue, 3,4-dehydro-L-proline, has several effects in addition to preventing the folding of the triple helix [6]. In the case of at least 4 proline analogues, however, the major effect is at the conformational level of the protein. It should be noted that proline analogues are also incorporated into proteins other than collagen, but there are at least 3 reasons for suggesting that effects of proline analogues may be relatively specific for collagen. One reason is that collagen contains far more amino acids as either proline or hydroxyproline than other proteins and consists of unusually large polypeptide chains. Therefore, if proline analogues are administered so that they replace proline to a small degree, there will be a higher proportion of collagen molecules containing the analogue than molecules of other proteins. The second reason for suggesting the effects may be relatively specific is that the role of proline and hydroxyproline residues in the triple helix of collagen is highly unusual and it seems likely, but by no means certain, that the presence of a proline analogue in most noncollagen proteins would not alter their native conformation. Finally, several experiments have suggested that proline analogues do not in fact have any effect on the synthesis and secretion of other macromolecules such as proteoglycans or elastin [7], and that they do not alter synthesis of non-collagen proteins in animals such as growing chick embryos [8]. For these and related reasons we, as well as others, have been interested in testing the effects of proline analogues in inhibiting collagen synthesis and accumulation in a number of experimental and disease conditions.

The second aspect of the rationale for using a proline analogue to prevent growth of cultured fibroblasts has come from work carried out by Kleinman, Liotta, Martin, andtheir associates at NIH. Their work [2], as well as the work of several other laboratories, has demonstrated that fibroblasts bind to the surface of culture dishes in part because the cells first bind to the cell surface-associated glycoprotein known as LETS or fibronectin. Fibronectin in turn binds to collagen films which have been

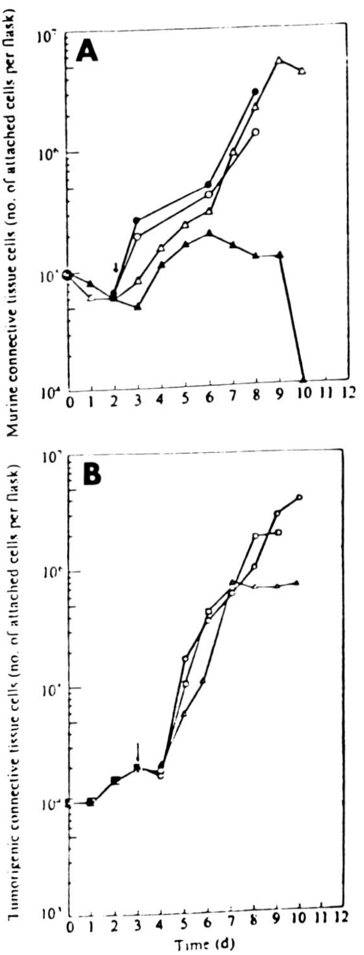

Fig. 4. Effect of *cis*-hydroxyproline on the proliferation of murine connective tissue cells and their spontaneously transformed counterparts. A) Connective tissue cells were prepared by enzymic digestion of subcutaneous tissue from 6-week-old mice. Passage-three cells were plated at low density (6×10^5 cells per 35-mm culture dish). Type I collagen was prepared from lathyritic rat skins and coated on bacteriologic plates. *cis*-Hydroxyproline at a concentration of 40 μg/ml was added to the cultures at the time indicated by the arrow. Cultures grown with *cis*-hydroxyproline on collagen-coated dishes (△). Cultures grown with *cis*-hydroxyproline on untreated plastic dishes (▲). Cultures grown without *cis*-hydroxyproline on collagen-coated plastic dishes (0). Cultures grown without *cis*-hydroxyproline on untreated plastic (●). B) Effects of *cis*-hydroxyproline on the growth of transformed cells. Cultures grown without *cis*-hydroxyproline (0). Cultures grown with 30 μg/ml of *cis*-hydroxyproline (□). Cultures grown with 100 μg/ml of *cis*-hydroxyproline (△). *cis*-Hydroxyproline was added to the cultures at the time indicated by the arrow. (From Liotta LA et al: Collagen required for proliferation of cultured connective tissue cells but not for their transformed counterparts. Nature 272:622, 1978, with permission.)

deposited on the surface of the dishes by the fibroblasts themselves. Evidence for this sequence of events was in part developed by using the proline analogue *cis*-hydroxyproline. As shown in Figure 4, the presence of *cis*-hydroxyproline inhibited the growth of fibroblasts obtained from 6-week-old BALB/c mice. The growth of the fibroblasts was not inhibited, however, if the plastic dishes were first coated with films of collagen. Also, growth of the cells was not inhibited by the analogue if the cells were transformed by repeated passage in vitro. The results of these experiments appear to demonstrate that *cis*-hydroxyproline prevents the growth of normal fibroblasts in culture by limiting the extent to which the cells can attach to the surface of the culture dishes.

As indicated above, we have not tested *cis*-hydroxyproline with epithelial cells and therefore the question of whether this technique will work with epithelial cells remains open. If it proves effective, it could prove highly useful. We might also point out, however, that if *cis*-hydroxyproline in moderate concentrations does not inhibit the growth of epithelial cells, this observation may provide clues as to the mechanism by which epithelial cells grow in culture and clues as to whether they synthesize collagen or related proteins. In this regard, it is of interest that Murray et al [12] have recently found that epithelial cells preferentially attach to basement membrane collagen compared to Type I or Type III collagen. Also, the attachment of epithelial cells to collagen films is not mediated by fibronectin. We have not tested the effects of *cis*-hydroxyproline on cells which synthesize basement membrane; therefore, if epithelial cells synthesize basement membrane collagen and depend on basement membrane films for their attachment to culture dishes, *cis*-hydroxyproline may also inhibit their growth in culture.

REFERENCES

1. Kao WW-Y, Prockop DJ: Proline analogue removes fibroblasts from cultured mixed cell populations. Nature 266:63-64, 1977.
2. Liotta LA, Vembu D, Kleinman HK, Martin GR, Boone C: Collagen required for proliferation of cultured connective tissue cells but not for their transformed counterparts. Nature 272:622-624, 1978.
3. Prockop DJ, Berg RA, Kivirikko KI, Uitto J: Intracellular steps in the biosynthesis of collagen. In Ramachandram GN, Reddi AH (eds): "Biochemistry of Collagen." New York: Plenum Press, 1976, pp 163–273.
4. Uitto J, Prockop DJ: Incorporation of proline analogues into collagen polypeptides. Effects on the production of extracellular procollagen and on the stability of the triple-helical structure of the molecule. Biochim Biophys Acta 336:234–251, 1974.
5. Uitto V-J, Uitto J, Kao WW-Y, Prockop DJ: Procollagen polypeptides containing *cis*-4-hydroxy-L-proline are overglycosylated and secreted as nonhelical pro-γ-chains. Arch Biochem Biophys 185:214–221, 1978.
6. Salvador RA, Tsai I, Marcel RJ, Felix AM, Kerwar SS: The in vivo inhibition of collagen synthesis and the reduction of prolyl hydroxylase activity by 3,4-dehydroproline. Arch Biochem Biophys 174:381–392, 1976.

7. Uitto J, Hoffmann H-P, Prockop DJ: Synthesis of elastin and procollagen by cells from embryonic aorta. Differences in the role of hydroxyproline and the effects of proline analogs on the secretion of the two proteins. Arch Biochem Biophys 173:187–200, 1976.
8. Dehm P, Prockop DJ: Biosynthesis of cartilage procollagen. Eur J Biochem 35:159–166, 1973.
9. Fowden L, Lewis D, Tristam H: Toxic amino acids: Their action as antimetabolites. Adv Enzymol 29:89–163, 1967.
10. Coulombre AJ, Coulombre JL: Corneal development. IV. Interruption of collagen excretion into the primary stroma of the cornea with L-azetidine-2-carboxylic acid. Dev Biol 28:183–190, 1972.
11. Galbraith DB, Kollar EJ: Effects of L-azetidine-2-carboxylic acid, a proline analogue, on the in vitro development of mouse tooth germs. Arch Oral Biol 19:1171–1175, 1974.
12. Murray JC, Stingl G, Kleinman HK, Martin GR, Katz SI: Epidermal cells adhere preferentially to type IV (basement membrane) collagen. J Cell Biol 80:197–202, 1979.

Epidermal Growth Factor: Biology and Mechanism of Action*

Graham Carpenter, PhD

The existence in both mouse [1] and man [2] of epidermal growth factors (EGF) having similar chemical characteristics and identical biologic activities indicates that this small polypeptide ($M_r \approx 6000$) has been retained throughout a long evolutionary process and probably has a function of general significance in nature [3–5]. When administered to experimental animals, EGF produces a variety of biologic responses, most of which involve enhanced proliferation and/or differentiation of epidermal or epithelial tissues (Table 1). Radioimmunoassays [23–25] have shown that EGF is present in various human body fluids: urine (88 ng/ml), saliva (12 ng/ml), breast milk (80 ng/ml), amniotic fluids (1 ng/ml), and plasma (2 ng/ml). Specific membrane receptors have been demonstrated not only in epidermal and epithelial tissues, but also in liver and placenta [26]. However, a natural function for EGF in mammalian biology has not been identified.

CELL CULTURE SYSTEMS: MITOGENIC RESPONSES TO EGF

EGF has been utilized as a mitogen in cell culture systems and displays growth-promoting activity for a wide variety of cell types, including fibroblasts [27–29], glia [30], mammary epithelia [31], vascular endothelia [32], chondrocytes [33], corneal endothelia [34], and granulosa [35]. The recorded responses of cultured cells to exogenous EGF (Table 2) include not only mitogenic activities but also the promotion of more specialized functions, such as the increased secretion of chorionic gonadotropin by choriocarcinoma cells [62]. The use of EGF in cell culture systems also offers certain technical advantages. For example, the serum requirement of normal cells such as diploid human fibroblasts may be considerably reduced by exogenous EGF, although growth regulating mechanisms, eg density-dependent inhibition of growth, may also be altered [53, 54]. In

*Supported by a Basil O'Connor Research grant from The National Foundation-March of Dimes and grant CA24071 from the National Cancer Institute.

Birth Defects: Original Article Series, Volume XVI, Number 2, pages 61–72

TABLE 1. Biologic Response to EGF In Vivo

Reference	Biologic effect
	Accelerated proliferation/differentiation
[6, 7]	of skin tissue
[8–10]	of corneal epithelial tissue
[11, 12]	of lung and tracheal epithelia
[13, 14]	Potentiation of methylcholanthrene carcinogenesis
[15, 16]	Increased activity of ornithine decarboxylase and accumulation of putrescine
[17]	Phosphorylation of nuclear protein
[18]	Formation of fatty liver
[19]	Increased disulfide group content in skin
[20]	Hepatic hypertrophy and hyperplasia
[21]	Potentiation of cleft palate
[22]	Inhibition of gastric acid secretion

TABLE 2. Response to EGF by Cultured Cells and Tissues

Reference	Biologic response
	Increased transport
[36]	α-aminobutyrate
[37]	deoxyglucose
[38]	potassium
[39]	lithium
[40]	uridine
[41]	putrescine
[42, 43]	Activation of glycolysis
[17]	Phosphorylation of nuclear protein
[44]	Increased activity of plasminogen activator
[15, 41]	Enhancement of ornithine decarboxylase activity
	Stimulation of macromolecular synthesis
[45]	hyaluronic acid
[28, 46, 47]	RNA
[46–48]	protein
[20, 27–36, 49–55]	DNA
[8, 27–31, 33–35, 49, 53–56]	Enhanced cell multiplication
[57–59]	Alteration of membrane properties and cell shape
[60, 61]	Increased replicative life-span
[62]	Increased secretion of HCG-α
[63]	Stimulation of LETS (large external transformation sensitive) protein biogenesis
[64]	Alteration of viral growth
[65]	Enhanced prostaglandin biosynthesis
[66]	Increased squame production
[67]	Inhibition of palate fusion

the case of tumor cells (HeLa) the serum requirement may be abolished by the addition of defined chemicals including EGF [68]. Work with cultured keratinocytes [60] and granulosa [61] cells indicates that growth in the presence of EGF will extend the in vitro life-span and allow much larger numbers of cells to be grown from a single explant.

The regulation of cell proliferation by EGF has been most extensively studied using cultured human fibroblasts [28, 29, 36, 53, 54] as a model system. These cells are considered "normal" as they maintain a diploid chromosome number in vitro and their growth is well regulated by mechanisms such as density-dependent inhibition of growth (DDIG), a high serum requirement, and anchorage-dependent growth. When human fibroblasts are cultured in the continuous presence of EGF (4 ng/ml), two of these growth controlling mechanisms are no longer evident [53, 54]. Cells grown in the presence of EGF continue to proliferate when the culture becomes confluent, forming a multilayered cell population that is not restricted by DDIG, and reaching population densities four- to sixfold higher than the controls [53]. Also, when human fibroblasts are incubated in media containing low or deficient serum (1% calf serum, 10% γ-globulin free serum or plasma), cell proliferation is normally restricted, but supplementation of these media with EGF yields cell growth equal to that obtained in the presence of optimal serum concentrations – 10% calf serum [54]. The apparent loss of sensitivity to these growth-regulating mechanisms by cells cultured in the presence of EGF bears some resemblance to the behavior of transformed cells in vitro. Transformed cells are frequently characterized by their insensitivity to normal growth-controlling mechanisms. Thus, EGF, while not transforming cells, does have the effect, under cell culture conditions, of creating an imbalance of homeostatic signals favoring cell proliferation.

The effects of EGF on the growth of cell populations is, of course, the end result of a complex series of biochemical and morphologic events. When quiescent cells are exposed to a mitogenic stimulus, a sequence of alterations in cell biochemistry occurs which appears to be similar regardless of the cell type or the mitogenic agent. These cellular reactions to mitogens have been collectively termed the pleiotropic response [69] and are listed in the first half of Table 2 according to their approximate temporal occurrence after the addition of EGF. Although some points on this temporal "map" have been established, it is clear that many other biochemical alterations have not been uncovered. In regard to the mechanism by which EGF elicits this complex series of biochemical changes, there is little information from which to propose a model. Tata [70] has suggested that polypeptide mitogens may enhance different cellular responses by different mechanisms. He has proposed one mechanism by which "early" changes, such as stimulated transport of nutrients, may be affected and a second mechanism for "late" changes, such as enhanced macromolecular synthesis. There is some evidence for this in the case of EGF. Experiments using antibodies to EGF to remove the growth factor from the media indicate that stimulation of DNA synthesis requires the continual presence of EGF in the media for at least 3–5 hours [53]. Since many of the "early" changes induced by EGF are maximally stimulated within 1–2 hours or less, the EGF-mechanism responsible for enhanced DNA synthesis may be slightly or substantially different from that required for "early" events.

BINDING AND METABOLISM OF EGF IN CELL CULTURE

Specific, saturable receptors for EGF have been demonstrated using ^{125}I-labeled EGF and a wide variety of cultured cells including corneal cells [71], human fibroblasts [29, 36, 72, 73] lens cells [55], human glial cells [74], human epidermoid carcinoma cells [75], 3T3 cells [76], granulosa cells [77], human vascular endothelial cells [32], and human choriocarcinoma cells [62].

For most cell types it has been estimated that each cell contains 40,000–100,000 binding sites for EGF, and apparent dissociation constants of $2–4 \times 10^{-10}$ M have been calculated [36, 72, 76].

Receptors for EGF were detected by O'Keefe et al [26] with crude membrane fractions prepared from a variety of mammalian tissues. These authors reported that placental and liver membranes have a high capacity to bind EGF. Specific binding of EGF has also been detected in liver membrane fractions of evolutionarily distant organisms, such as certain teleosts and the dogfish shark [78]. The specificity and high affinity of cells and membrane preparations for ^{125}I-EGF may be employed as the basis of competitive radioreceptor assays for EGF.

As a step toward understanding the biochemical mechanisms involved in the growth-stimulating effects of EGF, the fate of the cell-bound ^{125}I-EGF was examined using cultured human diploid fibroblasts. Carpenter and Cohen [73] postulated that subsequent to the initial binding of ^{125}I-EGF to specific plasma membrane receptors, the EGF:receptor complex is internalized and the hormone is ultimately degraded in lysosomes. These conclusions were drawn from the following series of observations: 1) Cell-bound ^{125}I-EGF is rapidly degraded to mono [^{125}I]iodotyrosine at 37°. 2) At 0°, cell-bound ^{125}I-EGF is not degraded but slowly dissociates from the cell. 3) When the binding of ^{125}I-EGF was carried out at 37° and the cells then incubated at 0°, almost no release of cell-bound radioactivity was detected. 4) The degradation, but not the binding, required metabolic energy. 5) The degradation was inhibited by drugs which inhibit lysosomal function, such as chloroquine and ammonium chloride. 6) When ^{125}I-EGF was bound to cells at 0°, the hormone was much more accessible to surface reactive agents, such as trypsin and antibodies to EGF, than when the hormone was bound at 37°. 7) Exposure of fibroblasts to EGF resulted in an apparent loss of plasma membrane receptors for EGF, suggesting that the receptor also is internalized. Internalization and degradation of ^{125}I-EGF has been confirmed with other cell types by workers in other laboratories.

The problem of direct visualization of the internalization of EGF has been approached in a number of laboratories using three procedures: the preparation and tracing of fluorescent derivatives of EGF, the tracing of ^{125}I-EGF by electron microscopic autoradiography, and the preparation and tracing of EGF-ferritin conjugates by electron microscopy.

Schlessinger et al [79] prepared a highly fluorescent rhodamine derivative of EGF and examined the binding and internalization of this derivative to 3T3 cells using image-intensified video fluorescence microscopy. Haigler et al [75] prepared fluorescein-conjugated EGF and examined the binding and internalization of this derivative by direct fluorescence microscopy using human epidermoid carcinoma cells (A-431) which are capable of binding much larger quantities of EGF than fibroblasts, thus rendering visualization possible. Both laboratories found that the initial binding of the derivatives to the cell surface was diffuse (except for a concentration of staining at the cell borders with the A-431 cells). Within 10–30 minutes at 37° the labeled hormone was found within the cells in endocytotic vesicles. An intermediary patching stage was seen in the 3T3 cells but was not detected in the A-431 cells; a "microclustering" of receptors was suggested for the latter cells.

Gorden et al [80] used quantitative electron microscopic autoradiography to localize ^{125}I-EGF in human fibroblasts. The initial binding of the labeled hormone was localized to the plasma membrane with some preference to coated pit regions. The membrane-bound ^{125}I-EGF was internalized by the cell in a time- and temperature-dependent fashion. The internalized grains were almost exclusively related to lysosomal structures.

Cohen and co-workers [81] have prepared a biologically active EGF-ferritin conjugate and have observed that at 4° the EGF-ferritin binds to the plasma membrane of A-431 cells. Within one minute at 37° the ferritin-EGF redistributed on the surface of the membrane to form an increased number of small clusters which were subsequently internalized into pinocytotic vesicles. Within 30 minutes approximately 90% of the ferritin was seen in lysosomes. All of these data directly confirm the original kinetic studies with ^{125}I-EGF [73].

MODULATION OF EGF RECEPTOR ACTIVITY

As plasma membrane receptors are crucial in determining the capacity of a cell to respond to a particular extracellular signal, an increasing area of investigation has been the study of mechanisms which control the level of receptors in the plasma membrane. The results of studies are summarized in Table 3.

Phosphorylation and Molecular Mechanisms

The evidence cited above clearly indicates that EGF forms a complex with plasma membrane receptors. This initiates an intricate series of biochemical and morphologic events within the cell, including internalization and degradation of

TABLE 3. Modulation of EGF Receptor Activity in Cultured Cells

Reference	Procedure	Increase (↑) or decrease (↓) of ^{125}I-EGF binding activity
[73, 82, 83]	"Down regulation" (incubation with unlabeled EGF)	↓
[73]	Addition of serum to "down-regulated" cells	↑
[84]	Inhibition of protein synthesis	↓
[84]	Reinitiation of protein synthesis	↑
[85]	Addition of tumor promoter TPA	↓
[86]	Transformation by murine of feline sarcoma viruses	↓
[87]	Addition of lectins	↓
[88]	Altered synthesis of cell surface carbohydrate	↓
[89]	Incubation of cells with glucocorticoids	↑

the hormone:receptor complex, which ultimately result in cell growth. It is reasonable to assume that the observed biochemical and morphologic alterations induced by EGF result from the generation, amplification, and propagation of a series of "signals." To understand the nature of these signals it would appear necessary to obtain cell-free systems which are responsive in vitro to the addition of either EGF, a fragment of EGF, or an EGF-induced cellular product.

Carpenter et al [90] have reported that membranes may be prepared from A-431 cells which retain the ability to bind ^{125}I-EGF in vitro, and that following the formation of EGF:receptor complexes the capacity of these membranes to phosphorylate endogenous proteins in the presence of γ-labeled [^{32}P]ATP is markedly enhanced. The A-431 membrane preparation appeared to have EGF-stimulated protein kinase activity toward exogenous substrates (histone, protamine) as well as toward membrane associated proteins.

Both the endogenous phosphorylation and EGF-stimulated phosphorylation were dependent on the presence of Mg^{2+} or Mn^{2+}; Ca^{2+} was ineffective. Partial acid hydrolysis and electrophoresis of the phosphorylated membranes showed that the major phosphorylated product, in both the presence and absence of EGF, was phosphothreonine. SDS polyacrylamide gel electrophoresis and autoradiography indicated that the phosphorylation of a number of membrane-associated proteins was enhanced in the presence of EGF, especially components with molecular weights of approximately 170,000; 150,000; 80,000; and 22,500.

The mechanism by which EGF enhances phosphorylation is not known; it is possible that the receptor is a protein kinase or a regulatory subunit of a kinase. Since neither the identity nor the function of the EGF-stimulated phosphorylated membrane components have been determined, it is currently not possible, however tempting, to relate these findings to specific metabolic alterations induced in intact cells by EGF. Possible biologic consequences of the EGF-induced phosphorylation might include the following: 1) alteration of the electrochemical potential across the membrane (hyperpolarization); 2) a signal for the clustering and/or internalization of receptors; 3) stimulation of specific membrane process, such as transport of nutrients, associated with the initiation of cell proliferation; 4) modification of cytoplasmic protein which may serve as "second messengers."

CONCLUSION

In the last five years there has been considerable progress toward understanding the mechanisms by which an extracellular signal (EGF) influences the proliferation of mammalian cells. These advances were critically dependent on the utilization of cell culture technology. Although less recognized but perhaps of equal importance have been studies of the action of EGF in developmental processes in vivo [11, 12, 21] and in organ culture systems [67]. These studies have suggested a role for EGF in the maturation of epithelia of the fetal respiratory system [11, 12] with some indication that the growth factor might be of use in preventing certain respiratory distress syndromes of the newborn.

It is important when considering what role exogenous signals or the lack thereof might have in producing birth defects to consider the mechanism of action of these polypeptides. Alterations of developmental processes might occur not only at the level of growth factor production but might also depend on the ability of cells to respond to the hormone. This latter category would include the presence of functional receptors, systems to couple binding to the generation of secondary signals, and metabolism of growth factor.

REFERENCES

1. Cohen S: Isolation of a mouse submaxillary gland protein accelerating incisor eruption eyelid opening in the new-born animal. J Biol Chem 237:1555–1562, 1962.
2. Cohen S, Carpenter G: Human epidermal growth factor: Isolation and chemical and biological properties. Proc Natl Acad Sci USA 72:1317–1321, 1975.
3. Carpenter G, Cohen S: Epidermal growth factors. In Litwack G (ed): "Biochemical Actions of Hormones." New York:Academic Press, 1978, vol 5, pp 203–247.
4. Carpenter G: The regulation of cell proliferation: Advances in the biology and mechanism of action of epidermal growth factor. J Invest Dermatol 71:283–287, 1978.
5. Carpenter G, Cohen S: Epidermal growth factor. Annu Rev Biochem 48:193–216, 1979.
6. Cohen S, Elliott GA: The stimulation of epidermal keratinization by a protein isolated from the submaxillary gland of the mouse. J Invest Dermatol 40:1–5, 1963.
7. Birnbaum JE, Sapp TM, Moore JB Jr: Effects of reserpine epidermal growth factor and cyclic nucleotide modulators on epidermal mitosis. J Invest Dermatol 66:313–318, 1976.
8. Savage CR Jr, Cohen S: Proliferation of corneal epithelium induced by epidermal growth factor. Exp Eye Res 15:361–366, 1973.

9. Frati L, Daniele S, Delogu A, Covelli I: Selective binding of the epidermal growth factor and its specific effects on the epithelial cells of the cornea. Exp Eye Res 14:135–141, 1972.
10. Ho PC, Davis WH, Elliott JH, Cohen S: Kinetics of corneal epithelial regeneration and epidermal growth factor. Invest Ophthalmol 13:804–809, 1974.
11. Sundell H, Serenius FS, Barthe P, Friedman Z, Kanerek KS, Escabedo MB, Orth DN, Stahlman MT: The effect of EGF on fetal lung maturation. (Abstract) Pediatr Res 9:371, 1975.
12. Catterton WZ, Escobedo M, Sexson WR, Gray ME, Sundell H, Stahlman MT: Effect of epidermal growth factor on lung maturation in fetal rabbits. Pediatr Res 13:104–108, 1979.
13. Reynolds VH, Boehm FH, Cohen S: Enhancement of chemical carcinogenesis by an epidermal growth factor. Surg Forum 16:108–109, 1965.
14. Rose SP, Stahn R, Passovoy DS, Herschman H: Epidermal growth factor enhancement of skin tumor induction in mice. Experientia 32:913–915, 1976.
15. Stastny M, Cohen S: Epidermal growth factor IV. The induction of ornithine decarboxylase. Biochim Biophys Acta 204:578–589, 1970.
16. Stastny M, Cohen S: The stimulation of ornithine decarboxylase activity in testes of the neonatal mouse. Biochim Biophys Acta 261:177–180, 1972.
17. Huff KR, Guroff G: Epidermal growth factor stimulates the phosphorylation of a specific nuclear protein in chick embryo epidermis. Biochem Biophys Res Commun 85:464–472, 1978.
18. Heimberg M, Weinstein I, LeQuire VS, Cohen S: The induction of fatty liver in neonatal animals by a purified protein (EGF) from mouse submaxillary gland. Life Sci 4:1625–1633, 1965.
19. Frati C, Covelli I, Mozzi R, Frati L: Mechanism of action of the epidermal growth factor. Effect on the sulfhydryl and disulphide groups content of the mouse epidermis during keratinization. Cell Differ 1:239–244, 1972.
20. Butcher NLR, Patel V, Cohen S: Hormonal factors and liver growth. Adv Enzyme Regul 16:205–213, 1978.
21. Bedrick AD, Ladda RL: Epidermal growth factor potentiates cortisone-induced cleft palate in the mouse. Teratology 17:13–18, 1978.
22. Bower JM, Camble R, Gregory H, Gerring EL, Willshire IR: The inhibition of gastric acid secretion by epidermal growth factor. Experientia 15:825–826, 1975.
23. Starkey RH, Orth DN: Radioimmunoassay of human epidermal growth factor (urogastrone). J Clin Endocrinol Metab 45:1144–1153, 1977.
24. Dailey GE, Kraus JW, Orth DN: Homologous radioimmunoassay for human epidermal growth factor (urogastrone). J Clin Endocrinol Metab 46:929–936, 1978.
25. Barka T, van der Noen H, Gresik EW, Kerenyi T: Immunoreactive epidermal growth factor in human amniotic fluid. Mt Sinai J Med NY 45:679–684, 1978.
26. O'Keefe E, Hollenberg MD, Cuatrecasas P: Epidermal growth factor. Characteristics of specific binding in membranes from liver, placenta, and other target tissues. Arch Biochem Biophys 164:518–526, 1974.
27. Armelin HA: Pituitary extracts and steroid hormones in the control of 3T3 cell growth. Proc Natl Acad Sci USA 70:2702–2706, 1973.
28. Hollenberg MD, Cuatrecasas P: Epidermal growth factor: Receptors in human fibroblasts and modulation of action by cholera toxin. Proc Natl Acad Sci USA 70:2964–2968, 1973.
29. Cohen S, Carpenter G, Lembach KJ: Interaction of epidermal growth factor (EGF) with cultured human fibroblasts. Adv Metab Disord 8:265–284, 1975.

30. Westermark B: Density dependent proliferation of human glia cells stimulated by epidermal growth factor. Biochem Biophys Res Commun 69:304–310, 1976.
31. Stoker MGP, Pigott D, Taylor-Papadimitriou J: Response to epidermal growth factors of cultured human mammary epithelial cells from benign tumours. Nature 264:764–767, 1976.
32. Gospodarowicz D, Brown KD, Bridwell CR, Zetter BR: Control of proliferation of human vascular endothelial cells. Characterization of the response of human umbilical vein endothelial cells to fibroblast growth factor, epidermal growth factor, and thrombin. J Cell Biol 77:774–788, 1978.
33. Gospodarowicz D, Mescher AL: A comparison of the responses of cultured myoblasts and chondrocytes to fibroblast and epidermal growth factors. J Cell Physiol 93:117–128, 1977.
34. Gospodarowicz D, Mescher AL, Birdwell CR: Stimulation of corneal endothelial cell proliferation in vitro by fibroblast and epidermal growth factors. Exp Eye Res 25:75–89, 1977.
35. Gospodarowicz D, Ill CR, Birdwell CR: Effects of fibroblast and epidermal growth factors on ovarian cell proliferation in vitro. I. Characterization of the response of granulosa cells to FGF and EGF. Endocrinology 100:1108–1120, 1977.
36. Hollenberg MD, Cuatrecasas P: Insulin and epidermal growth factor. Human fibroblast receptors related to deoxyribonucleic acid synthesis and amino acid uptake. J Biol Chem 250:3845–3853, 1975.
37. Barnes D, Colowick SP: Stimulation of sugar uptake in cultured fibroblasts by epidermal growth factor (EGF) and EGF-binding arginine esterase. J Cell Physiol 89:633–640, 1976.
38. Rozengurt E, Heppel LA: Serum rapidly stimulates ouabain-sensitive $^{86}Rb^{+}$ influx in quiescent 3T3 cells. Proc Natl Acad Sci USA 72:4492–4495, 1975.
39. Smith JB, Rozengurt E: Lithium transport by fibroblastic mouse cells: Characterization and stimulation by serum and growth factors in quiescent cells. J Cell Physiol 97:441–450, 1978.
40. Rozengurt E, Mierzejewski K, Wigglesworth N: Uridine transport and phosphorylation in mouse cells in culture; Effect of growth-promoting factors, cell cycle transit and oncogenic transformation. J Cell Physiol 97:241–252, 1978.
41. DiPasquale A, White D, McGuire J: Epidermal growth factor stimulates putrescine transport and ornithine decarboxylase activity in cultivated human fibroblasts. Exp Cell Res 116:317–323, 1978.
42. Diamond I, Legg A, Schneider JA, Rozengurt E: Glycolysis in quiescent cultures of 3T3 cells. Stimulation by serum, epidermal growth factor, and insulin in intact cells and persistence of the stimulation after cell homogenization. J Biol Chem 253:866–871, 1978.
43. Schneider JA, Diamond I, Rozengurt E: Glycolysis in quiescent cultures of 3T3 cells. Addition of serum, epidermal growth factor, and insulin increases the activity of phosphofructokinase in a protein synthesis-independent manner. J Biol Chem 253: 872–877, 1978.
44. Lee LS, Weinstein IB: Epidermal growth factor, like phorbol esters, induces plasminogen activator in HeLa cells. Nature 274:696–697, 1978.
45. Lembach KJ: Enhanced synthesis and extracellular accumulation of hyaluronic acid during stimulation of quiescent human fibroblasts by mouse epidermal growth factor. J Cell Physiol 89:277–288, 1976.
46. Hoober JK, Cohen S: Epidermal growth factor. I. The stimulation of protein and ribonucleic acid synthesis in chick embryo epidermis. Biochim Biophys Acta 138:347–356, 1967.

47. Cohen S, Stastny M: Epidermal growth factor. III. The stimulation of polysome formation in chick embryo epidermis. Biochim Biophys Acta 166:427–437, 1968.
48. Hoober JK, Cohen S: Epidermal growth factor II. Increased activity of ribosomes from chick embryo epidermis for cell-free protein synthesis. Biochim Biophys Acta 138: 357–368, 1967.
49. Cohen S: The stimulation of epidermal proliferation by a specific protein (EGF). Dev Biol 12:394–407, 1965.
50. Bertsch S, Marks F: Effect of foetal calf serum and epidermal growth factor on DNA synthesis in explants of chick embryo epidermis. Nature 251:517–519, 1974.
51. Turkington RW: The role of epithelial growth factor in mammary gland development in vitro. Exp Cell Res 57:79–85, 1969.
52. Richman RA, Claus TH, Pilkis SJ, Friedman DL: Hormonal stimulation of DNA synthesis in primary cultures of adult rat hepatocytes. Proc Natl Acad Sci USA 73:3589–3593, 1976.
53. Carpenter G, Cohen S: Human epidermal growth factor and the proliferation of human fibroblasts. J Cell Physiol 88:227–238, 1976.
54. Carpenter G, Cohen S: Biological and molecular studies of the mitogenic effects of human epidermal growth factor. In Papaconstantinou J, Rutter WJ (eds): "Molecular Control of Proliferation and Differentiation." New York: Academic Press, 1978, pp 13–31.
55. Hollenberg MD: Receptors for insulin and epidermal growth factor: Relation to synthesis of DNA in cultured rabbit lens epithelium. Arch Biochem Biophys 171:371–377, 1975.
56. Lembach KJ: Induction of human fibroblast proliferation by epidermal growth factor (EGF): Enhancement by an EGF-binding arginine esterase and by ascorbate. Proc Natl Acad Sci USA 73:183–187, 1976.
57. Brunk U, Schellens J, Westermark B: Influence of epidermal growth factor (EGF) on ruffling activity, pinocytosis and proliferation of cultivated human glia cells. Exp Cell Res 103:295–302, 1976.
58. Aharonov A, Vlodavsky I, Pruss RM, Fox CF, Herschman HR: Epidermal growth factor induced membrane changes in 3T3 cells. J Cell Physiol 95:195–202, 1978.
59. Gospodarowicz D, Greenburg G, Birdwell CR: Determination of cellular shape by the extracellular matrix and its correlation with the control of cell growth. Cancer Res 38:4155–4171, 1978.
60. Rheinwald JG, Green H: Epidermal growth factor and the multiplication of cultured human epidermal keratinocytes. Nature 265:421–424, 1977.
61. Gospodarowicz D, Bialecki H: The effects of the epidermal and fibroblast growth factors on the replicative lifespan of cultured bovine granulosa cells. Endocrinology 103: 854–865, 1978.
62. Benveniste R, Speeg KV Jr, Carpenter G, Cohen S, Lindner J, Rabinowitz D: Epidermal growth factor stimulates secretion of human chorionic gonadotropin by cultured human choriocarcinoma cells. J Clin Endocrinol Metab 46:169–172, 1978.
63. Chen LB, Gudor RC, Sun TT, Chen AB, Mosesson MW: Control of a cell surface major glycoprotein by epidermal growth factor. Science 197:776–778, 1977.
64. Knox GE, Reynolds DW, Cohen S, Alford CA: Alteration of the growth of cytomegalovirus and herpes simplex virus type 1 by epidermal growth factor, a contaminant of crude human chorionic gonadotropin preparations. J Clin Invest 61:1635–1644, 1978.
65. Levine L, Hassid A: Epidermal growth factor stimulates prostaglandin biosynthesis by canine kidney (MDCK) cells. Biochem Biophys Res Commun 76:1181–1187, 1977.
66. Green H: Terminal differentiation of cultured human epidermal cells. Cell 11:405–416, 1977.

67. Hassell JR: The development of rat palatal shelves in vitro. An ultrastructural analysis of the inhibition of epithelial cell death and palate fusion by the epidermal growth factor. Dev Biol 45:90–102, 1975.
68. Hutchings SE, Sato GH: Growth and maintenance of HeLa cells in serum-free medium supplemented with hormones. Proc Natl Acad Sci USA 75:901–904, 1978.
69. Hershko A, Mamont P, Shields R, Tomkins GM: Pleiotypic response. Nature [New Biol] 232:206–211, 1971.
70. Tata JR: Growth-promoting actions of peptide hormones. Ciba Found Symp 41: 297–312, 1976.
71. Covelli I, Rossi R, Mozzi R, Frati L: Synthesis of bioactive ^{131}I-labeled epidermal growth factor and its distribution in rat tissues. Eur J Biochem 27:225–230, 1972.
72. Carpenter G, Lembach KJ, Morrison MM, Cohen S: Characterization of the binding of ^{125}I-labeled epidermal growth factor to human fibroblasts. J Biol Chem 250: 4297–4304, 1975.
73. Carpenter G, Cohen S: ^{125}I-labeled human epidermal growth factor. Binding, internalization, and degradation in human fibroblasts. J Cell Biol 71:159–171, 1976.
74. Westermark B: Local starvation for epidermal growth factor cannot explain density-dependent inhibition of normal human glial cells. Proc Natl Acad Sci USA 74:1619–1621, 1977.
75. Haigler H, Ash JF, Singer SJ, Cohen S: Visualization by fluorescence of the binding and internalization of epidermal growth factor in human carcinoma cells A-431. Proc Natl Acad Sci USA 75:3317–3321, 1978.
76. Das M, Miyakawa T, Fox CF, Pruss RM, Aharonov A, Herschman HR: Specific radio-labeling of a cell surface receptor for epidermal growth factor. Proc Natl Acad Sci USA 74:2790–2794, 1977.
77. Vlodavsky I, Brown KD, Gospodarowicz D: A comparison of the binding of epidermal growth factor to cultured granulosa and luteal cells. J Biol Chem 253:3744–3750, 1978.
78. Naftel J, Cohen S: Epidermal growth factor receptors in lower vertebrates. J SC Med Assoc 74:53, 1978.
79. Schlessinger J, Shechter Y, Willingham MC, Pastan I: Direct visualization of binding, aggregation, and internalization of insulin and epidermal growth factor on living fibroblastic cells. Proc Natl Acad Sci USA 75:2659–2663, 1978.
80. Gorden P, Carpentier JL, Cohen S, Orci L: Epidermal growth factor: Morphological demonstration of binding, internalization, and lysosomal association in human fibroblasts. Proc Natl Acad Sci USA 75:5025–5029, 1978.
81. Haigler H, Cohen S: Direct visualization of the binding and internalization of a ferritin conjugate of epidermal growth factor in human carcinoma cells A-431. J Cell Biol (in press).
82. Aharonov A, Pruss RM, Herschman HR: Epidermal growth factor: Relationship between receptor regulation and mitogenesis in 3T3 cells. J Biol Chem 253:3970–3977, 1978.
83. Das M, Fox CF: Molecular mechanisms of mitogen action: Processing of receptor induced by epidermal growth factor. Proc Natl Acad Sci USA 75:2644–2648, 1978.
84. Carpenter G: Regulation of epidermal growth factor (EGF) receptor activity during the modulation of protein synthesis. J Cell Physiol 99:101–106, 1979.
85. Lee LS, Weinstein IB: Tumor-promoting phorbol esters inhibit binding of epidermal growth factor to cellular receptors. Science 202:313–315, 1978.
86. Todaro GJ, DeLarco JE, Cohen S: Transformation by murine and feline sarcoma viruses specifically blocks binding of epidermal growth factor to cells. Nature 264:26–31, 1976.
87. Carpenter G, Cohen S: Influence of lectins on the binding of ^{125}I-labeled EGF to human fibroblasts. Biochem Biophys Res Commun 79:545–552, 1977.

88. Pratt RM, Pastan I: Decreased binding of epidermal growth factor to BALB/c 3T3 mutant cells defective in glycoprotein synthesis. Nature 272:68–70, 1978.
89. Baker JB, Barsh GS, Carney DH, Cunningham DD: Dexamethasone modulates binding and action of epidermal growth factor in serum-free cell culture. Proc Natl Acad Sci USA 75:1882–1886, 1978.
90. Carpenter G, King L Jr, Cohen S: Epidermal growth factor stimulates phosphorylation in membrane preparations in vitro. Nature 276:409–410, 1978.

In Vitro Histotypic Reaggregation of Fetal Rat Lung Cells Following Cryopreservation and Storage in Liquid Nitrogen*

James A. McAteer, PhD and William H.J. Douglas, PhD

INTRODUCTION

The technique of freezing cultured cells for storage in liquid nitrogen provides a distinct advantage toward broadening the research potential of the cell culture laboratory. Frozen cells may be stored for extended periods prior to retrieval. This provides the opportunity to bank cells for future study, providing a source of replicate cultures bearing similar characteristics. Various techniques are available for freezing and storing cells [1, 2]. Common well-established methods employ treatment of dissociated cells with a cryoprotectant [3], such as dimethyl sulfoxide or glycerol followed by freezing to extremely low temperature ($<-70°C$) at a constant slow rate (1–5°C per min) or some controlled stepwise cooling program [4–8]. Subsequent retrieval from frozen storage must be accomplished by very rapid thawing [9]. The effectiveness of the freezing procedure is assessed not only by viability upon recovery but, more critically, by the capacity of the cells to exhibit their normal culture characteristics, function, and replicative potential [10].

Cryopreservation is applied most commonly to cells raised in culture; however, the same principles extend to cells derived from fresh organs. Methods have been reported for the cryopreservation of primary tissue dissociates [11, 12], minced organs [13, 14], and entire early stage mammalian embryos [15]. Indeed, as a principle application of many of these studies is the development of methods to preserve whole organs for transplantation, so attempts have also been made to freeze and revive intact mammalian organs [16–19].

*This work was funded by grants from the National Heart, Lung and Blood Institute (HL23969, HL21008, HL19513), and The United Cerebral Palsy Research and Education Foundation, Inc.

Birth Defects: Original Article Series, Volume XVI, Number 2, pages 73–83

Most frozen cell preparations are used as a source of cells for monolayer culture. To our knowledge there are no reports of the establishment of reaggregate organotypic cultures with previously frozen cells. We have investigated the effects of freezing upon enzymatically dissociated fetal rat lung cells in order to develop a method of cryopreservation that will provide large numbers of viable cells capable of selective reaggregation in vitro. Our observations indicate that cells from frozen storage will undergo histotypic reaggregation when inoculated onto a Gelfoam collagen sponge substrate. These cultures possess morphologic characteristics similar to organotypic cultures derived from freshly dissociated fetal lung [20–22]. This report describes our experience in using frozen cells to establish fetal rat lung organotypic cultures and discusses the application of the technique to in vitro studies of type II alveolar epithelial cell function and pulmonary surfactant production.

MATERIALS AND METHODS

Cell Dissociation and Establishment of Organotypic Cultures

Fetal rat lung organotypic cultures were established by methods detailed elsewhere [20–23]. The technique involved the preparation of a monodisperse cell suspension by progressive enzymatic digestion of finely minced lung fragments. Fetal lungs (16–19 days gestational age [ga]) were dissected free of the airways and great vessels, and minced into small pieces (1 mm^3). The fragments were rinsed with serum-free culture medium (F12K, Gibco) containing antibiotics (penicillin 100 U/ml; kanamycin sulfate 100 μg/ml; amphotericin B 6.25 μg/ml), and then treated with enzyme solution (CTC: collagenase 0.1%; trypsin 0.1%; chicken serum 1%, in Moscona's saline [24]). Each enzyme treatment consisted of a 15-minute incubation on a reciprocal shaker bath at 37°C. Following each incubation, the liberated cells were harvested and fresh enzyme solution was added. The cell suspension was collected, filtered through a nylon screen (Nitex 41 μm, Tetko), and diluted with chilled culture medium containing serum (10% v/v fetal bovine serum [FBS]), to inhibit further enzymatic activity. The harvested cells were stored on ice. This procedure was repeated successive times until the lung fragments were reduced to residual connective tissue. Trituration with a syringe and cannula (14 gauge) following each enzyme incubation (after the fourth incubation) enhanced the dissociation.

Following the completion of the dissociation procedure the harvested cells were passed through 25 μm nylon screening and pooled. A sample was collected for a determination of cell viability by erythrocin B dye exclusion [25]. The cell suspension was then centrifuged (160 $\times$ g) to form a pellet, which was incubated at 37°C for 1 hour. At the conclusion of this incubation the cells were resuspended in a volume of medium to give 10^7 viable cells per 50 μl.

Control cultures were established by inoculating individual pieces (2 $\times$ 2 cm) of media-hydrated Gelfoam sponge with 10^7 viable cells. The cultures were placed in Petri dishes containing 20 ml of medium (F12K + 10% FBS) and incubated under 5% CO_2 in air at 37°C. On the second day in vitro the cultures were placed on a rocker platform set at 3 cycles per min. The culture medium was replaced every second day.

Cryopreservation and Retrieval of Cells From Frozen Storage

Following the final 1-hour incubation step of the cell dissociation procedure, cells to be frozen were resuspended in cold (4°C) culture medium containing 20% FBS and 10% dimethyl sulfoxide (DMSO), to give 2.5×10^6 viable cells per ml. Aliquots (5 ml, 1.25×10^7 cells) of the cell suspension were then added to polypropylene screw cap freezing vials (Cryotube No. 1086, Vangard). The cells were allowed to equilibrate in the cryoprotectant medium (4°C) for 5 minutes and were then frozen at a rate of 1–2°C per min using a Linde BF-6 controlled rate biological freezer. Following the attainment of –80°C, the vials were transferred to storage in the vapor phase of liquid nitrogen.

Cells were retrieved from frozen storage by rapidly thawing the vials through immersion and agitation in water at 37°C. The contents of the vials were pooled in a flask and an equal volume of standard culture medium (F12K + 10% FBS) was added. A sample was collected for cell counting to determine the percent viability of the cell population. The cell suspension was transferred to 50-ml tubes which were then centrifuged to pellet the cells. The cells were then immediately resuspended in culture medium to give 10^7 viable cells per 50 μl. Organotypic cultures were established as described above.

Morphologic Analysis

TTC Staining. A one-step vital staining procedure [26] was used to assess the degree of reaggregation in intact organotypic cultures. Cultures were incubated in medium containing 0.05–0.1% 2, 3, 5′-triphenyl-tetrazolium chloride for 1 hour at 37°C. Cellular aggregates stained bright red and could be visualized macroscopically.

Light and Electron Microscopy. TTC-stained organotypic cultures were trimmed to remove excess Gelfoam surrounding the tissue area. The cultures were then fixed in 2.5% glutaraldehyde in 0.1 M cacodylate buffer, cut into smaller pieces (1×3 mm) and postfixed in buffered 1% osmium tetroxide. The specimens were then dehydrated in graded acetones and embedded in Epon-Araldite. Thick sections for light microscopy were stained with 0.5% toluidine blue. Thin sections for electron microscopy were stained with uranyl acetate and lead citrate.

RESULTS

Organotypic cultures established from previously frozen cells were in many ways comparable to cultures derived from freshly dissociated lung. Cryopreserved cells reaggregated in vitro (Fig. 1) forming the histotypic alveolar-like structures

(ALS) (Fig. 2) characteristic of the fetal rat lung organotypic culture system [20–22]. These epithelial cells also differentiated in culture, the majority developing the morphologic characteristics of type II alveolar epithelial cells (Figs. 3 and 4). In many cases experimental and control cultures were morphologically indistinguishable. However, some differences were observed that characterized cultures of frozen cell stocks from those established from freshly dissociated tissue. Those differences consisted of a brief lag in the reaggregation phase of culture development and the occurrence of a substantially larger number of damaged cells in frozen cell organotypic cultures.

In cultures established under standard conditions cellular reaggregation is evident during the first 24 hours of culture. During this time epithelial cells from the monodisperse cell inoculum have begun to associate, forming unstructured cell aggregates and histotypic ALS. The ALS (Figs. 2 and 3) consist of discrete aggregates in which adjacent epithelial cells enclose a central lumen. The ALS thus resemble the epithelium-lined peripheral pulmonary passages (presumptive alveolar spaces) of the intact fetal rat lung. The epithelial cells of the ALS possess a distinct polarity. The apical surface faces the lumen, and the basal surface interfaces with subjacent fibroblastic cells that surround the aggregates.

Reaggregation continues throughout the first 4–5 days of culture. During this period morphogenetic changes take place. The ALS increase in size, change in overall form, and the epithelial cells undergo cytodifferentiation. The disposition of the surrounding fibroblastic cell population also changes. Initially these cells are loosely organized, forming a sparse mesenchymal matrix that occupies the

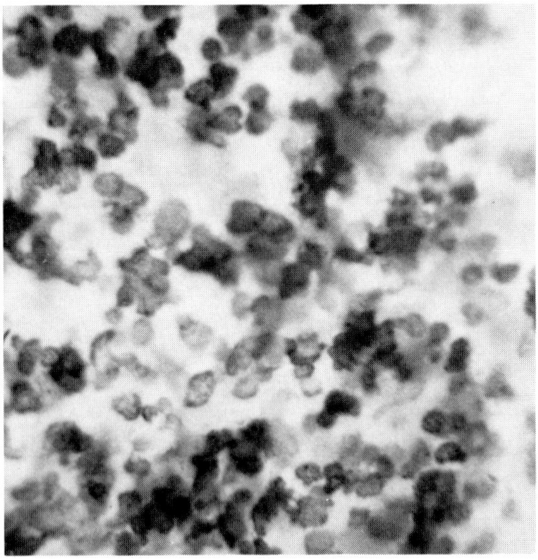

Fig. 1. Fetal rat lung organotypic culture (5 days in vitro) established from cryopreserved cells. This is the view through the dissecting microscope of a portion of the intact culture stained by TTC. Numerous discrete aggregates have formed, visible against the light background of the Gelfoam substrate (× 10.5).

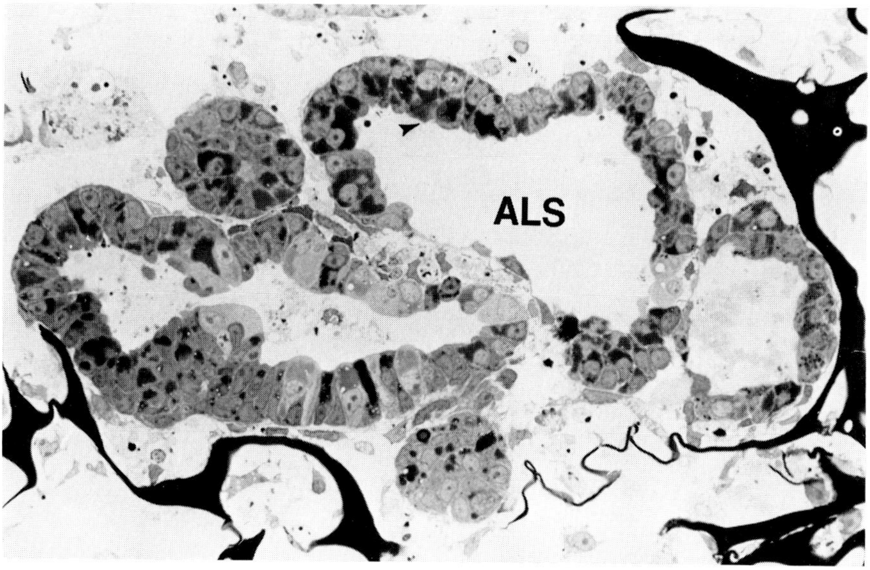

Fig. 2. Light micrograph of the organotypic culture shown in Fig. 1 (5 days in vitro). The histologic appearance of the culture is comparable to that of control cultures. Several alveolar-like structures (ALS) are present in the field. Many cells (▲) contain large dark staining areas in the apical cytoplasm. Electron microscopy shows these cells to contain glycogen deposits. This indicates that the cells have not yet differentiated. Several cells (↗) possess dense staining granules characteristic of type II cells (× 520).

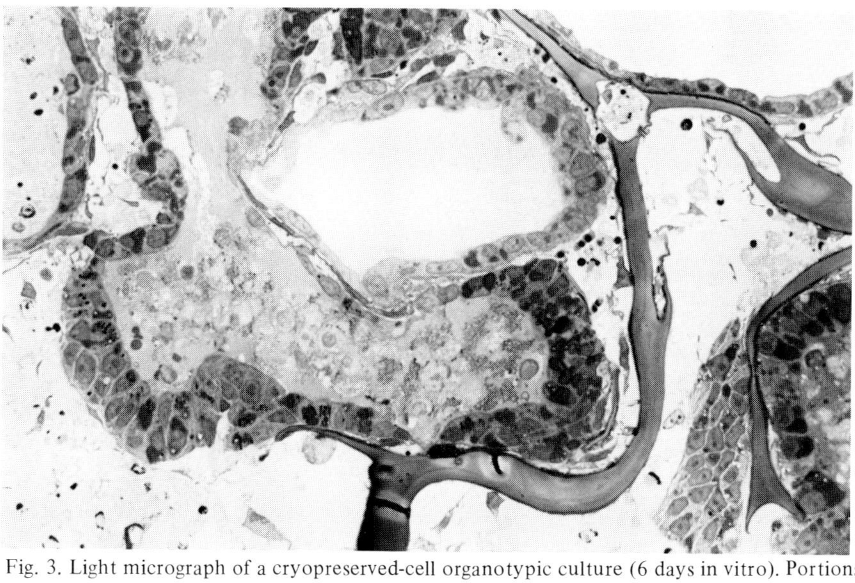

Fig. 3. Light micrograph of a cryopreserved-cell organotypic culture (6 days in vitro). Portions of several ALS in the field contain large amounts of cell debris. Many cells (▲) also bear dense staining granules (× 520).

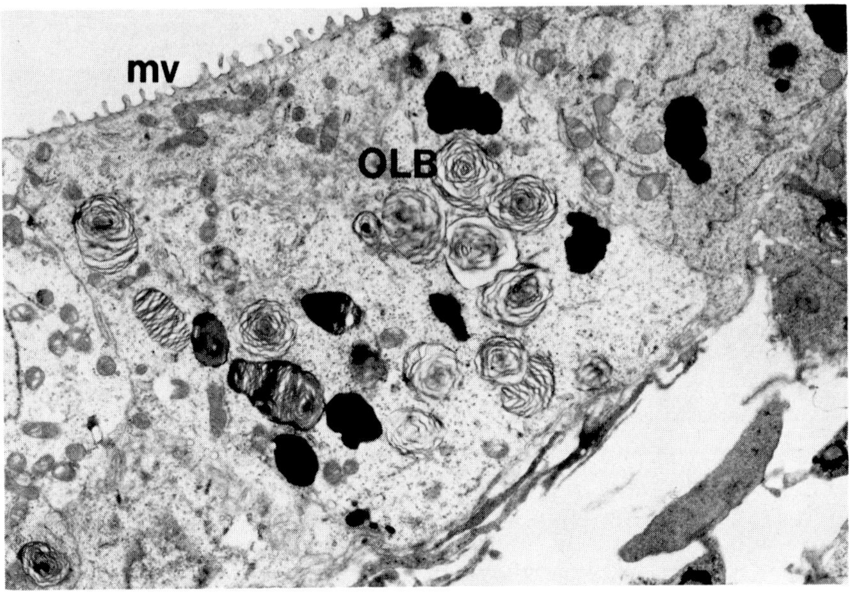

Fig. 4. Electron micrograph of type II cells lining an ALS of an organotypic culture derived from previously frozen cells. These cells are cuboidal, possess microvilli (mv) at the apical surface, and contain numerous osmiophilic lamellar bodies (OLB) (× 8,800).

space between the aggregates and the Gelfoam. By the end of the first week in culture these cells have formed a far more condensed cell mass immediately surrounding the ALS.

Type II cell differentiation in organotypic cultures accompanies the extensive morphogenetic development that takes place during the first week of culture. Cultures derived from fetal rat lung during late gestation (19–20 days ga) often possess identifiable type II cells in the first ALS that form. This is since type II cells may occur in the lungs at the time of collection and dissociation. When established from lung at an earlier period in fetal development (16–17 days ga) ALS form from undifferentiated cells. The epithelial cell composition and, thus, the time course of subsequent cytodifferentiation may then be considered gestation dependent. Regardless of the embryonic age of the starting lung material (16–20 days ga) organotypic cultures develop a predominantly differentiated cell population by the end of one full week in culture. During the differentiation process the undifferentiated cells lose their large content of cytoplasmic glycogen (Fig. 2) and acquire morphologic features (Fig. 4) that include cuboidal form, apical surface microvilli, and the osmiophilic lamellar bodies characteristic of the type II cell in vivo.

Organotypic cultures established following retrieval of cells from frozen storage possessed the morphologic characteristics described above for standard cultures, yet exhibited a somewhat altered pattern of in vitro development. Reaggregation occurred more slowly in these cultures than under standard conditions. ALS were rarely evident until about 48 hours in culture. At this time, TTC staining patterns disclosed a sparse population of aggregates that proved to be similar in histologic structure to the ALS observed in 24 hour control cultures. The number of ALS increased rapidly during the following several days, and aggregate formation appeared to continue through about day 5. The morphologic appearance of experimental cultures at any point during the first week in vitro more closely resembled standard cultures of a younger in vitro age than cultures of the same relative age. This apparent lag in the reaggregation process was accompanied by a similar delay in the appearance of differentiated type II cells in the ALS. As with control cultures, some type II cells occurred in the first aggregates to form. However, during subsequent development ALS bearing large numbers of type II cells were rarely observed until after 6–7 days in culture. Control cultures on the other hand often possessed a large complement of type II cells by day 5–6.

After 7 days in vitro, experimental and control cultures were often indistinguishable in morphology. One uncommon feature of cultures from previously frozen cells was the presence of a large number of damaged cells in the population (Fig. 3). Within routine cultures, damaged cells and debris indicative of autolysis are commonly observed at all stages of the in vitro period. Cellular debris is most prevalent during the first several days of culture, and again after 5–6 weeks when cell viability normally attenuates. Early in culture, cells damaged during the dissociation procedure litter the culture matrix surrounding newly formed aggregates of healthy cells. These damaged cells apparently undergo further degeneration, since substantially fewer disrupted cells are normally observed at the conclusion of the reaggregation period. It may be noted that macrophages containing large amounts of ingested material are commonly observed in organotypic cultures, both within and outside the ALS. These cells may function in sequestering some of the cell debris. Degenerative cells apparently derived from the epithelium of the ALS are also occasionally observed within the lumen. ALS often contain these disrupted cells but rarely in large number. It is, however, common especially in cultures with a large type II cell population to observe ALS that contain an accumulation of dense staining osmiophilic material. Luminal contents in this case contain cellular debris and often whole cells. The contents consist predominantly of amorphous material observed at the ultrastructural level to be lamellar bodies secreted by the type II cells.

Damaged cells were abundant in cultures from cryopreserved cells. Large numbers of disrupted cells were commonly present within the lumen of ALS (Fig. 3). Occasionally each ALS in a given field was filled with cells. It was not uncommon, however, to find ALS within the same culture that did not contain damaged cells.

DISCUSSION

This study demonstrates that enzymatically dissociated fetal rat lung cells frozen and stored in liquid nitrogen retain their capacity for histotypic reaggregation and subsequent cytodifferentiation in vitro. Morphologic analysis indicates that the structure and cellular composition of ALS in the two systems is comparable. Slight differences were observed, however, in the culture characteristics of organotypic cultures derived from frozen cells as compared to standard cultures. A noticeable lag in the time course of aggregate formation suggests that frozen cells require a recovery period prior to regaining the capacity to reaggregate. The ability of these cells to reaggregate was not permanently impaired since the number of ALS that eventually formed from previously frozen cells was comparable to standard cultures.

Another explanation for this latency of reaggregation might be found in the fact that the cellular composition of the initial inoculum was not equivalent in each case. Both standard and experimental cultures were seeded with 10^7 viable cells; however, the number of damaged cells within the initial cell preparations was vastly different. Following the dissociation procedure, cell viability was determined to be 90–95%. Following retrieval from frozen storage the cell suspension contained, at best, only 50% viable cells. Thus, experimental cultures were seeded with an almost equivalent number of nonviable as viable cells. The inclusion of such a large number of cells incapable of participating in reaggregation may have in some way influenced the capactiy of the viable epithelial cell population to associate. We have found through experimentation with a variety of culture substrates that reaggregation is influenced by the physical form of the culture matrix. In concept, efficient reaggregation requires unhindered cell movement to maximize cell-cell contact and provide the proper frequency and quality of cell interactions. A large population of nonparticipatory cells within the inoculum might thus conceivably interfere physically, or otherwise, with cell movement, cell-cell contact, or some other aspect of cell association.

The purpose of this study was to determine whether cell freezing techniques could be used to generate fetal rat lung organotypic cultures bearing an enriched population of differentiated type II cells. Morphologic analysis indicates that methods were successful in this regard. Cultures after one full week in vitro possessed ALS in which type II cells were the predominant epithelial cell type.

It must be acknowledged that this study did not attempt to assess type II cell function in the cryopreserved organotypic cultures. Fetal rat lung organotypic cultures have previously been shown to exhibit a variety of type II cell specific functions related to the synthesis and secretion of pulmonary surfactant [27–30]. These cultures have also been used to examine aspects of prostaglandin synthesis and metabolism by the type II cell [31]. The demonstration of similar type II cell specific functions in cultures from cryopreserved cells will be essential before cell banking techniques can be effectively applied to surfactant related studies with this culture system.

We have demonstrated that cell freezing techniques can be applied to a differentiating reaggregate cell culture system. A principle disadvantage seen in the cryopreservation technique we have described is the relatively poor viability (<50%) realized upon retrieval of cells from frozen storage. It is hoped that refinements in the various parameters known to influence cell survival during cryopreservation will increase the effectiveness of the technique.

SUMMARY

Enzymatically dissociated fetal rat lung cells were frozen in medium containing dimethyl sulfoxide (DMSO) as the cryoprotectant, and stored at liquid nitrogen temperature. The cells were retrieved from frozen storage and seeded into Gelfoam collagen sponges. The cultures were examined morphologically using tetrazolium chloride (TTC) vital staining, light microscopy, and transmission electron microscopy, at various points throughout a two-week in vitro period. Fetal rat lung organotypic cultures established from previously frozen cells posessed the characteristics of cultures derived from freshly dissociated lung. Though the percent recovery of viable cells following freezing was low (< 50%), those cells that survived the cryopreservation procedure exhibited histotypic reaggregation. These pulmonary epithelial cells formed alveolar-like structures (ALS) in which the cells associated to enclose a central lumen. The majority of these epithelial cells differentiated in vitro, developing the morphologic characteristics of type II alveolar epithelial cells. It is suggested that cryopreservation methods are applicable to in vitro studies on the pulmonary surfactant system.

REFERENCES

1. Perry VP, Kroener CA, Martin JL: Protected freezing of cell suspensions. Procedure No 76161. Tissue Culture Association (TCA) Manual 1:119–120, 1975.
2. Hay RJ: Preservation of cell-culture stocks in liquid nitrogen. Procedure No. 18601. TCA Manual 4:787–790, 1978.
3. Karow AM Jr: Cryoprotectants – A new class of drugs. J Pharm Pharmacol 21: 209–223, 1969.
4. Leibo SP, Mazur P: The role of cooling rates in low-temperature preservation. Cryobiology 8:447–452, 1971.
5. Alink GM, Verheul CC, Offerijns FGJ: The effect of cooling rate and dimethyl sulfoxide concentration on low temperature preservation of neonatal rat heart cells. Cryobiology 13:295–304, 1976.
6. Scheiwe MW, Schwindke P: Improvements of the deepfreezing of biological cell suspensions by automatic detection of the thermal history of the sample. Biomed Tech (Stuttg) 23:144–151, 1978.

7. Harris LW, Griffiths JB: Relative effects of cooling and warming rates on mammalian cells during the freeze-thaw cycle. Cryobiology 14:662–669, 1977.
8. McGann LE, Farrant J: Survival of tissue culture cells frozen by a two-step procedure to −196°C. I. Holding temperature and time. Cryobiology 13:261–268, 1976.
9. McGann LE, Farrant J: Survival of tissue culture cells frozen by a two-step procedure to −196°C. II. Warming rate and concentration of dimethyl sulphoxide. Cryobiology 13:269–273, 1976.
10. Harris LW, Griffiths JB: An assessment of methods used for measuring the recovery of mammalian cells from freezing and thawing. Cryobiology 11:80–84, 1974.
11. Wollenberger A, Halle W, Kallabis E, Kleitke B, Hinterberger U, Schulze W: Cultivation of beating heart cells from frozen heart cell suspensions. Naturwissenschaften 54:174, 1967.
12. Price PJ, Anderson BP, Bell MR: The freezing and processing of human embryonic kidney cells. Cryobiology 3:85–87, 1966.
13. Stenchever MA, Hempel JM, Macintyre MN: Maintenance of in vitro growth ability and chromosome integrity following the deep freezing of minced fetal tissue. Cryobiology 1:240–241, 1965.
14. Janiszewski E, Wollenberger A: Low-temperature preservation of heart cells and heart fragments. Acta Biol Med Ger 29:135–147, 1972.
15. Wilmut I: The effect of cooling rate, warming rate, cryoprotective agent and stage of development on survival of mouse embryos during freezing and thawing. Life Sci 11:1071–1079, 1972.
16. Robertson RD, Jacob SW: The preservation of intact organs. Adv Surg 3:75–159, 1968.
17. Barner HB, Rivers RJ, Cady B, Watkins E Jr: Survival of the canine ureter after freezing. Surgery 53:344–347, 1963.
18. Barner HB, Schenk EA: Autotransplantation of the frozen-thawed spleen. Arch Pathol 82:267–271, 1966.
19. Offerijns FGJ, Krijnen HW: The preservation of the rat heart in the frozen state. Cryobiology 9:289–295, 1972.
20. Douglas WHJ, Teel RW: An organotypic in vitro model system for studying pulmonary surfactant production by type II alveolar pneumonocytes. Am Rev Respir Dis 113: 17–23, 1976.
21. Douglas WHJ, Moorman GW, Teel RW: The formation of histotypic structures from monodisperse fetal rat lung cells cultured on a three-dimensional substrate. In vitro 12: 373–381, 1976.
22. Douglas WHJ, Del Vecchio P, Teel RW, Jones RM, Farrell PM: Culture of type II alveolar lung cells. In Bouhuys A (ed): "Lung Cells in Disease." New York:Elsevier/North-Holland Biomedical Press, 1976, pp 53–68.
23. Douglas WHJ, McAteer JA, Cavanagh T: Organotypic culture of dissociated fetal rat lung cells on a collagen sponge matrix. Procedure No 44166. TCA Manual 4:749–753, 1978.
24. Moscona A: Cell suspensions from organ rudiments of chick embryos. Exp Cell Res 3:535–539, 1952.
25. Tolnai S: A method for viable cell count. Procedure No. 70111. TCA Manual 1:37–38, 1975.
26. Douglas WHJ, McAteer JA, Dell'Orco RT, Phelps D: The use of 2, 3, 5′ -triphenyl tetrazolium chloride for the visualization of cellular aggregates cultured on a three dimensional collagen sponge matrix. In vitro (Submitted for publication).

27. Engle MJ, Sanders RL, Douglas WHJ: Synthesis of surfactant phospholipids (PLs) in isolated type II cells. (Abstract) Fed Proc 37:719, 1978.
28. Sanders RL, Engle MJ, Douglas WHJ: Use of an organotypic type II cell culture system for the study of surfactant synthesis. (Abstract) Am Rev Respir Dis 117 (Suppl):391, 1978.
29. Sanders RL, Engle MJ, Douglas WHJ: Response of type II cells to insulin treatment. (Abstract) Fed Proc 38:1436, 1979.
30. Engle MJ, Sanders RL, Douglas WHJ: Type II alveolar cells in organotypic culture: A model system for the study of surfactant synthesis. Biochim Biophys Acta (Submitted for publication).
31. Taylor L, Polgar P, McAteer J, Douglas WHJ: Prostaglandin production by cultured type II alveolar epithelial cells. Biochim Biophys Acta 572:502–509, 1979.

Culture of Urinary Cells

Fritz Herz, PhD

As pointed out by other contributors to this volume, the utilization of cultured epithelial cells for the detection of birth defects would represent a significant advance, provided an adequate source and simple techniques were available for this purpose. Although several methods have been proposed for obtaining pure epithelial cultures, most of them are tedious, requiring an inordinate amount of manipulation of the tissue of origin and/or the cultured cells. Even with such procedures as the selective enzymatic digestion of intracellular materials [1], there is no guarantee that the resulting cultures will not be an admixture of epithelial and fibroblastic cells. In addition, it is well known that the latter tend to overgrow epithelial cells after repeated passages of the cultures. Among the various techniques suggested for obtaining pure cultures of epithelial cells are 1) the use of cloning cylinders to select epithelial colonies from mixed cultures [2, 3]; 2) replacing D-valine for L-valine in the culture medium [4]; 3) starting cultures with epithelial cells spilled from sliced tumor tissues [5], from tissues dissected in such a manner as to remove the connective tissue elements [6], from a proliferating carcinoma [7] and hoping that its cells will eventually overgrow the normal cells, and by placing explants in collagenase-containing medium [8]; 4) adding thimerosal [9] or cis-4-hydroxy-L-proline [10] to mixed cultures; 5) short-term exposure of cultures to trypsin-EDTA [8], etc. From this brief enumeration it is obvious that other possibilities for the cultivation of epithelial cells should be forcefully explored. The reports on the use of human postweaning milk [11], semen [12], and amniotic fluid [13] represent attempts in this direction. However, it is evident that these sources place restrictions in regard to sex, age, and physiologic status of the sample donor. Thus, if it were possible, it would be preferable to obtain epithelial cells capable of multiplying in vitro from a common, noninvasive, easily available source. It would appear that urine may fulfill this requisite.

Birth Defects: Original Article Series, Volume XVI, Number 2, pages 85–93

Despite several attempts to employ urinary sediments for the initiation of short-term cultures of epithelial cells, it seems that this nonconventional source of viable cells has heretofore not been fully explored, and/or that, with some exceptions [12], negative results were not deemed necessary to report. A review of the literature indicates that Jacobson and Barter [14], in an effort to document the origin of amniotic fluid cells, initiated cultures with sheep urine and bladder aspirates of human fetuses. They obtained a single successful culture with sheep urine that was slow growing; the proliferating cells had epithelioid appearance. Sutherland and Bain [15] cultured the urines of newborn infants of less than 2 days of age and used the multiplying cells for chromosomal analysis. Seven out of 8 cultures yielded primary cell "strains," one of which was subcultured 6 times. However, a small number of urinary cultures from older children failed to grow. Hoehn et al [16] obtained outgrowth of cells from the urines of 4 human fetuses between the 12th and 16th weeks of gestation. In all instances the proliferating cells displayed epithelioid morphology and were similar to the type of cells cultured from amniotic fluid. No fibroblast-like cells were observed. These findings would suggest that fetal urine contributes to some extent to the population of viable cells present in amniotic fluids. The in vitro cultivation of urine cells from 5 adult individuals was attempted by Linder [17]. Of 28 cultures initiated, 21 resulted in the outgrowth of one or more colonies of epithelial cells. Growth was evident as early as 3 days in some instances and as late as 18 days in others; in some cases the cells could be subcultured up to 2 times. Felix and Littlefield [18, 19] recently reported the outgrowth of epithelial cells with 54% of urinary specimens from newborn infants between 1–7 days of age and with 20% from infants older than 1 week. Upon subculture the cells doubled every 24 hours, until after several divisions the cultures showed signs of senescence. Some cultures could be transferred for up to 6 times and it was estimated that the cells had undergone a maximum of up to 25 doublings. With urines from normal adults the frequency of initial colony formation was less than with specimens from newborns, but 50% of the samples yielded at least one colony.

We have verified and extended some of these observations. However, because of our interest in cultured cells derived from human bladder tumors [20], our experience has been limited to urinary specimens from adult individuals. We have obtained proliferation of epithelial-like cells with 70% of the urines from normal adult males and from patients with an indwelling catheter. In some instances we have also observed outgrowth of malignant cells from urines of patients with urothelial carcinoma.

URINE CELL CULTURE

We have explored several modifications of various culturing techniques in order to enhance the proliferative abilities of urinary cells. However, because none of them proved superior to the simple method initially employed, we will describe the latter in some detail.

Midstream urines are collected in sterile 5-ml centrifuge tubes or 250-ml Erlenmeyer flasks. Samples obtained through catheter are collected in centrifuge tubes. No preservatives are employed. The volume of urine from which we have obtained successful cell outgrowth varies widely (5–250 ml). Following an initial centrifugation at 250 X g for 10 minutes, the supernatant is discarded; the urinary sediments are combined into one tube (if necessary) and resuspended in 12 ml of Eagle's Minimal Essential Medium supplemented with fetal bovine serum (20%), penicillin (100 U/ml), streptomycin (100 μg/ml), and amphotericin B (0.25 μg/ml). After washing by repeated inversion, the cells are sedimented again. After centrifugation, the supernatant medium is removed and the cells are resuspended in fresh medium. The volume of medium employed at this step depends on the dimensions of the culture containers to be used. To inoculate a 30-ml T flask, we use 2 ml; for a 35-mm Petri dish, a culture/chamber slide, or a coverslip-containing Leighton tube, we use 1 ml. The cultures are incubated at 37°C in a humidified atmosphere of 5% CO_2 in air and left undisturbed for the initial 24 hours. Afterwards they are examined daily for cellular attachment and growth. Cultures contaminated with bacteria and/or fungi are discarded as soon as they are noticed. The initial microscopic examination of cultures from individuals with gross hematuria is best accomplished by tilting the flask. We replace the culture medium as soon as cellular attachment is evident or 7–10 days after culture initiation when no attachment is microscopically apparent. After determining that cell proliferation is occurring, the medium is changed twice or thrice a week. Cultures not exhibiting growth are kept in the incubator for up to 4–6 weeks.

By using the procedure outlined above, we have observed primary outgrowth of colonies of epithelial-like cells from the urines of adult males within 5–20 days. Growth has been obtained with 37 out of 55 normal individuals. The proliferating cells are flat, and they spread and form relatively densely packed colonies. Frequently round (mitotic?) cells are seen. Occasionally colonies of smaller cells forming dense whorls are also observed. In no instance have we seen outgrowth of typical fibroblasts. Figure 1 depicts the proliferating urinary cells of a normal adult male 7 days after initiation of the culture. Figure 2 shows the same area of the culture flask 3 days later. Figure 3 is an example of growing cells derived from the urine of another individual 11 days after starting the culture.

We have obtained growth with the sediment of as little as 25 ml of normal male urine and 5 ml of urine collected through a catheter. Figure 4 shows the proliferating cells derived from the sediment of 5 ml of urine obtained through an indwelling catheter from an individual with benign nodular overgrowth of the prostate. This picture was taken 10 days after initiation of the culture. No significant differences in frequency of colony formation were seen between spontaneously voided urines and that obtained from patients with an indwelling catheter. No correlation

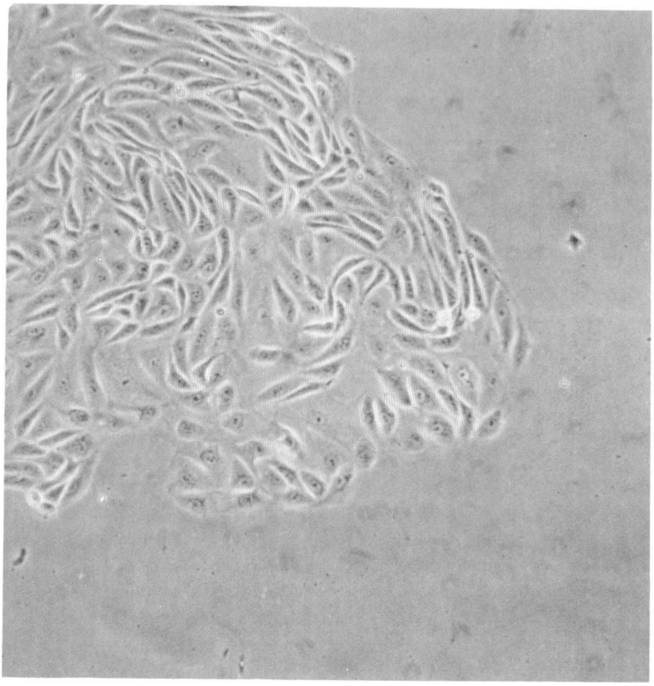

Fig. 1. Cells cultured from the urine of a 43-year-old normal male, 7 days after initiation of the culture. Phase contrast of living cells (× 97).

was noted between the age of the urine donor and the degree of cell proliferation. As a rule the specimens were processed immediately, but in some cases we kept them experimentally for up to 6 hours at room temperature. Outgrowth from these samples was as good as that seen with their control counterparts worked up immediately.

Less than 10% of the urinary cultures from male individuals have been contaminated by bacteria and/or fungi. By contrast the proportion of contaminated cultures from normal females was close to 90%. Understandably our success rate with the latter has been accordingly smaller. We have tried to overcome this problem by increasing up to fivefold the concentration of the antibiotic-antimycotic mixture (this concentration did not affect cellular outgrowth from male urines) in the

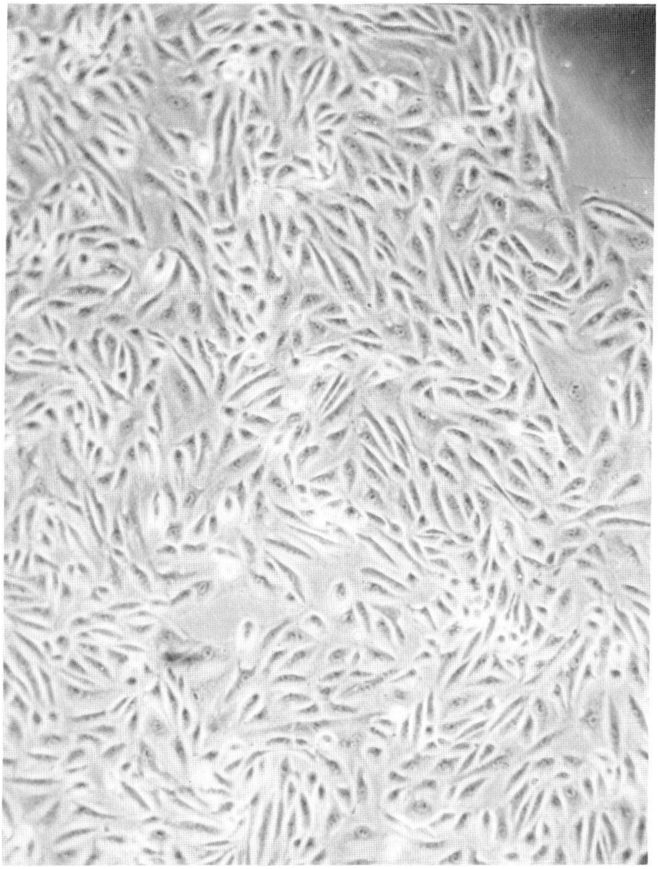

Fig. 2. Cultured urinary cells derived from the same individual as Fig. 1, 10 days after starting the culture. Phase contrast (× 97).

medium, but no significant improvement was seen. A more systematic study of the contaminating flora in female specimens and their antibiotic sensitivity is certainly indicated.

Because around 30% of the cultures initiated from the urinary sediments of normal male subjects failed to grow, the suitability of more complex media (Waymouth's 752/1; McCoy's 5A; RPMI-1640; M-199) and several other variables (30% fetal calf serum, human serum, urine itself) were tested. However, in similarity to the experience of others [19] in no instance was an improvement in the culture outcome observed. Our attempts in subculturing the proliferating cells have not been very encouraging. Occasionally we have had success in transferring cells twice and

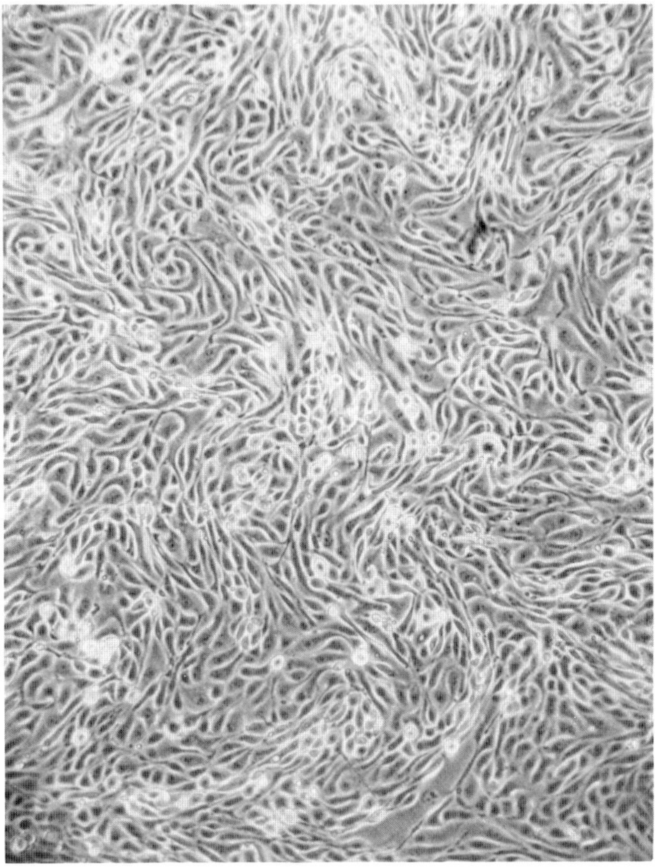

Fig. 3. Proliferating cells from the urine of a 30-year-old normal male, 11 days after culture initiation. Phase contrast (× 97).

maximally thrice. Others [17, 19] have reported similar experience and Felix and Littlefield [19] found that only colonies that were in culture for less than 2 weeks could be subcultured. The reason for this behavior is unknown, but it would appear that the growth potential of the exfoliated urinary cells from adult individuals is limited once they reach maximal proliferation in primary culture.

COMMENTS

It is evident that some epithelial cells recovered from urine are capable of in vitro proliferation, but nothing is known about their anatomic site(s) of origin [17, 19, 21]. The cells could originate from anywhere along the urinary tract: kidney, ureter, bladder, urethra. In the female there may be an admixture of cells,

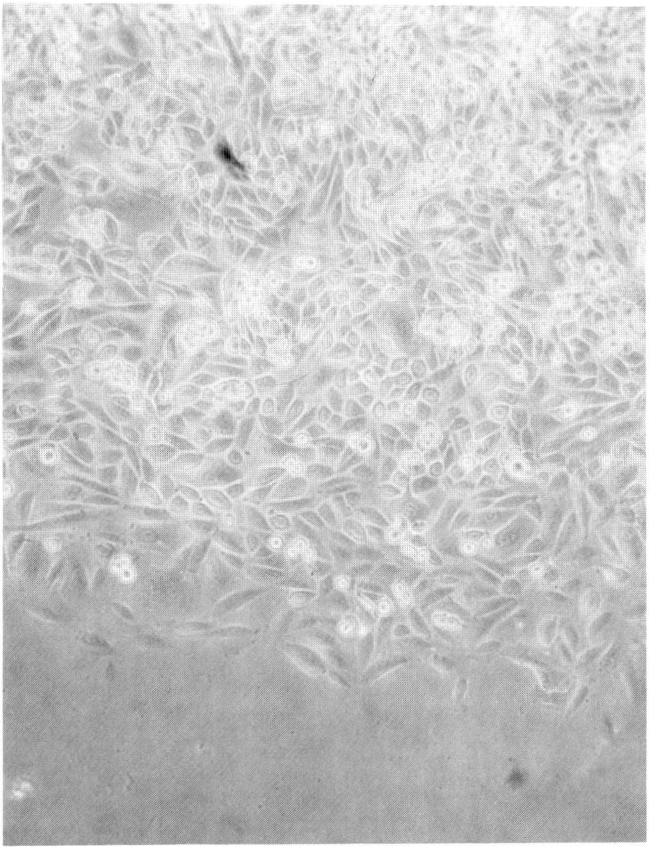

Fig. 4. Cells cultured from the urinary sediment of a catheterized 66-year-old male, 10 days after initiating the culture. Many rounded (mitotic?) cells can be seen. Phase contrast (× 97).

including those of vaginal origin, and in the male the urinary sediment may also contain prostatic cells. In the absence of disease the urine usually contains few urothelial and squamous cells, but in lithiasis, inflammatory disorder, neoplastic diseases, or after catheterization their number increases considerably [22].

We have attempted to answer some questions regarding the origin of the proliferating cells. Our observation that the urine collected from the bladder through an indwelling catheter contains cells capable of proliferating in vitro would support that in these instances they may come from the bladder or above. As another approach, perhaps too naive, we initiated repeated urine cultures from a male renal transplant patient who received a kidney from a female donor. Unfortunately in no instance did we observe cell growth, but the idea was to perform karyologic analysis on the proliferating cells.

Although many problems remain to be solved, urine cell culture appears to be a promising approach for the study of epithelial cells. It might be possible to use this system for both diagnostic and research purposes. For the former, the proliferating cells might be used especially in those instances where the proportion of cells of interest in the urinary sediments is minimal and the multiplying cells retain in culture distinguishing diagnostic characteristics.

SUMMARY

Cellular proliferation takes place when sediments from voided or catheterized urines are cultured. Outgrowth of epithelial-like cells has been obtained with 70% of the urines from normal adult males. In no case was outgrowth of fibroblast-like cells observed. Because of the large proportion of contaminated cultures, the cultivation of urinary cells from females has been less successful. The proliferating cells have a limited life-span; only occasionally could they be subcultured. Although the site (s) of origin of the urinary cells capable of multiplying in vitro remains unknown, they may represent a potentially useful tool for diagnostic and research purposes.

REFERENCES

1. Lasfarques EY, Moore DH: A method for the continuous cultivation of mammary epithelium. In Vitro 7:21–25, 1971.
2. Yasumura Y, Tashjian AH Jr, Sato GH: Establishment of four functional clonal strains of animal cells in culture. Science 154:1186–1189, 1966.
3. Brown AM: In vitro transformation of submandibular gland epithelial cells and fibroblasts of adult rats by methycholanthrene. Cancer Res 33:2779–2789, 1973.
4. Gilbert SF, Migeon BR: D-Valine as a selective agent for normal human and rodent epithelial cells in culture. Cell 5:11–17, 1975.
5. Lasfarques EY, Ozzello L: Cultivation of human breast carcinomas. J Natl Cancer Inst 21: 1131–1147, 1958.
6. Wigley CB, Franks LM: Salivary epithelial cells in primary culture: Characterization of their growth and functional properties. J Cell Sci 20:149–165, 1976.
7. Kondo T, Muragishi H, Imaizumi M: A cell line from a human salivary gland mixed tumor. Cancer 27:403–410, 1971.
8. Owens RB, Smith HS, Nelson-Rees WA, Springer EL: Epithelial cell cultures from normal and cancerous human tissues. J Natl Cancer Inst 56:843–849, 1976.
9. Braaten JT, Lee MJ, Schenk A, Mintz DH: Removal of fibroblastoid cells from primary monolayer cultures of rat neonatal endocrine pancreas by sodium ethylmercurithiosalicylate. Biochem Biophys Res Commun 61:476–482, 1974.
10. Kao, WW-Y, Prockop DJ: Proline analogue removes fibroblasts from cultured mixed cell populations. Nature 266:63–64, 1977.
11. Russo J, Furmanski P, Rich MA: An ultrastructural study of normal human mammary epithelial cells in culture. Am J Anat 142:221–232, 1975.
12. Phillips SG, Phillips DM, Kabat EA, Miller OJ: Human semen as a source of epithelial cells for culture. In Vitro 14:639–650, 1978.

13. Hoehn H, Bryant EM, Karp LE, Martin GM: Cultivated cells from diagnostic amniocentesis in second trimester pregnancies. I. Clonal morphology and growth potential. Pediat. Res 8:746–754, 1974.
14. Jacobson CB, Barter RH: Intrauterine diagnosis and management of genetic defects. Am J Obstet Gynecol 99:796–807, 1967.
15. Sutherland GR, Bain AD: Culture of cells from the urine of newborn children. Nature 239:231, 1972.
16. Hoehn H, Bryant EM, Fantel AG, Martin GM: Cultivated cells from diagnostic amniocentesis in second trimester pregnancies. III. The fetal urine as a potential source of clonable cells. Humangenetik 29:285–290, 1975.
17. Linder D: Culture of cells from the urine and bladder washings of adults. Somatic Cell Genet 2:281–283, 1976.
18. Felix JS, Littlefield JW: Epithelial cells cultured form human urine. (Abstract) Am J Hum Genet 21:41A, 1977.
19. Felix JS, Littlefield JW: Urinary tract epithelial cells cultured from human urine. Int Rev Cytol (In press).
20. Herz F, Barlebo H, Koss LG: Modulation of alkaline phosphatase activity in cell cultures derived from human urinary bladder carcinoma. Cancer Res 34:1943–1946, 1974.
21. Kern WH: Epithelial cells in urine sediments. Am J Clin Path 56:67–72, 1971.
22. Koss LG: "Diagnostic Cytology and Its Histopathologic Bases," 3rd Ed. Philadelphia: JB Lippincott, 1979, pp 711–748.

Characterization of Cells in Suspension From Normal Rat Colonic Mucosa*

Theresa P. Pretlow, PhD and Thomas G. Pretlow II, MD†

Mammalian epithelial tissues are composed of many different cells in addition to the epithelial cells. The likelihood of obtaining pure epithelial cells in culture might be greatly enhanced if the starting inoculum were exclusively epithelial cells rather than a mixture of cells that included red blood cells, lymphocytes, granulocytes, endothelial cells, fibroblasts, and macrophages. In this paper we shall discuss our attempts to purify viable epithelial cells from rat colons and the cytologic appearances of some unusual cells we have observed in low concentrations in our suspensions of rat colonic cells. Similar methods can be used to purify a wide variety of epithelial cells. The specific details of tissue disaggregation and subsequent purification, however, must be worked out for each specific tissue and species and will be dependent upon the goals of the investigator. We have recently discussed the purification of cells from solid tissues in more detail [1–3].

METHODS AND RESULTS

Tissue Dissociation

Colons were removed from female, 55- to 65-day-old Fischer rats (Charles River Breeding Laboratories, North Wilmington, MA), cooled to 4°C in Joklik's modification of minimum essential medium (Grand Island Biological Co., Grand Island, NY), cut into 5-cm segments, and weighed. The colonic segments were pinned to paraffin-filled culture dishes (60 × 15 mm; Falcon Plastics, Cockeysville, MD) that contained 10% fetal calf serum (FCS) in cold medium. The tissue was washed for 3, successive, 10-minute periods in 5-ml changes of this medium with

*Supported by grants CA-16764 and CA-23922 from the National Cancer Institute, and by grant PDT-126 from the American Cancer Society.

†Supported by NIH Research Career Development Award K4-CA-70584.

Birth Defects: Original Article Series, Volume XVI, Number 2, pages 95–107

gentle rotation on a Thomas Rotating Apparatus (Arthur H. Thomas Co., Philadelphia, PA). The washing medium was replaced with citrate [4], 0.05% collagenase (type II; Sigma Chemical Co., St. Louis, MO) in medium with 10% FCS [5, 6], 0.1% Pronase (EM Laboratories, Elmsford, NY) in medium without serum [7, 8], or 0.25% trypsin (Flow Laboratories, Inc. Rockville, MD) in medium without serum [7, 9, 10]. The mucosal surface was exhaustively digested during 12, successive, 20-minute incubations at room temperature. The suspended cells from each period of digestion were cooled for 5 minutes in an ice bath, sedimented at 97 g for 7.5 minutes, resuspended in medium with 10% FCS, and stored in an ice bath. Cells from the first 2 periods of digestion were discarded since they contained many red blood cells and many cells that failed to exclude trypan blue. Cells from digestions 3–12 were combined, filtered through single layers of Nitex (TETKO, Inc., Elmsford, NY) with pore diameters of 100 and 48 μm, respectively, centrifuged at 97 g for 7.5 minutes, and resuspended in medium with 10% FCS.

With this method we obtained manyfold fewer cells with citrate (0.25 to 0.5×10^6 cells/gm) than with any of the enzymes. From the proximal 5 cm of colon we obtained $2.9 \pm 0.7 \times 10^6$ cells/gm with trypsin, $7.6 \pm 3.7 \times 10^6$ cells/gm with collagenase, and $37.7 \pm 11.0 \times 10^6$ cells/gm with Pronase. We obtained significantly more cells from the proximal 5 cm of colon ($37.7 \pm 11.0 \times 10^6$ cells/gm) than from the distal 5 cm of colon ($7.1 \pm 3.2 \times 10^6$ cells/gm) with Pronase. Consequently, all of the subsequent data are from suspensions of cells obtained from the proximal colon with Pronase. Viability, as assessed by trypan blue exclusion, was $96.5 \pm 1.5\%$.

Types of Cells

Our suspensions of cells from normal rat colon contained many, cytologically different kinds of cells (Fig. 1). In preliminary experiments we attempted to classify the cells observed in our suspensions with a large number of histochemical procedures. Of all the examined procedures, Wright's stain was the most useful to us for the classification of cells from the proximal colon. Since each type of cell has not been unequivocally located in the intact colon, we have assigned a number to each type that we believe can be recognized in the suspensions of rat colonic cells after Wright's stain (Table 1). Type 1 cells are characterized by a very palely staining nucleus and numerous inclusions (Fig. 1A and B). Type 2 cells, the predominant cell type, have a darkly staining nucleus and foamy cytoplasm with variable numbers of clear vacuoles (Fig. 1C–F). Type 2 cells with a single nucleus (Fig. 1C and D) comprised over 82% of the cells in our suspensions of colon cells, but binucleated and multinucleated type 2 cells (Fig. 1C and F) were observed occasionally. An intensely basophilic cytoplasm (Fig. 1G and H) characterizes type 3 cells, while type 4 cells have a less basophilic cytoplasm and their nuclei appear to contain large, irregular, clear vacuoles (Fig. 1I–L). In type 5 cells, the nucleus is displaced peripherally by a large central vacuole (Fig. 1M). Type 6 cells

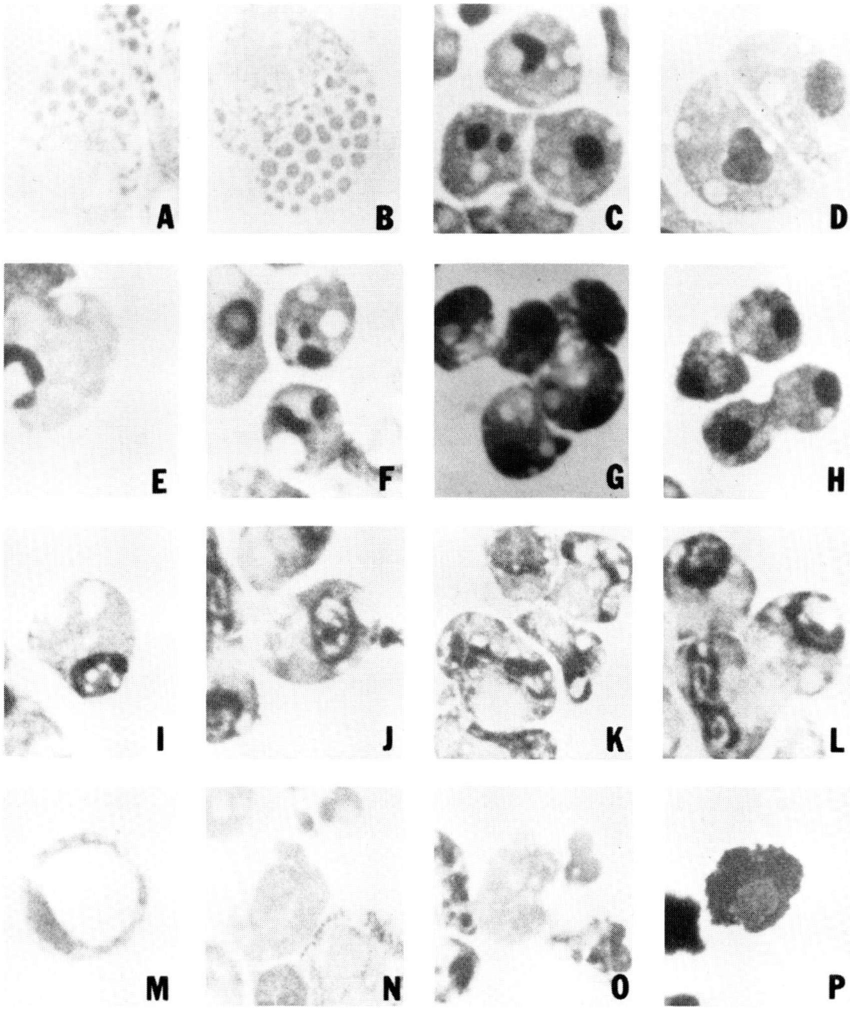

Fig. 1A–P. All cells are stained with Wright's stain and photographed with an original magnification of × 800. The cells are described in detail in Table 1 and include: A and B) type 1 ("giraffe") cells, C-F) type 2 cells, G and H) type 3 cells, I-L) type 4 cells, M) type 5 cells ("signet ring"), N and O) type 6 cells, and P) mast cells.

have an intensely eosinophilic cytoplasm (Fig. 1N and O). Although types 1–6 may represent variants or different maturational stages of the same cell type(s), it seems best to give a separate designation to each identifiable type of cell until the relationships among these kinds of cells are clarified. The frequency of each type

TABLE 1. Suspensions of Colon Cells*

Cell type	Frequency (%)†	Description of cell	Illustrated in Fig. 1, Part:
1	1.9 ± 1.6	These cells, "giraffe cells," are very distinct from other types of colon cells in that their cytoplasm is filled with numerous inclusions which are 0.5 to 2.0 μm in diameter in preparations made with the Cytocentrifuge. These inclusions are red when the cells have been stained with Wright's stain. The nuclei of these cells frequently fail to stain with Wright's stain and are apparent only because they displace the cytoplasmic granules; when the nuclei of these cells do stain, they stain with a pale, reddish-blue color. The chromatin may be homogeneous or slightly reticulated.	A and B
2	84.9 ± 4.5	When stained with Wright's stain, these cells have a foamy cytoplasm which contains variable numbers of clear vacuoles 0.5 to 4.0 μm in diameter. When these vacuoles overlie the nuclei, they appear as clear defects (Fig. 1F) in the basophilic nuclei. The nuclei of these cells generally stain homogeneously dark blue but may be slightly reticulated. They are generally oval but may be somewhat angular. Approximately 2% of these cells are binucleated, and 0.5% have 3 or more nuclei. When there are multiple nuclei, some of the nuclei are frequently extremely small. Occasionally, the nucleus is lobated (Fig. 1E) as though part of the nucleus were being pinched off to form those nuclei which are extremely small.	C–F
3	3.5 ± 2.4	The most unique feature of this cell is the intense basophilia of its cytoplasm. In the Wright-stained preparation, it is approximately half as great in diameter as the type 1 and type 2 cells. There may be a small, clear vacuole located peripherally in the cytoplasm.	G and H
4	1.8 ± 1.7	The cytoplasm of these cells stains less basophilically than that of type 3 cells. The nuclei appear to contain large, irregular, clear vacuoles.	I–L
5	0.6 ± 0.3	These cells are the common signet-ring cells with a large central vacuole which displaces the nucleus peripherally.	M
6	1.4 ± 0.6	The cytoplasm of these cells is intensely eosinophilic. The nucleus may be oval and solid or may be shaped like a doughnut.	N and O
Mast cells	1.0 ± 0.5		P

*In addition to these cells, suspensions of cells from the rat colon contain lymphocytes (1.7 ± 0.4% and red blood cells (3.5 ± 2.1%).

†Values are means ± standard deviation.

of cell in our suspensions of colonic cells is found in Table 1. Note that most of the cells illustrated in Fig. 1A–O, including the binucleated and multinucleated type 2 cells, individually were less than 4% of the total cells and together comprised less than 12% of the cells in the suspensions of colonic cells prior to the separation of cells in density gradients. Cells from the proximal and distal segments of colon showed different staining properties both in situ and in suspension. One such difference was the staining of mucus in sections of distal colon with both PAS and Alcian blue at pH 2.5 [11]. Mucus-containing cells in sections of proximal colon stained with Alcian blue but failed to stain with PAS.

Velocity Sedimentation

Velocity sedimentation in an isokinetic gradient is a widely applicable means of purifying cells from many mammalian tissues [2, 12]. Linear density gradients of Ficoll (polysucrose; average molecular weight, 400,000; Pharmacia Fine Chemicals, Piscataway, NJ) in tissue culture medium were constructed with a previously described [3, 13], 2-chambered gradient generator (Lido Glass, Stirling, NJ) in 100-ml polycarbonate centrifuge tubes (#2806; International Equipment Co., Needham Heights, MA). The solutions for isokinetic gradients were sterilized by filtration (Millipore Corp., Bedford, MA) prior to gradient formation. The isokinetic gradient [14], used in these experiments varied linearly from 2.7% (wt/wt) Ficoll at the sample-gradient interface, 13.7 cm from the center of revolution, to 5.5% (wt/wt) Ficoll at the gradient-cushion interface, 26.7 cm from the center of revolution. Velocity sedimentation in the isokinetic gradient was performed in a Mistral 6L centrifuge (Measuring and Scientific Equipment, Ltd., London, England); the speed of the centrifuge was monitored continuously during the experiment with an electronic stroboscope (General Radio Co., Concord, MA). Suspensions of rat colon cells were sedimented in the isokinetic gradient for 18 minutes at 4°C with a centrifugal force of 38 g measured at the sample-gradient interface.

Fractions were collected from the density gradients with a tapping cap described previously [3]. Each fraction contained 4 ml except for the first fraction from each gradient which comprised the 7-ml starting sample volume. Cell counts were done in hemocytometer chambers. The refractive indexes of all fractions were measured with an Abbe-3L refractometer (#33-45-58-01; Bausch and Lomb, Rochester, NY). Slides of each gradient fraction were made with the Cytocentrifuge (Shandon Southern Instruments, Inc., Sewickley, PA) and stained with Wright's stain. Differential cell counts were performed by counting 500 cells from each fraction and from the starting sample.

Suspensions of cells from rat colons always contained large amounts of a mucoid, gelatinous material that we had not observed in suspensions of cells from many other tissues. When the suspensions of cells were sedimented in the isokinetic gradient, the gel was frequently found in fractions 2 or 3 near the top of the gradient. This gel appeared to trap many cells and prevent them from sedimenting with their characteristic, unimpeded velocities. Several methods previously described for the elimination of gels were evaluated. Prior to sedimentation, an aliquot of cells was incubated in medium with 0.05% lysozyme [15] for 10 minutes at 25°C. A second aliquot of the same suspension was incubated with 0.001% DNase [16] for 10 minutes at 25°C. A third aliquot was centrifuged through a neutral density column of FCS (K. Shortman, personal communication), and a fourth aliquot was washed 3 times with medium that contained 10% FCS (G. Sachs, personal communication). The mucoid material that impeded the sedimentation of cells was greatly reduced by all 4 methods; this is evident by the relatively small number of cells found in fractions 2 or 3 after isokinetic sedimentation (Fig. 2). However, all 4 methods resulted in some loss of cells and some degree of cellular aggregation. Large aggregates have larger diameters than single cells and are found in fraction 22 (Fig. 2). The amount of aggregation varied enormously in the 4 experiments conducted to compare these procedures, but seemed to be greatest after centrifuging through neutral density columns of FCS and least after repeated washings in medium with 10% FCS.

If mucoid material was present in large amounts, then variable but often large numbers of cells were found in fraction 2 (Fig. 3, before washing); the locations of other modal populations of cells were not consistent from experiment to experiment. Repeatable separations were obtained by washing the colonic cells 3 times in medium with 10% FCS. This washing procedure eliminated all of the visible gel in the gradients, reduced the number of cells in fractions 2 and 3, and increased the number of cells that sedimented to the location (fraction 10 ± 1 fraction) of the modal population of type 2 cells (Fig. 3, after washing). This modal fraction contained 93.0 ± 5.4% type 2 cells. Due to small amounts of gel, type 2 cells were still frequently found in fraction 2. Also, type 2 cells aggregate readily; the larger aggregates were found at the gradient-cushion interface. Type 2 cells comprised 93.1 ± 3.1% of the cells in fraction 2 and 95.7 ± 1.2% of the cells in the purest fraction at or adjacent to the gradient-cushion interface (fraction 21 or 22). Lymphocytes and red blood cells sedimented more slowly; their modal populations were located in fraction 4 ± 1 fraction. This fraction contained 18.4 ± 12.1% lymphocytes and 32.7 ± 26.3% red blood cells. The modal population of mast cells was in fraction 8 where mast cells comprised 4.9 ± 3.9% of the cells. The remaining less common types of cells in our suspensions of colonic cells were not significantly concentrated.

The total recovery after isokinetic sedimentation was 66.1 ± 12.3% of all cells layered over the gradients. This included recovery of 58.5 ± 19.0% of the type 2 cells, 46.1 ± 24.9% of the type 3 cells, and 78.2 ± 8.2% of the red blood cells. The several other types of cells in our suspensions were individually less than 2% of the cells. Differential counts of 500 cells did not constitute an adequate sample for accurate assessment of the recovery of these types of cells.

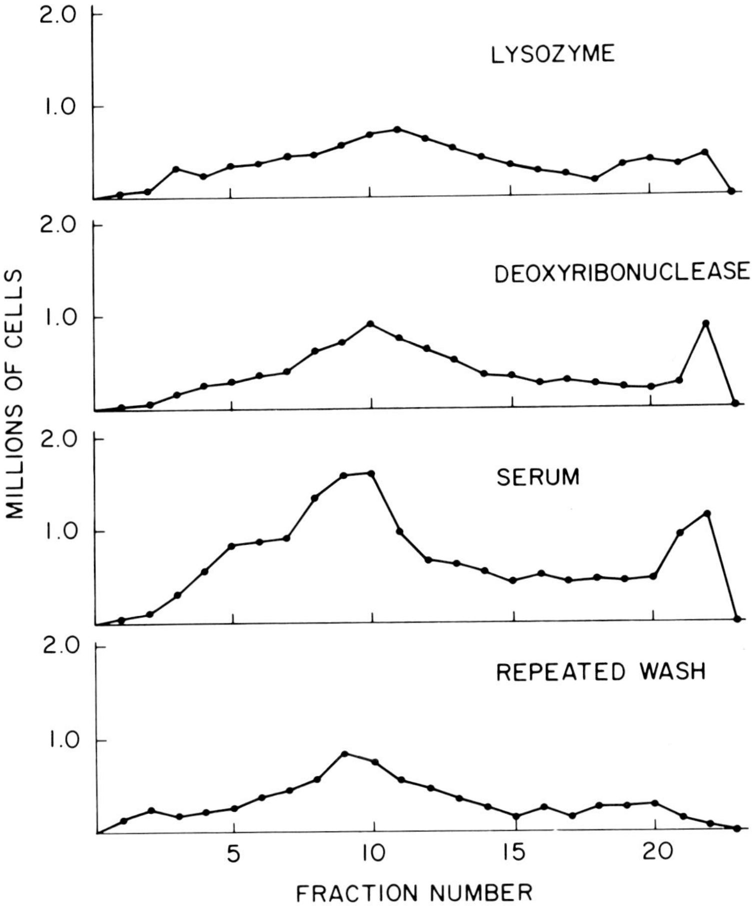

Fig. 2. Distribution of cells from the proximal colon in the isokinetic gradient after treatment with lysozyme, treatment with DNase, centrifugation through a column of FCS, or washing 3 times with medium with 10% FCS. All 4 methods were effective in greatly reducing the mucoid material which hampered the sedimentation of cells; this is reflected by the relatively small numbers of cells found in fractions 2 and 3. However, all 4 methods caused some degree of aggregation of cells; the large aggregates are found in fraction 22. The amount of aggregation appeared to be least when the cells were washed 3 times in medium with 10% FCS. Conditions for sedimentation were the same as described in Fig. 3.

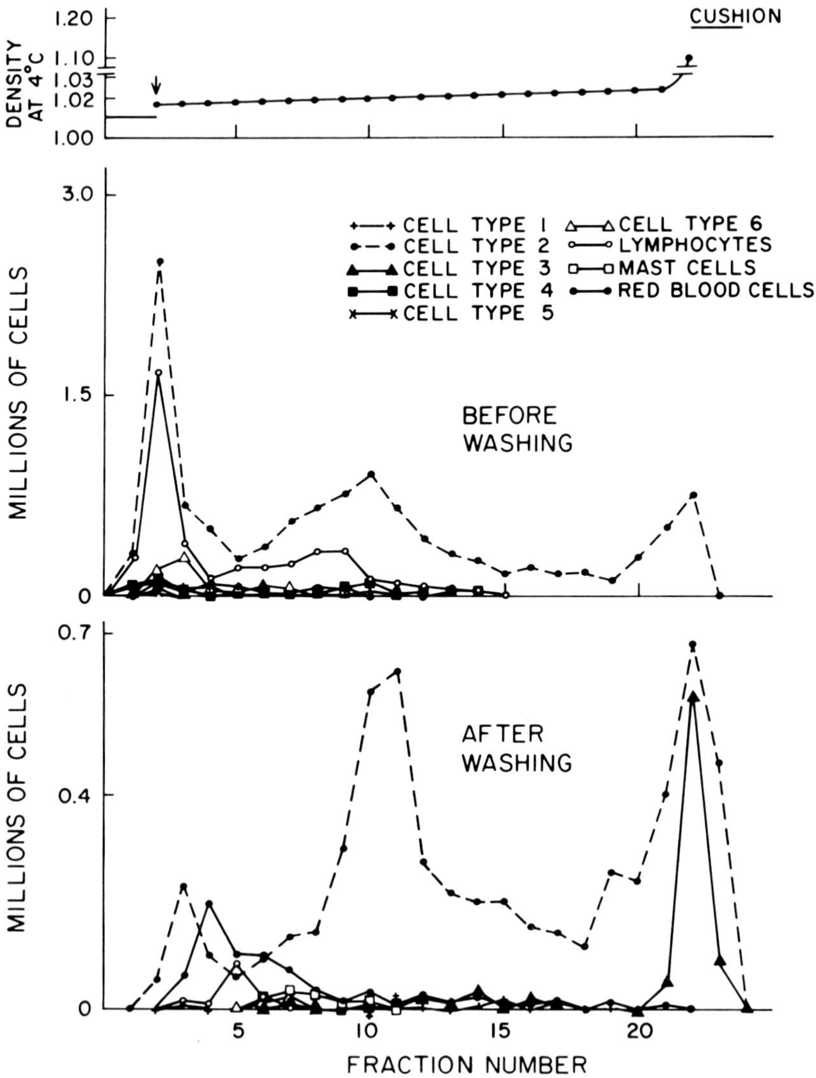

Fig. 3. Distribution of cells after velocity sedimentation in an isokinetic gradient before and after washing the suspensions of cells 3 times in medium with 10% FCS. Velocity sedimentation was carried out for 18 minutes at 4°C with a centrifugal force of 38 g measured at the sample-gradient interface. An arrow marks the sample-gradient interface on the density plot.

Culture of Cells

Our work in the culture of colonic epithelial cells is very preliminary; however, we have found a method that generally prevents bacterial overgrowth of the cultures. After velocity sedimentation in a sterile gradient, colonic epithelial cells can be maintained in culture with 50 μg gentamicin/ml (Shering Pharmaceutical Corp., Kenilworth, NJ) for several days without overgrowth of the cultures by bacteria. This medium can be replaced with medium without gentamicin after 3 days, and the cultures will remain sterile. In our experience, this has not been possible prior to separation of the cells in a sterile gradient. Since bacteria are considerably smaller than mammalian cells, they are expected to sediment less rapidly in the isokinetic gradient than mammalian cells. In work with human colonic carcinomas [17], fractions that contain purified cells with the capacity to form colonies in soft agar are widely separated from fractions near the top of the gradient that contain microorganisms as demonstrated by culture on blood agar.

DISCUSSION

The choice of methods for obtaining cells in suspension is of great importance. The most sophisticated studies of colonic epithelial cells can be of little value in augmenting our understanding of the normal or diseased colon if the cells studied are not representative of the cells in the intact tissue. It is desirable to destroy as few of the cells in the tissue as possible and to cause the least possible alterations in the isolated cells. Citrate has the advantage over proteolytic enzymes that it should not cleave proteins on the cell surface. However, our application of citrate, as used previously in work with intestine [4], yielded less than 1.4% of the cells per gram of tissue that we obtained with Pronase. Viability, as assessed by the exclusion of trypan blue is 96.5 ± 1.5% after dissociation with Pronase. While it is possible that the cells obtained with Pronase are chemically altered by the Pronase, the much greater yield leads us to prefer Pronase over citrate. Also, the ability to culture Pronase-dissociated cells after sedimentation in the isokinetic gradient further establishes that the Pronase-dissociated cells are still intact. The fivefold more cells per gram of tissue from the proximal colon than from the distal colon is unexpected; examination of the histology of the proximal and distal colon does not suggest an explanation for this difference.

The morphology and kinetics typical of epithelial cells in the colonic epithelium have been studied by many [18–25]. Although we have studied some plastic-embedded, 0.5 to 1.0 μm sections, much more work will be required to relate the types of cells that we have observed in low frequencies in suspensions of colonic cells to the kinds of cells that have been seen in the colon prior to its disaggregation. Currently, we think that type 1 cells are found in the lamina propria and that types 2–5 are colonic epithelial cells. Type 6 cells probably represent blood granulocytes in various stages of differentiation.

Many of the cytologically unusual cells were observed first in suspensions of cells from normal human colons. The nuclear morphology of some type 2 and type 4 cells, ie multiple "micronuclei" and fragmented nuclear material, suggested nuclear pyknosis and karyorrhexis. We wondered if these cellular types were present in human colonic mucosa in vivo or if they were merely artifacts produced in the surgical specimens by hypoxia. Since we could control the rapid removal and cooling of tissues more precisely with laboratory animals than with human surgical specimens, we began studies on the normal rat colon. Cell suspensions from normal rat colons that were rapidly removed and cooled in tissue culture medium still contained several cytologically unusual types of cells (Fig. 1A–O). Similar types of cells have been observed in cultures of cell lines from human colonic carcinoma [26–29], as well as in material directly from human colonic carcinoma and transplantable rat and mouse colonic carcinomas [30, 31]. Much evidence supports the hypothesis that these cells are present in vivo and are not artifacts: they are observed in imprints of colonic carcinoma, they have not been seen in the many other tumors [2, 32–37] and normal tissues [3, 12] examined in our laboratory by similar techniques, and they sediment like viable cells. Dead cells sediment more slowly than viable cells [3], whereas these cytologically unusual cells are found in fractions that contain more than 99% viable cells. Even if these are degenerating cells which still behave and sediment like viable cells, they appear to be uniquely characteristic of colonic epithelial tissue in vivo and not the consequence of our laboratory procedures. While we have not observed more than 2 nuclei in semi-thin sections or sections for electron microscopy, it is unlikely that more than 2 (of 2 to 6) small particles would be included in a plane of one micron or less when one considers the geometry of a cell. Consequently, cells with multiple "micronuclei" are more likely to be evident in Cytocentrifuge preparations of whole cells than in sections of cells one micron or less in thickness.

Although we have encountered gels previously in our work with cell suspensions [3], we have encountered much more difficulty with gels in our work with colonic epithelial cells than in our work with any previously studied cell. Stern [16] used DNase to combat gel in preparations of colonic epithelial cells. As described above, repeated washings was the most effective method in our hands.

In addition to normal rat colon, epithelial cells from a wide variety of tissues have been obtained in greater than 90% purity after sedimentation in the isokinetic gradient. These include hamster pancreas [8], hamster proximal tubule [38], lactating rat mammary gland [39], hamster prostate [40], and hamster parotid gland [41]. The control of infection is possible when colonic epithelial cells are cultured after separation in a sterile isokinetic gradient. The control of infection has been a major problem in the culture of colonic tissue. Consequently, most of the work has been conducted with very short-term (24–48 hours) cultures that are probably less plagued with obvious contamination than longer-term cultures.

Corbett et al [42] have found that colonic tumors are even more difficult to transplant in syngeneic hosts than most tumors. They suggest that the primary reason for this difficulty with the primary transplantation of colonic carcinomas may be related to the fact that transplanted tissue is obtained from an area that contains numerous kinds of microorganisms. Overgrowth of the cultures with fibroblasts is another problem that appears to be eliminated by the availability of relatively pure colonic epithelial cells for the culture inoculum.

In this report we have attempted to define the problems that we encountered in our work with the dissociation and characterization of colonic epithelial tissue. While our problem with gels (DNA, colonic mucus, or other gel) was not solved to our complete satisfaction, we have included the methods that we tested in the hope that others will not have to invest as much time with this problem as we have invested. Our methods for obtaining colonic cells in suspension and for separating colonic epithelial cells from red blood cells, lymphocytes, bacteria, and debris provide a means of preparing relatively homogeneous colonic epithelial cells for in vitro studies. Similar methods can be applied to a wide variety of mammalian tissues [2, 3, 12] to obtain pure epithelial cells for culture.

SUMMARY

Pronase gave a larger number of viable epithelial cells per gram of colon than other tested agents. Proximal colon yielded fivefold more cells per gram of tissue than distal colon. Several cytologically different cells were described. Epithelial cells were separated from most bacteria and could be maintained in culture after separation in a sterile isokinetic gradient.

REFERENCES

1. Pretlow TP, Pretlow TG II: Principles of cell separation. In Karow AM, Pegg D (eds): "Organ Preservation for Transplantation," 2nd Ed. New York: Marcel Dekker Publishing Corp. (In press).
2. Pretlow TG II, Pretlow TP: Separation of indivudual kinds of cells from tumors. Contemp Top Immunobiol, vol 10. (In press).
3. Pretlow TG II, Weir EE, Zettergren JG: Problems connected with the separation of different kinds of cells. Int Rev Exp Pathol 14:91–204, 1975.
4. Stern BK, Jensen WE: Active transport of glucose by suspensions of isolated rat intestinal epithelial cells. Nature 209:789–790, 1966.
5. Hilfer SR, Brown JM: Collagenase. Its effectiveness as a dispersing agent for embryonic chick thyroid and heart. Exp Cell Res 65:246–249, 1971.
6. Pretlow TG II, Luberoff DE, Hamilton LJ, Weinberger PC, Maddox WA, Durant JR: Pathogenesis of Hodgkin's disease: Separation and culture of different kinds of cells from Hodgkin's disease in a sterile isokinetic gradient of Ficoll in tissue culture medium. Cancer 31:1120–1126, 1973.
7. Mills DM, Zucker-Franklin D: Electron microscopic study of isolated Kupffer cells. Am J Pathol 54:147–166, 1969.
8. Blackmon J, Pitts A, Pretlow TG II: Separation of lipase-positive cells from suspensions

of pancreas cells in an isokinetic gradient of Ficoll in tissue culture medium. Am J Pathol 72:417–426, 1973.

9. Moscona A: Cell suspensions from organ rudiments of chick embryos. Exp Cell Res 3:535–539, 1952.
10. Wilson JKV, Pretlow TG II, Zaremba JL, Brattain MG: Heterogeneity among preparations of crude trypsin used to disaggregate the human tonsil. Immunology 30:157–160, 1976.
11. Luna LG (ed): "Manual of Histologic Staining Methods of the Armed Forces Institute of Pathology," 3rd Ed. New York: McGraw, 1968, pp 168–169.
12. Pretlow TG II, Pretlow TP: Separation of viable cells by velocity sedimentation in an isokinetic gradient of Ficoll in tissue culture medium. In Catsimpoolas N (ed): "Biological Separations. Methods of Cell Separation." New York: Plenum Publishing Corp, 1977, vol 1, pp 171–191.
13. Pretlow TG II, Boone CW: Separation of mammalian cells using programmed gradient sedimentation. Exp Mol Pathol 11:139–152, 1969.
14. Pretlow TG: Estimation of experimental conditions that permit cell separations by velocity sedimentation on isokinetic gradients of Ficoll in tissue culture medium. Anal Biochem 41:248–255, 1971.
15. Hommes FA, Draisma MI, Molenaar I: Preparation and some properties of isolated rat liver cells. Biochim Biophys Acta 222:361–371, 1970.
16. Stern BK: Some biochemical properties of suspensions of intestinal epithelial cells. Gastroenterology 51:855–867, 1966.
17. Brattain MG, Kimball PM, Pretlow TG II, Pitts AM: Partial purification of human colonic carcinoma cells by sedimentation. Br J Cancer 35:850–857, 1977.
18. Lipkin M, Deschner E: Comparative analysis of cell renewal in the gastrointestinal tract of newborn hamster. Exp Cell Res 49:1–12, 1968.
19. Moe H: The goblet cells, Paneth cells, and basal granular cells of the epithelium of the intestine. In Felts WJL, Harrison RJ (eds): "International Review of General and Experimental Zoology." New York: Academic Press, 1968, vol 3, pp 241–287.
20. Chang WWL, Leblond CP: Renewal of the epithelium in the descending colon of the mouse. I. Presence of three cell populations: Vacuolated-columnar, mucous and argentaffin. Am J Anat 131:73–100, 1971.
21. Chang WWL, Leblond CP: Renewal of the epithelium in the descending colon of the mouse. II. Renewal of argentaffin cells. Am J Anat 131:101–110, 1971.
22. Chang WWL: Renewal of the epithelium in the descending colon of the mouse. III. Diurnal variation in the proliferative activity of epithelial cells. Am J Anat 131:111–120, 1971.
23. Eidelman S, Lagunoff D: The morphology of the normal human rectal biopsy. Hum Pathol 3:389–401, 1972.
24. Lipkin M: Proliferation and differentiation of gastrointestinal cells. Physiol Rev 53:891–915, 1973.
25. Chang WWL, Nadler NJ: Renewal of the epithelium in the descending colon of the mouse. IV. Cell population kinetics of vacuolated-columnar and mucous cells. Am J Anat 144:39–56, 1975.
26. Tompkins WAF, Watrach AM, Schmale JD, Schultz RM, Harris JA: Cultural and antigenic properties of newly established cell strains derived from adenocarcinomas of the human colon and rectum. J Natl Cancer Inst 52:1101–1110, 1974.

27. Drewinko B, Romsdahl MM, Yang LY, Adhearn MJ, Trujillo JM: Establishment of a human carcinoembryonic antigen-producing colon adenocarcinoma cell line. Cancer Res 36:467–475, 1976.
28. Leibovitz A, Stinson JC, McCombs WB III, McCoy CE, Mazur KC, Mabry ND: Classification of human colorectal adenocarcinoma cell lines. Cancer Res 36:4562–4569, 1976.
29. Tom BH, Rutzky LP, Jakstys MM, Oyasu R, Kaye CI, Kahan BD: Human colonic adenocarcinoma cells. I. Establishment and description of a new line. In Vitro 12:180–191, 1976.
30. Brattain MG, Pretlow TP, Pretlow TG II: Cell fractionation of large bowel cancer. Cancer 40:2479–2486, 1977.
31. Pretlow TP, Glover GL, Pretlow TG II: Purification of malignant cells and lymphocytes from a rat transplantable mucinous adenocarcinoma of the colon by isokinetic sedimentation in gradients of Ficoll. J Natl Cancer Inst 59:981–987, 1977.
32. Pretlow TG II, Boone CW: Separation of malignant cells from transplantable rodent tumors. Exp Mol Pathol 12:249–256, 1970.
33. Stewart MJ, Pretlow TG II, Hiramoto R: Separation of ascites myeloma cells, lymphocytes and macrophages by zonal centrifugation on an isokinetic gradient. Am J Pathol 68:163–182, 1972.
34. Zettergren JG, Luberoff DE, Pretlow TG II: Separation of lymphocytes from disaggregated mouse malignant neoplasms by sedimentation in gradients of Ficoll in tissue culture medium. J Immunol 111:836–840, 1973.
35. Helms SR, Pretlow TG II, Bueschen AJ, Lloyd KL, Murad TM: Separation of cells with histochemically demonstrable acid phosphatase activity from suspensions of cells from human prostatic carcinomas in an isokinetic gradient of Ficoll in tissue culture medium. Cancer Res 36:481–486, 1976.
36. Pretlow TG II, Jones CM, Pretlow TP: Separation of tumor cells by density gradient centrifugation: Recent work with human tumors and a discussion of the kind of quantitation needed in cell separation experiments. Biophys Chem 5:99–106, 1976.
37. Pretlow TP, Glover GL, Pretlow TG II: Separation of lymphocytes and mast cells from the Furth transplantable mast cell tumor in an isokinetic gradient of Ficoll in tissue culture medium. Cancer Res 37:578–584, 1977.
38. Pretlow TG II, Jones J, Dow S: Separation of cells having histochemically demonstrable glucose-6-phosphatase from suspensions of hamster kidney cells in an isokinetic density gradient of Ficoll in tissue culture medium. Am J Pathol 74:275–286, 1974.
39. Pretlow TG II, Dow SR, Murad TM, Jones J: Separation of acinar cells from lactating mammary gland using velocity sedimentation in an isokinetic gradient of Ficoll in tissue culture medium. Am J Pathol 76:95–106, 1974.
40. Dow SH, Pretlow TG II: Separation of cells exhibiting acid phosphatase activity from disaggregated hamster prostate cells in an isokinetic gradient of Ficoll in tissue culture medium. J Natl Cancer Inst 54:147–150, 1975.
41. Aspray DW, Pitts A, Pretlow TG II: Separation of epithelial cells from suspensions of cells from the hamster parotid gland in an isokinetic density gradient of Ficoll in tissue culture medium. Anal Biochem 66:353–364, 1975.
42. Corbett TH, Griswold DP Jr, Roberts BJ, Peckham JC, Schabel FM Jr: Tumor induction relationships in development of transplantable cancers of the colon in mice for chemotherapy assays, with a note on carcinogen structure. Cancer Res 35:2434–2439, 1975.

A New Approach for Establishment of Human Epithelial Lines: Suspension Cultures*

B. Shannon Danes, MD, PhD

In vitro studies on human epithelium have been curtailed due to a lack of human epithelial lines. Techniques to establish epithelial lines from isolated cells or sheets of cells which migrate from primary tissue explant have not produced any culture lines of normal epithelium from any human tissue.

Sluffing of epithelial cells from the surface of such epithelial sheets in primary cultures has long been recognized [1]. The purpose of this paper is to describe two methods for establishing epithelial suspension lines from such primary explant cultures.

MATERIALS AND METHODS

Method 1 – Buccal Mucosal Suspension Lines

Samples of buccal mucosal cells were obtained by cleansing the surface of the inner cheek pouch with alcohol and then scrapping this surface with a tip of a 1 ml plastic pipette. The tip of the pipette became filled with cells and tissue fragments. This plug was immediately dispersed into 2 ml of medium (reinforced Eagle's medium containing 10% (vol) fetal bovine serum and 50 μg gentamicin/ml medium) at pH 7.4. Weekly, 1 ml medium was added and the culture gassed with 100% CO_2 to maintain pH 7.4. When the total volume of the culture medium was 10 ml, the cells were removed by centrifugation (80 rpm for 5 min) and resuspended in 2 ml medium.

Method 2 – Buccal and Colonic Mucosal Suspension Lines

Biopsies (5 × 5 mm) of buccal mucosa and colonic mucosa from the ascending colon were obtained from surgical and postmortem specimens (Fig. 1). Some colonic

*Supported by a grant from the National Large Bowel Cancer Project of the National Cancer Institute Division of Cancer Research (CA 15973), and supported in part by the Danes Medical Research Fund, Cornell University Medical College, and the Zemurray Foundation.

Birth Defects: Original Article Series, Volume XVI, Number 2, pages 109–120

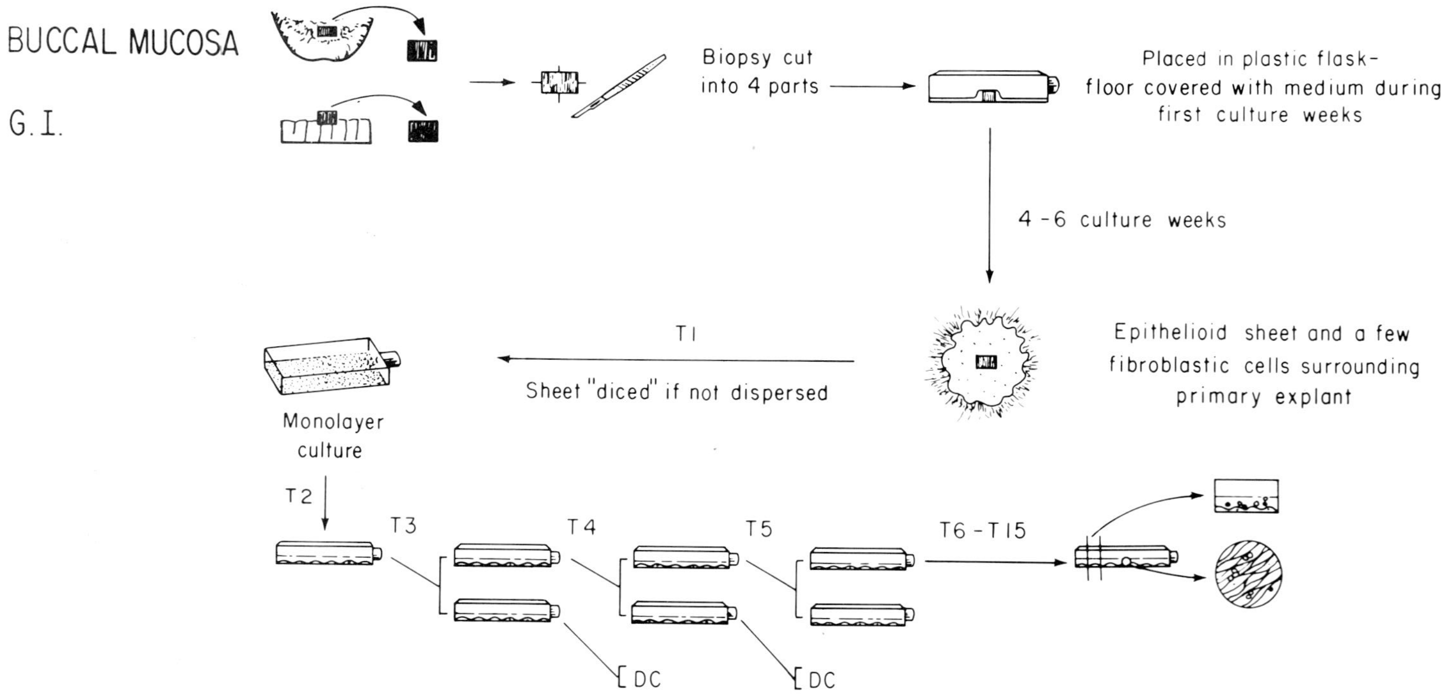

Fig. 1. Methodology used in the establishment of diploid human epithelial suspension lines from tissue biopsies of buccal mucosa and colonic mucosa.

specimens were taken during colonoscopy. All biopsies were cut into small fragments (<1 mm × 1 mm) and placed in a culture tube containing reinforced Eagle's medium with 10% (vol) fetal bovine serum, 50 μg/ml medium of gentamicin, and Fungizone, at pH 7.4 and stored at 4°C for 24–48 hours.

Primary cultures were then set up by placing 4 such tissue fragments in Falcon plastic Petri dish in Eagle's Minimum Essential Medium with 20% (vol) in a humidified atmosphere of 5% CO_2 in air [2]. To enhance the migration of epithelial cells from the tissue explant, a minimum amount of medium (approximately 1 ml) was used in the first culture weeks (just enough to cover the biopsy and floor of the culture dish). The pH of the medium was kept between 7.0 and 7.4 during the culture period. After 2 culture weeks the initial explant culture was examined microscopically to verify that both sheets of epithelial cells and fibroblasts were present in the migration zone surrounding the explant before trypsinization. Medium used in monolayer cultures was reinforced Eagle's medium containing 10% (vol) fetal bovine serum without antibiotics. The medium was completely changed every 7 days; each monolayer was split by trypsinization into 2 cultures monthly. When cells were observed in the culture medium, only half the media was removed and replaced to minimize loss and disturbance of these suspension cells.

The following analyses were done to compare in vivo and in vitro cell properties. Living cells were examined under light and phase contrast microscopy. Cells were fixed in methanol and stained with hematoxyline and eosin for microscopy. Specimens for scanning electron microscopy (EM) were prepared by critical point freeze-dry methodology [3]. Resistance to sodium dodecyl sulfate [4] was used as an index of the presence of cornified cellular envelopes seen in the keratinocyte and squame cell. Chemical assay for keratin was determined [5]. Karyotypes were analyzed [6]. These analyses were repeated at the end of the first culture year to determine any change in either morphology or differentiated function of the cultured suspension population.

Anchorage requirement was determined by plating cells in culture medium containing 1.2% methyl cellulose over a layer of 0.9% agar. To test for tumorigenicity 0.2 ml containing 10^4 cells was subcutaneously injected into a male athymic mouse (4–8-week-old BALB/c *nu/nu*); treated mice were checked weekly for tumor development over a 6-month period.

OBSERVATIONS

Cultured Epithelial Cells From Buccal Mucosal Scrappings

The buccal cells remained in suspension as either single cells or in small clumps (Fig. 2). If the pH was maintained at approximately 7.4 and the media renewed every 7 days, cell morphology remained unchanged for over 1 culture year (Fig. 3).

The suspension population was composed of one cell type (Fig. 2): a cylindric

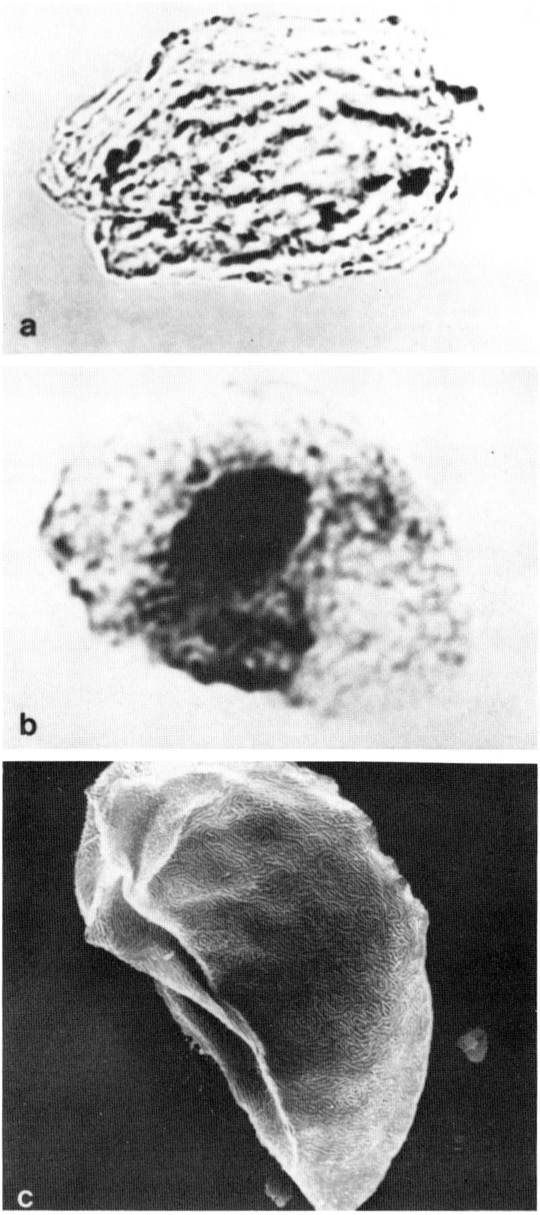

Fig. 2. Cultured keratinocytes derived from buccal mucosal scrappings grown in suspension culture for over 12 months. Single keratinocytes observed a) in the living state under light microscopy (magnification, × 1,500), b) after fixation in methanol and stained with hematoxylin (magnification, × 1,500), and c) after critical point freeze-dry preparation under the scanning EM showing surface topography (magnification, × 2,000).

cell with a single nucleus and a few cytoplasmic granules. Surface topography by scanning EM (Figs. 3 and 4) showed blebs (stubby microvilli), smooth microridges, and pore-like depressions. The blebs and microvilli were either in patches or interspersed (Figs. 3 and 4). The pore-like depressions appeared to be randomly distributed. Through the 12-month culture period there was no apparent alteration in surface topography (Figs. 2–4).

Mitoses were observed in cultures but rarely. The karyotypes examined were diploid having 46 human chromosomes.

These cells had the characteristics of epidermal cells: 1) resistance to sodium dodecyl sulfate indicating cornified layer or presence of keratin and 2) presence of keratin by chemical assay. All cells appeared to be keratinocytes, a nucleated cell containing keratin and having a low mitotic activity. Terminal differentiation of the keratinocyte to a squame, an anucleated cell containing keratin and no mitotic activity, did not occur.

Suspension Cultures From Primary Explant Cultures

Buccal mucosal cultures. In monolayer sublines established from tissue biopsies of buccal mucosa, a uniform population of round cells (Fig. 5), either single or in aggregates, was invariably seen as free-floating cells or attached loosely to the monolayer surface (freed by gentle agitation of the medium) after a variable culture period (from 1 1/2–6 months). The underlying monolayer maintained its integrity with the round cell appearing to "cycle."

The monolayer underwent senescence after 8–12 culture months. The suspension population could be subcultured without the presence of the monolayer only after several months of growth over parent monolayers.

The suspension population was composed of one cell type (Fig. 5): a round cell (average diameter 32 μm) with a single nucleus and lightly staining cytoplasm. Its cell surface (as shown by scanning EM of critical point freeze-dry preparations) had many stubby microvilli. On this basis this cell was considered to be an epidermal basal cell.

These cells had none of the characteristics of differentiated epidermal cells: There was no sign of differentiation either morphologic (evidence of keratinocytes or squames) or chemical (resistance to sodium dodecyl sulfate indicating cornified layer or presence of keratin).

They did not have the characteristics associated with cultured fibroblasts: spindle-shaped, surface topography (smooth with occasional microvilli), or dependency on surface adherence for survival. The karyotypes examined showed that the cells in suspension were diploid having 46 chromosomes.

This cell suspension population showed the morphology of an epidermal basal cell, the ability to grow without monolayer support, and an apparent unlimited life-span, but did not show growth in semisolid media nor tumor formation in athymic nude mice.

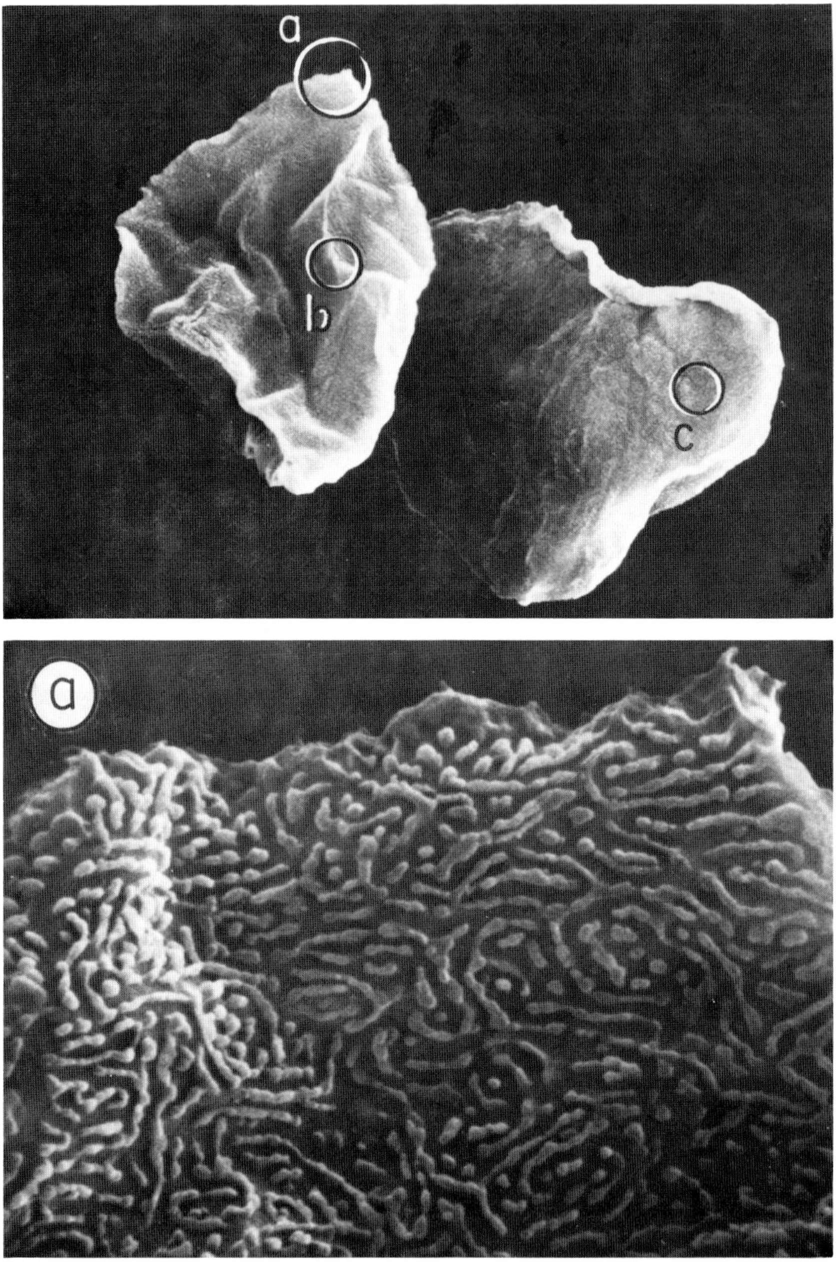

Fig. 3. A scanning EM of two human keratinocytes taken from a 3-month-old suspension culture of keratinocytes obtained from buccal mucosal scrappings from a normal 35-year-old male (magnification, × 1,500). Higher magnifications (× 10,000) of areas showing a) stubby microvilli arranged either singly or in rows, b) microvilli adjacent to one containing primarily linear smooth ridges, and c) smooth ridges in looped patterns.

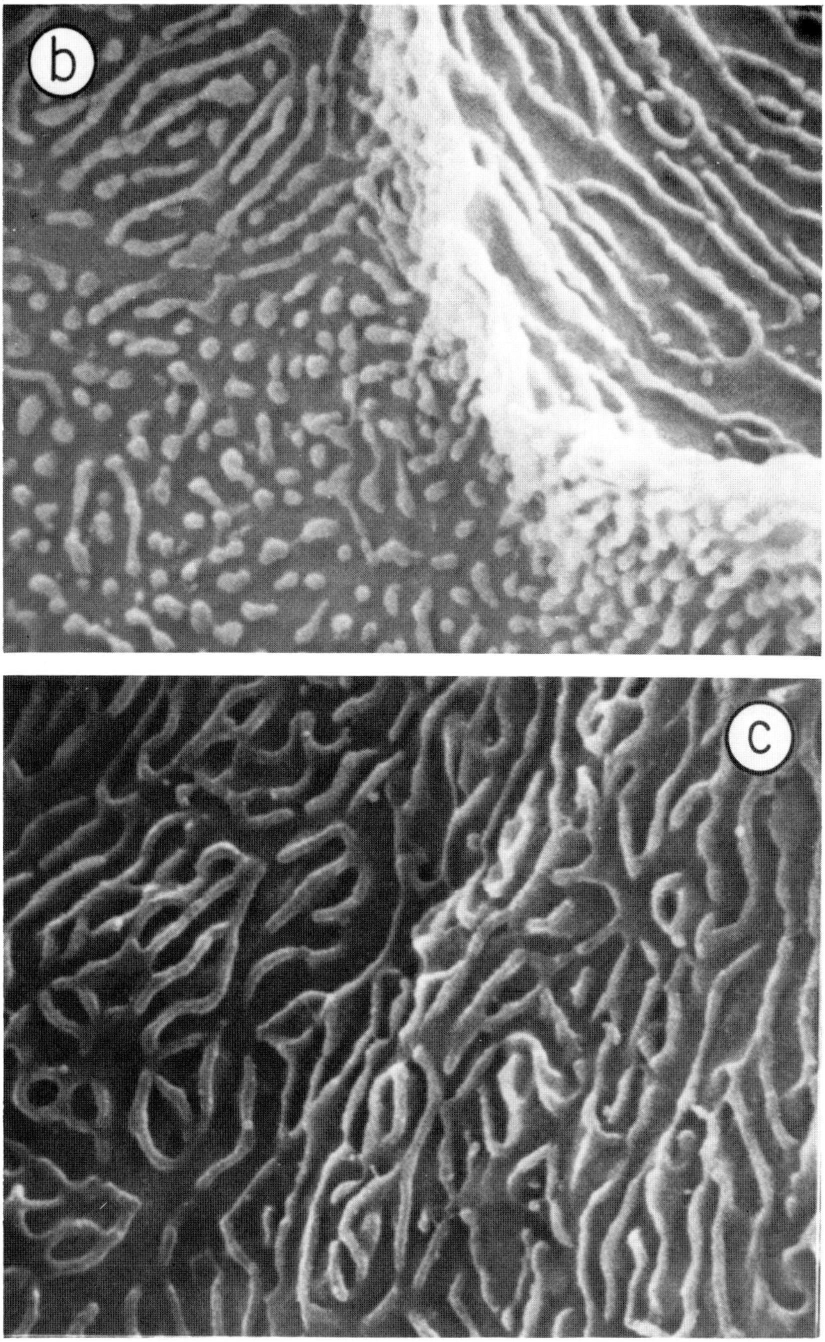
b
c

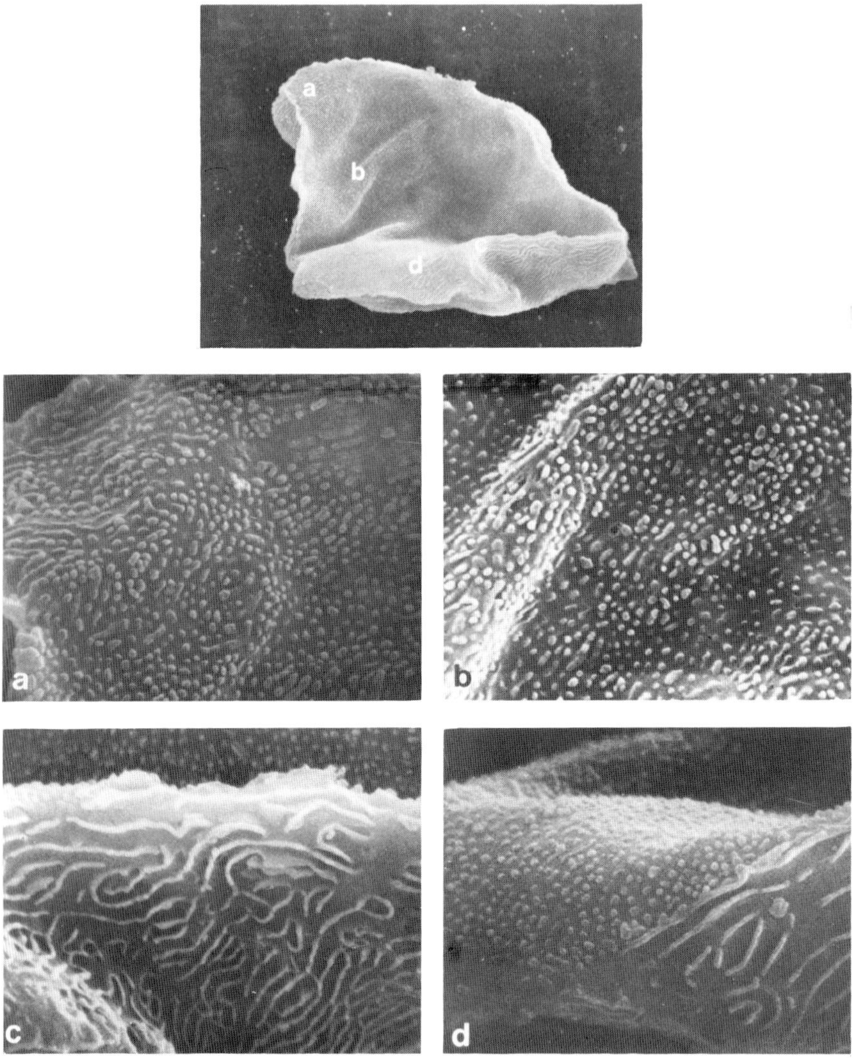

Fig. 4. A scanning EM of a single human keratinocyte taken from a 1-year-old suspension culture of keratinocytes obtained from buccal mucosal scrappings from a normal 35-year-old male (magnification, × 1,000). Higher magnifications (× 5,000) of areas showing a) blebs (stubby microvilli), b) pore-like depressions interspersed between microvilli, c) smooth microridges arranged in linear and circular patterns, and d) an area of sharp demarcation between blebs and microridges.

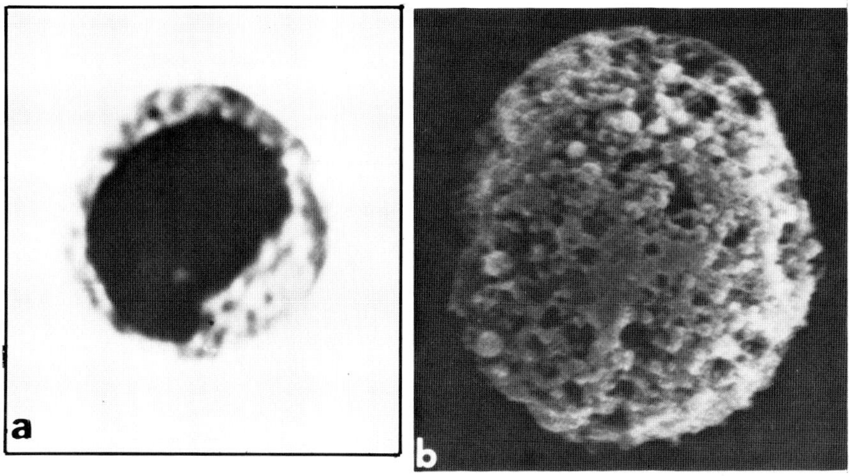

Fig. 5. Single cells from a suspension culture derived from a primary explant culture established from a biopsy of buccal mucosa from a normal 1-year-old male. A single cell observed a) after fixation in methanol and stained with hematoxylin (magnification, × 5,000) and b) after critical point freeze-dry preparation under the scanning EM showing surface topography (magnification, × 5,000).

Colonic mucosal cultures. In the primary cultures, cells were observed to constantly slough off the surface of the epithelial sheets surrounding the explant. These cells did not reattach to the culture floor but stayed in suspension. Only half of the medium was removed and renewed weekly to avoid loss of these cells. When the primary culture was trypsinized to establish monolayer cultures, the culture media containing the suspension population was centrifuged and the cell pellet introduced into the monolayer culture. Weekly, half of the media was removed and replaced allowing the suspension population to grow with minimum manipulations.

The cells in suspension were primarily in clumps of two to several cells (Fig. 6). On the basis of morphology, it was considered to be a columnar epithelial cell (Fig. 6). These cells did not grow in semisolid medium nor form tumors in athymic mice.

DISCUSSION

Research on human birth defects expressed in epithelium has been limited by the availability of either uncultured epithelial cells or derived culture lines. Pure epithelial populations have been found to be difficult to derive from tissue biopsies due to contamination with fibroblast and the inability to transfer the cells for

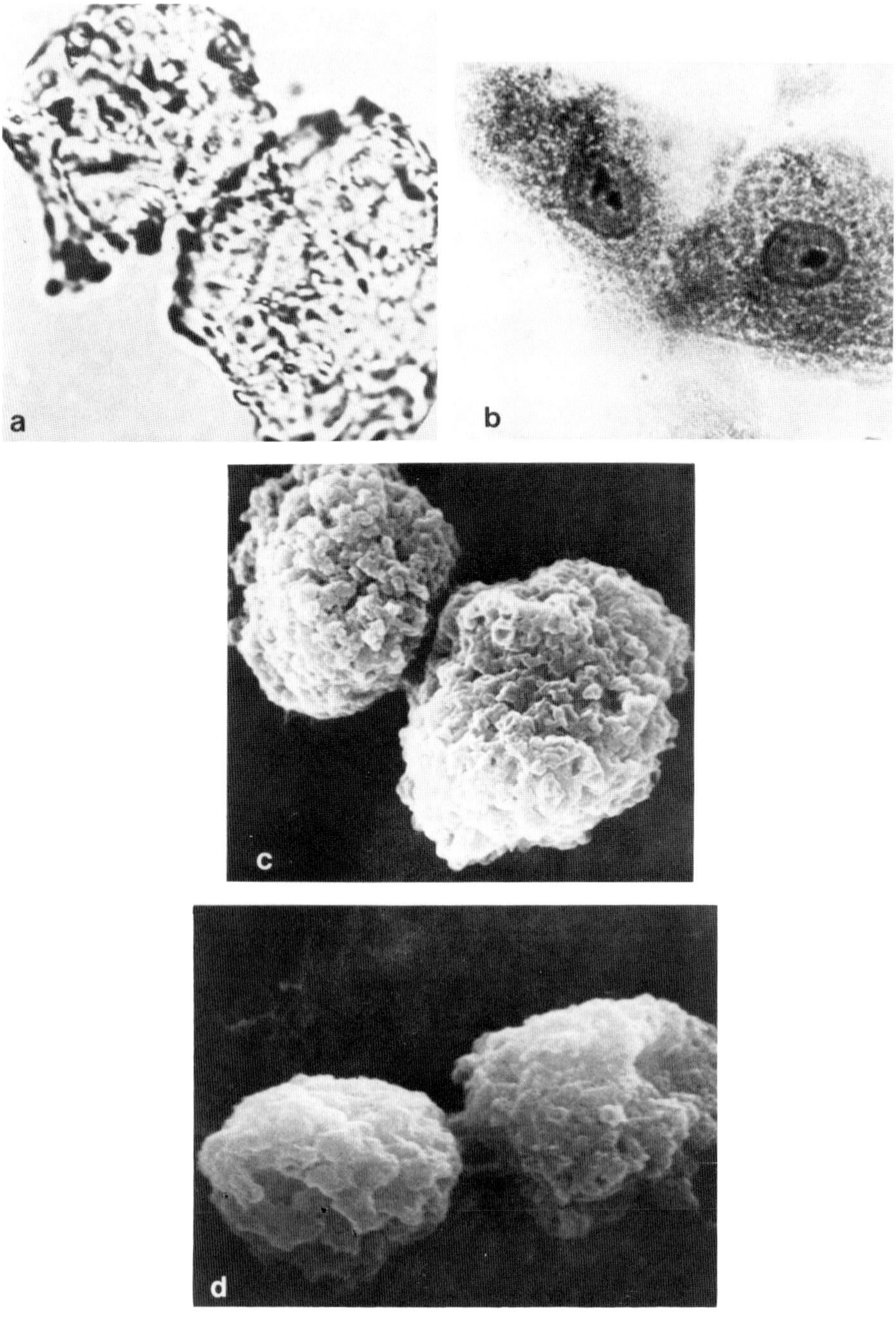
a
b
c
d

subculture. The two methods described in this paper overcome these limitations.

Scrappings of buccal mucosa are an epithelial source which has several advantages: 1) specimens could be obtained easily without any surgical procedure; 2) the primary cell samples contained no contaminating fibroblasts; 3) only one cell type, the keratinocyte, was present rather than a mixed cell population; 4) as in vivo [7] terminal differentiation of keratinocytes to squames (evidenced by loss of nucleus) did not occur (as it has been observed to occur in suspension cultures derived from epidermis [7, 8]); 5) the suspension culture was maintained over a year without evidence of cell death (low mitotic activity with a stable total cell number per culture).

A possible use of such suspension cultures of keratinocytes would be in the study of alterations in the surface topography of the plasmalemma. An example was the scanning EM study on cultured buccal mucosal cells from individuals with and without the cystic fibrosis (CF) genotype [8] which has shown differences in: 1) the organization of microridges and blebs (more orderly in the cells from individuals without the CF genotype), 2) the relative size and number of blebs (stubby microvilli), 3) the quality of the microridges (smoother and more homogeneous in cells without the CF genotype; relatively more irregular in those cells with the CF genotype), and 4) possibly the size and quantity of the pore-like depressions.

Although establishment of suspension populations from primary explant cultures took months, the lines obtained contained only one cell type: the basal cell from buccal mucosa and a columnar cell from colonic mucosa. As terminal differentiation was not observed in any of these lines, this appears to be a methodology by which cell samples of one epithelial type could be obtained for studies on human epithelial structure and/or function.

The ability to grow in suspension might have been interpreted as a phenotypic change due to a somatic mutation. It was concluded that this ability to grow in suspension was a characteristic of the epithelial cell in culture and not due to a somatic mutation because: 1) Epithelial cells were observed to sluff off the surface of the epithelial sheet as soon as the epithelial sheet appeared. This process has been long recognized and named "spillage" by Lasfargues and Ozzello [1]. 2) These cells had the morphologic characteristics recognized for each cell type in vivo. 3) The criteria for in vitro transformation due to mutation were absent – a) shift in chromosome number as the mitoses studied had normal human diploid

---

Fig. 6. Two-cell clumps from a 15-month-old suspension culture derived from a primary explant culture established from a biopsy of normal colonic mucosa from a normal 42-year-old male. Two-cell clumps observed a) in the living state under light microscopy (magnification, × 3,000), b) after fixation in methanol and stained with hematoxylin (magnification, × 2,500), and under the scanning EM c) after air-dry fixation and d) after critical point freeze-dry preparations to show surface topography (magnification, × 3,000).

karyotypes, b) tumorigenicity when injected into athymic nude mice, and c) anchorage independency (inability to grow in semisolid medium). It appeared that single cells did not have this property as no growth was obtained when single cells were cultured in semisolid medium. Although mitoses were observed in single cells in suspension, it appeared that growth occurred mainly in cell clumps adherent to the monolayer or within aggregates. Such cell-cell contacts presumably substituted for cell-substrate contacts, allowing growth to occur in such suspension populations.

The approach to establish human epithelial lines from primary explant cultures by propagating the epithelial cells which spill off the epithelial sheets that migrate from the primary explant has only been attempted for 2 tissues, buccal and colonic mucosa. As each tissue yielded a cell type which was specific for the mucosa of origin, it was presumed that application of this approach to other epithelial-containing tissue would yield epithelial-type specific lines.

ACKNOWLEDGMENTS

The author wishes to acknowledge the invaluable assistance of Erika Sutanto and Irene Tsalapatanis.

REFERENCES

1. Lasfargues EY, Ozzello L: Cultivation of human breast carcinoma. J Natl Cancer Inst 21: 1131–1147, 1958.
2. Danes BS, Bearn AG: Cystic fibrosis of the pancreas. A study in cell culture. J Exp Med 129:775–793, 1969.
3. Anderson TF: Techniques for the preservation of three-dimensional structure in preparing specimens for the electron microscope. Trans NY Acad Sci 13:130–134, 1951.
4. Sun TT, Green H: Cultured epithelial cells of cornea, conjunctiva and skin: Absence of marked intrinsic divergence of their differentiated states. Nature 269:489–493, 1977.
5. Young EG: Occurrence, classification, preparation and analysis of proteins. In Florkin M, Stotz EH (eds): "Comprehensive Biochemistry." New York: Elsevier Publishing Co, 1963, vol 7, pp 1–55.
6. Danes BS: The Gardner syndrome: Increased tetraploidy in cultured skin fibroblast. J Med Genet 13:52–56, 1976.
7. Flaxman BA, Lutzner MA, Van Scott EJ: Cell maturation and tissue organization in epithelial outgrowths from skin and buccal mucosa in vitro. J Invest Dermatol 49:322–332, 1967.
8. Danes BS, Sutanto E: Pathogenesis of cystic fibrosis: Possible importance of alteration in epithelial surface. Med Hypotheses 5:289–295, 1979.

Measurement of Epithelial Cell Adhesion During the Transition From Suspension to Stationary Culture

Ronald D. Fletcher, PhD and MaryAnn C. Labant, BS

Epithelial cell suspension cultures would provide greater quantities of cells for various enzymatic studies of birth defects. However, in most cases these cells aggregate or adhere to inanimate materials preventing adaptation to the suspended state. In an effort to determine more about the transition of cells from the suspended to the attached state, we have quantitatively measured the rate of cell adhesion.

Attramadal [1] has shown that the exclusion of Ca^{++} and Mg^{++} from Hanks' balanced salt solution resulted in rapid epithelial cell detachment from a glass substratum. We found that the gingival epithelial cells could be detached by similar methods; also, we observed these cells to grow best in the attached state. In order to simulate the transition of cells from the suspended to the attached state, cells were grown on a primary surface; they were later attached to a second surface, and debond pressures were measured. This appears to demonstrate an attachment process similar to that of suspension to the monolayer stage, yet allows quantitative measurements of cell-substratum adhesion.

This technique for measuring cell adhesion could also be applied to cellular adhesion selectivity as it relates to the role of determining or maintaining the positions of cells in organs. This adhesive selectivity was described by Buultjens and Edwards [2] using embryonic chick retina. Our technique allows for an accurate measure of cell adhesiveness and therefore should provide a more reliable indication of this selectivity.

Epithelial cells which usually form sheets or strands in the animal seem to require a solid substrate for growth unless they have undergone transformation. In an effort to understand this phenomenon better, we have experimented with a gingival epithelial cell line [3]. These cells were described as epithelial-like cells from a 19-year-old healthy white female. Evidence of their epithelial-like nature

Birth Defects: Original Article Series, Volume XVI, Number 2, pages 121–127

has been based in part on the demonstration of desmosomes [4]. These cells are characterized as having a pleomorphic nucleus; little, if any, contact inhibition; and a chromosome modal number of 57. There is good continuity between cells with good cell clarity and distinct nuclei. The passage number of these cells during the course of this study was between 980 and 1,020.

The gingival cells were plated at 250,000 cells/ml in Earle's Medium (BME) (Grand Island Biological Co., Grand Island, NY) supplemented with bovine serum (10%), penicillin (100 U/ml), streptomycin (100 μg/ml), Fungizone (25 μg/ml), and sodium bicarbonate (0.085%), at pH 7.5. The cells were incubated at 37°C in 5% CO_2 until confluent monolayers or desired cell numbers were obtained.

For comparison Flow skin and muscle cells (Flow 1000) were utilized. These fibroblasts were grown in Earle's Medium (MEM) with fetal calf serum and tested in the medium under the conditions described above. In an attempt to determine

In an attempt to determine the rate of cell attachment from the suspended state, cell counts were made of the cell suspensions at different times (0, 0.5, 1, 2, and 4 hours). The viable cell count was determined with trypan blue. Cells excluding the stain were counted and calculated as viable cells/ml. This system, cells in suspension converting to the attached state, lent itself well to cell counts but not to adhesion measurements. This was due to low adhesion levels at zero time of contact with a suitable substratum. As a result of this difficulty, cells were attached to a primary surface of polystyrene (10 × 35-mm Corning Petri dish) for 24 hours or until confluent cell monolayers were formed. These primary growing surfaces were fitted with a central aperture (the aperture was sealed with masking tape during the cell growth state), and the monolayers were then overlaid with polystyrene or with agar (Fig. 1). Incubation was continued for the indicated times before debonding was attempted. This debonding simulated the adhesion observed during the transition from the cell suspension to the attached state, as cells remained preferentially attached to the primary surface and debonded from the secondary growing surface.

Before determining the pressure required for cell-substratum debonding, the masking tape was removed from the bottom of the Petri dish and the systems (Fig. 1) were examined to be sure the aperture in the Petri plate was clear of debris. The cell monolayer-overlay systems were then debonded on the pressure-producing apparatus which included a constant volume air reservoir compressed by a uniform flow rate from a water column as described by Fletcher et al [5]. The pressure change was determined by a capacitance pressure transducer (Serta Systems, Inc., Model 204E; 0-25 psi), the output of which was measured by a strip chart recorder.

Using this technique, skin-muscle fibroblasts and gingival epithelial cells were compared. Cell monolayers were grown on a polystyrene substratum and then were overlaid with a 15-mm polystyrene disk for 0.5, 1, 2, and 4 hours before cell-substratum debonding was accomplished.

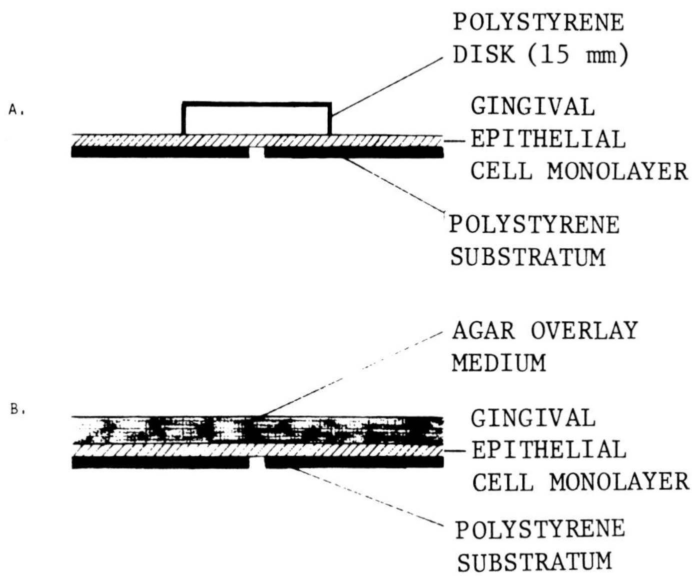

Fig. 1. Diagram of adhesion test systems. Monolayers are overlaid with A) polystyrene or B) agar.

A study was also conducted utilizing different concentrations of the epithelial cells which were grown on a polystyrene surface for 24 hours before being overlaid for an additional 24 hours with an agar growth medium. The final cell concentrations were 5.80, 12.75, 20.80, 35.75, 54.50, 90.35, and 132.00 $\times 10^3$ cells/cm^2. From this study the γa/cell was calculated.

RESULTS

In order to promote attachment, the gingival epithelial cells were tested in a complete growth medium as described. The cell suspension contained 250,000 cells/ml before exposure to the polystyrene substratum. Within 30 minutes, over 20% of the cells had attached, increasing to 50% within 1 hour (Table 1). After 4-hour incubation, only 15% of the cells remained in suspension and of these cells the majority were not recoverable in a viable state.

Transition from suspension cell culture to attached cell culture was simulated using cell monolayers on a primary substratum that was debonded from a second substratum. The cells were grown on polystyrene for 24 hours, or until confluent, and then overlaid with a polystyrene disk for 0.5, 1, 2, and 4 hours. The gingival cells showed a progressive adhesion with 40 cm H_2O required for debond at 0.5

TABLE 1. Depletion of Viable Gingival Epithelial Cells From a Suspention Culture as a Result of Attachment to a Polystyrene Substratum

Time (hr)	Viable cell count (cells/ml)	Percent attached (%)
zero	250,000	–
0.5	199,500	20.2
1.0	125,000	50.0
2.0	66,250	73.5
4.0	38,500	84.6

hour and 54 cm H_2O required at 4 hours (Fig. 2). The fibroblasts adhered more rapidly and maintained their level of adhesiveness throughout the 4-hour test. Adhesive strength (γa) was not calculated on these debond pressures due to the unavailability of moduli on the polystyrene substratum.

Cell adhesion was also measured using an agar overlay because of the availability of moduli readings [5] by which the adhesive strength (γa) could be calculated. Agar has been described as a low energy colloidal surface [6]. In this study, the γa was similar from 5,800 to 35,750 cells/cm^2 and increased with 54,500 to 132,000 cells/cm^2 (Table 2). The average γa value was 107.13 erg/cm^2 for the range of 54,500 to 132,000 cells/cm^2. The final cell concentration per cm^2 and the adhesive strength (γa) were utilized to calculate the γa/cell (Fig. 3). It can be seen that from 25 to 150 $\times$ 10^3 cells/cm^2 are required to give a relatively constant γa/cell. Cells/cm^2 of 25 $\times$ 10^3 or less gave erroneously high γa values because of background agar-substratum adhesion.

DISCUSSION

For many investigations the ideal way to grow cells is in suspension. This type of culture provides uniform conditions permitting more accurate sampling and, therefore, provides the ideal system for biochemical and kinetic studies. Most continuous cell lines can be grown in this way. However, certain primary cell cultures and epithelial cells which adhere to glass or plastic will not grow in suspension. This appears to be due, in part, to the need for a solid substrate for growth unless the cells have undergone transformation. The epithelial-like gingival cells described here grow in suspension culture if the medium is depleted of divalent cations; however, the cell concentration is only equal to or slightly less than that obtained by an equal volume grown in stationary culture. It is probably that the divalent cations, such as Ca^{++}, influence the adhesiveness of cells by a weakening of the repulsive forces of the cells [7].

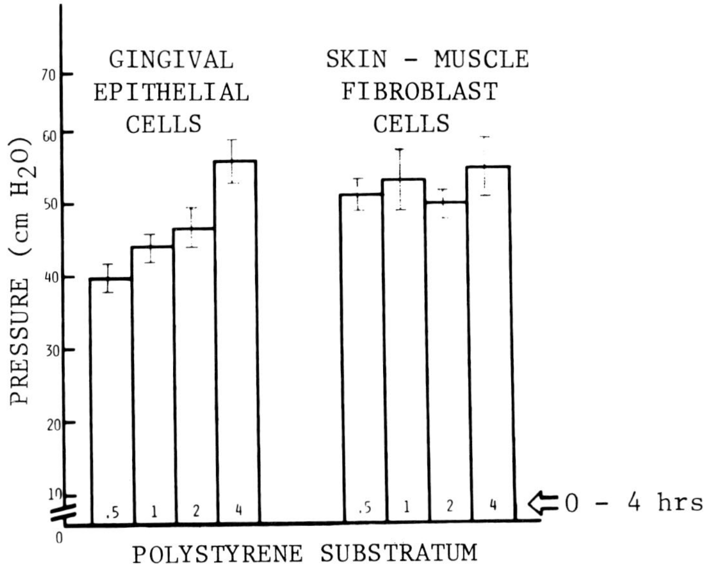

Fig. 2. The pressure (cm H_2O) of debond of gingival epithelial cells and human skin-muscle fibroblast cells from a polystyrene substratum at selected times. Standard errors were calculated on 4 experiments.

In an effort to understand better why certain cells (not transformed) grow best in the presence of a solid substratum, we developed a method to evaluate the adhesiveness of cells from the suspended state. By using this technique, it is possible to measure parameters affecting cell adhesion that can be detected before the loss of cell viability. In this regard, alteration of HeLa cell membrane architecture was observed during suspension and monolayer culturing [8]. The suspended cells were spherical and covered with microvilli, whereas the attached cells had surface blebs and large processes, but no microvilli. The gingival cells appeared to produce microvilli during the stationary phase.

Cell counts of suspension cultures demonstrated the rapid rate of adhesion for the gingival epithelial cells with 50% of the cells attaching within 1 hour. This method is not as sensitive as a measurement of the adhesive strength for determining factors that influence the maintenance of a suspended state. In growth medium these cells showed a progressive increase in the pressure required to cause a debond from polystyrene. In comparison, the fibroblast cells immediately required high pressures to debond and this level was maintained throughout the test period. It would appear that fibroblast attachment was more electrostatic by its rapid nature, whereas the gingival cells may produce a substance

TABLE 2. Measurement of Adhesive Strength (γa) as Affected by Cell Concentration (cells/cm^2) on an Agar Substratum*

Cell Concentration (cells/cm^2)	γ_a (erg/cm^2)	Standard error
5,800	69.8	± 3.2
12,750	70.9	± 7.2
20,800	69.5	± 3.6
35,750	73.2	± 3.9
54,500	93.8	± 6.6
90,350	108.5	± 8.2
132,000	119.1	± 8.9

*The cell-agar substratum contact time was 24 hours. (From Fletcher RD et al: Improvements of in vitro cell-material adhesion measurements. J Periodont Res vol 14, 1979.)

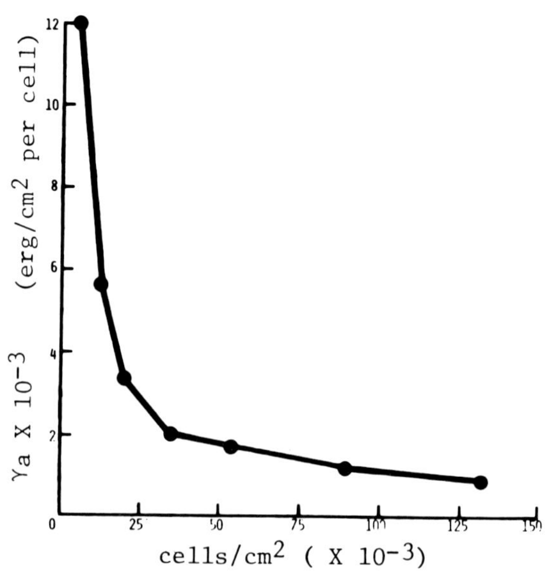

Fig. 3. The adhesive strength (γa) per cell as indicated by the total cell concentration per cm^2.

that is necessary before firm attachment. This may be similar to the cell spreading factor described by Grinnell [9] and also reported to be produced by certain other cells [10].

Cell adhesion to agar allowed for longer incubation periods due to the replenishment of nutrients by the agar growth medium and the dilution of waste products. Because of the longer incubation period, greater adhesion was observed. By plating different cell concentrations, it was observed that a critical number of cells ($\geq 54.5 \times 10^3$ cells/cm^2) was necessary before maximum cell attachment to the agar overlay. The γa/cell also indicated the need for these cell concentrations to demonstrate reliable adhesive strength values calculated on an individual cell basis. This might indicate that in a suspension culture high concentrations of these gingival epithelial cells favor adhesiveness. By constantly removing cells and adding fresh medium it may be possible to produce larger cell yields in suspension culture.

SUMMARY

In order to better understand why epithelial cells prefer to grow in the attached state, the adhesiveness of a continuous gingival cell line was measured. Based on cell counts, 50% of the cells in suspension attached to a suitable substratum within 1 hour. Simulation of this process (suspension to attached cells) with 2 growth surfaces allowed adhesion measurements. Gingival epithelial cells showed progressive adhesion with time and appeared dependent on a critical cell concentration for uniform adhesive strength (γ_a) measurements/cell.

REFERENCES

1. Attramadal A: The effect of divalent cations on cell adhesion. J Periodont Res 4: 281–285, 1969.
2. Buultjens TEJ, Edwards JG: Adhesive selectivity is exhibited in vitro by cells from adjacent tissues of the embryonic chick retina. J Cell Sci 23:101–116, 1977.
3. Smulow JB, Glickman I: An epithelial-like cell line in continuous culture from normal adult human gingiva. Proc Soc Exp Biol Med 121:1294–1296, 1966.
4. Fletcher RD, Shoemaker R, Albertson JN Jr: Desmosomes observed in a gingival cell line. J Dent Res 56:1106, 1977.
5. Fletcher RD, Breitling SM, Adamiak JK, Williams ML Jr: Measurement of the adhesive strength of a gingival cell line to agar. In Vitro 13:857–860, 1977.
6. Grinnell F, Milam M, Srere PA: Studies on cell adhesion. Arch Biochem Biophys 153: 193–198, 1977.
7. Deman JJ, Bruyneel A: A correlation between the effects of calcium on intercellular adhesion and electrostatic repulsion between cells. Arch Int Physiol Biochim 85:117–124, 1977.
8. Springer EL, Hackett AJ, Nelson-Rees WA: Alteration of the cell membrane architecture during suspension and monolayer culturing. Int J Cancer 17:407–415, 1976.
9. Grinnell F: Cell spreading factor. Exp Cell Res 102:51–62, 1976.
10. Moore EG: Cell to substratum adhesion-promoting activity released by normal and virus-transformed cells in culture. J Cell Biol 70:634–647, 1976.

Morphologic and Biosynthetic Modulations of HeLa Cells Mediated by Sodium Butyrate*

Robert J. Fallon, BS, MS,† Nimai K. Ghosh, PhD, FRIC, and Rody P. Cox, MD

INTRODUCTION

The focus of this volume is the cultivation of differentiated cells of epithelial origin. The presentations clearly indicate that it is now possible to culture epithelial cells from a variety of normal tissues. These cells retain their characteristic phenotypes and provide model systems for investigating gene expression and differentiated function. A complementary approach to understanding regulation of gene expression and perhaps the development of the differentiated phenotype is to induce morphologic and biosynthetic modulation in tumor cells derived from epithelium. HeLa cells [1] derived over 25 years ago from a human cervical carcinoma, have been used for our initial investigations since these cells have been intensively studied both at the cellular and molecular level by many investigators and more is known about their fundamental biology than is known of most other cell types. Our laboratory has found that HeLa cells produce several polypeptides that are normally synthesized only in trophoblastic cells. These include the placental or fetal form of alkaline phosphatase [2, 3] and human chorionic gonadotropin [4, 5]. Recently, we have found that gonadotropic hormones previously believed to be normally produced exclusively in pituitary cells, for example follicle-stimulating hormone [6] and luteinizing hormone [7] are also synthesized in HeLa cells. The production of fetal proteins and glycopeptide hormones is markedly increased by certain aliphatic monocarboxylates and by agents that block DNA synthesis and cell multiplication at specific sites of the cell cycle [5, 8]. More-

*Supported by grant GM26072 from the NIH and by the Samuel A. Berger Foundation.
†Medical Scientist Trainee (5 T32 GMO 7308).

Birth Defects: Original Article Series, Volume XVI, Number 2, pages 129–143

over, the biosynthetic "differentiation" induced in HeLa cells by sodium butyrate is accompanied by morphologic alterations at the ultrastructural level in which structures (tonofilaments and desmosomes) that are associated with epithelial cells appear [9].

ULTRASTRUCTURAL MODULATIONS OF HeLa CELLS MEDIATED BY SODIUM BUTYRATE

HeLa cells grown with sodium butyrate (1 mM) exhibit a striking increase in the number of microfilaments that are arranged in conspicuous bundles, similar to bundles of tonofilaments that are observed in squamous epithelium [9]. Moreover, HeLa cells grown in the presence of sodium butyrate demonstrate well-developed desmosomes in contrast to HeLa cells grown in medium without monocarboxylate in which the intercellular attachment zones show merely a thickening of the plasma membrane [9]. These findings are of considerable interest in view of the controversy over whether HeLa cells were derived from a squamous cell carcinoma as originally proposed by Gey et al [1], or whether the tumor was an adenocarcinoma, as a recent review of the initial biopsy specimen suggested [10]. The appearance of well-developed tonofilaments and desmosomes in HeLa cells grown with sodium butyrate strongly supports a squamous epithelial derivation of HeLa cells.

PRODUCTION OF ONCOFETAL PROTEINS BY HeLa CELLS

The inappropriate production by neoplasms of specialized proteins and polypeptides that are normally produced by differentiated cells from another germ line or at a particular stage of embryonic development, provides a useful model for investigating the control of gene activity and for possibly understanding the expression of the differentiated phenotype. HeLa cells grown with sodium butyrate have the morphologic characteristics of epithelial cells. The enzymatic and biosynthetic properties of HeLa cells are remarkably similar to human trophoblasts. The alkaline phosphatase present in many strains of HeLa cells is nearly identical to the fetal form of the enzyme found in trophoblasts of the human placenta [2, 3]. Placental alkaline phosphatase is a polymorphic protein whose phenotype is determined by a single genetic locus of the fetus. There are multiple alleles at this locus that alter the electrophoretic mobility of placental alkaline phosphatase [11]. HeLa cells appear heterozygous for 2 of these alleles, F which determines a fast moving isozyme and S which determines a slow component [2]. The electrophoretic mobilities of the HeLa isozymes are slightly different from the authentic placental variants. These slight differences may reflect altered post-translational modifications which are often observed when peptides from tumors are compared to their normal counterparts. Immunologic studies also show that the HeLa and placental alkaline phosphatases are very similar though probably not identical [2, 3].

Other fetal proteins are also produced by HeLa cells. Richter [12] has shown that ferritin synthesis can be induced in HeLa cells by adding iron to the medium. The apoferritin induced by iron resembles the placental form of the protein [13]. HeLa cells exclusively synthesize the A form of aldolase similar to that found in placenta, while human fibroblasts in culture have a mixture of the A, B, and perhaps the C forms of this enzyme [14]. The ectopic synthesis by HeLa cells of several fetal forms of proteins normally produced in placental trophoblasts suggested that perhaps HeLa cells might produce or might be induced to synthesize other proteins characteristic of this specialized epithelial cell.

INDUCTION OF HUMAN CHORIONIC GONADOTROPIN (HCG) SYNTHESIS IN ASYNCHRONOUS HeLa CELL CULTURES

One of the earliest proteins synthesized by the trophoblast is HCG. This glycopeptide hormone is believed to play a role in implantation of the zygote [15] and perhaps in altering the maternal immune response so as to accept the fetal allograft [16]. Initial attempts to detect HCG in a strain of HeLa cells ($HeLa_{65}$) had equivocal results. We carried out a series of studies aimed at activating this fetal locus. Cortisol, other hormones, and cyclic AMP did not affect HCG synthesis. However, as a control for experiments utilizing dibutyryl cyclic AMP, butyric acid was added to replicate cultures. This aliphatic monocarboxylate was found to produce a coordinate effect on HeLa cells, causing reduced cell multiplication, morphologic alterations, increased activity of the fetal form of alkaline phosphatase [9, 17, 18] and 5′-nucleotidase [9], and the increased production of several glycopeptide hormones including HCG [4–7]. This finding is of additional importance because butyrate is not only a normal metabolic substrate but it is commonly used as a food additive for its antimicrobial properties.

Figure 1 shows the effects of increasing concentrations of butyrate on HCG production in HeLa cells [4]. Approximately 90–95% of the hormone synthesized is secreted into the medium. HCG is composed of 2 dissimilar subunits, an α–chain that is common to glycopeptide hormones – follicle-stimulating hormone (FSH), luteinizing hormone (LH), thyroid-stimulating hormone (TSH), and HCG – and a unique β-subunit for each hormone that confers biologic specificity [19, 20]. In this and subsequent studies, HCG was measured by radioimmunoassay (RIA) using antiserum against the purified β-chain of HCG [21]. Figure 2 shows the kinetics of induction of HCG synthesis by 1 mM sodium butyrate in asynchronous HeLa cell cultures. Cells grown without butyrate (control) 18 hours after subculture produce relatively high levels of HCG. As they enter the exponential

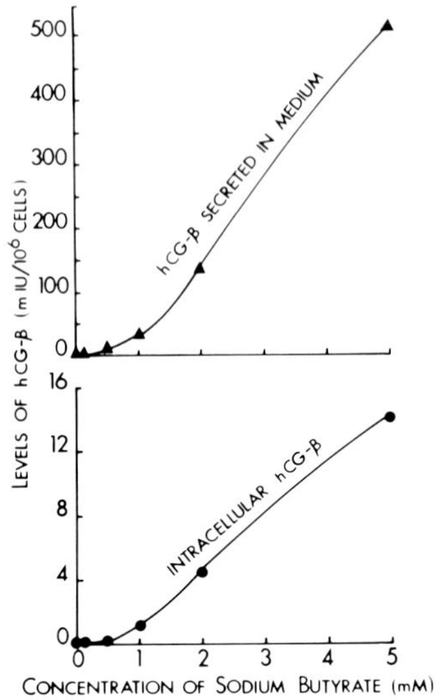

Fig. 1. Production of HCG-β by $HeLa_{65}$ cells grown for 120 hours in the presence of different concentrations of sodium butyrate. HCG-β was determined by RIA using polyethylene glycol as a precipitant for ^{125}I-labeled antigen-antibody complex. (From Ghosh NK, Cox RP: Production of human chorionic gonadotropin in HeLa cell cultures. Nature 259:416–417, 1976, with permission.)

growth phase the synthesis of HCG declines and later increases as the cultures become confluent at 120 hours. In contrast to controls, HeLa cells grown with 1 mM sodium butyrate maintain HCG synthesis for the first 48 hours (Fig. 2) and then show a marked increase in synthesis. Addition of cycloheximide, an inhibitor of protein synthesis, to culture medium at 48 hours inhibits the further increase in HCG induced by butyrate (Fig. 2).

The structural requirements for aliphatic monocarboxylate induction of HCG are quite stringent as shown in Figure 3. The C_4 butyrate is most effective but propionate (C_3), pentanoate (C_5), and hexanoate (C_6) also increase HCG synthesis but with lesser potency. Other alterations of butyrate by conversion into a branched chain or substitution of the methyl groups markedly decrease HCG induction relative to n-butyrate [5]. The addition of a terminal amino group, the introduction of a double bond, or hydroxyl group on any of the carbon atoms abolishes the capacity of butyrate to mediate increased HCG synthesis, further emphasizing the structural specificity of the "inducer" [5].

The mechanism by which aliphatic monocarboxylates modulate HCG synthesis in HeLa cells is not known although the extent of induction was correlated with their inhibition of HeLa cell multiplication. However, inhibition of cell replica-

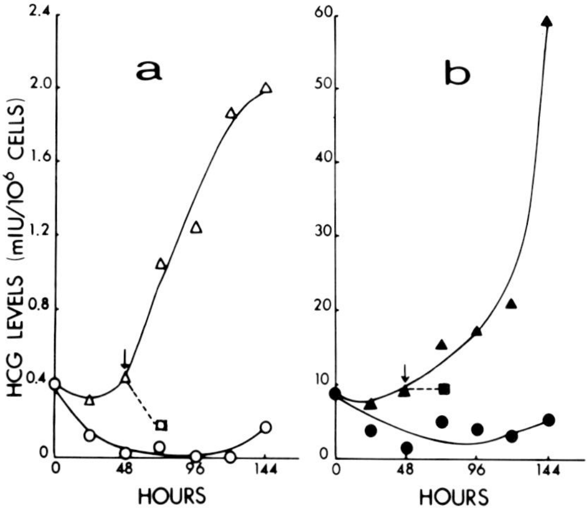

Fig. 2. Kinetics of choriogonadotropin induction by sodium butyrate and its inhibition by cycloheximide. HCG was measured by RIA using antiserum directed against the β-chain. a) Intracellular choriogonadotropin concentrations (mIU/10^6 cells): ○ – cells grown without butyrate (controls); △ – cells grown with 1 mM sodium butyrate; □ – cells grown with 1 mM sodium butyrate for 48 hours and 1 μg cycloheximide/ml for the subsequent 24 hours. The arrow indicates the time of addition of cycloheximide. b) Extracellular choriogonadotropin concentrations (mIU/10^6 cells): ● – secreted into medium by cells grown without butyrate (controls); ▲ – secreted into medium by cells grown with 1mM sodium butyrate; ■ – secreted into medium by cells grown with 1 mM sodium butyrate for 48 hours and 1 μg cycloheximide/ml for the next 24 hours. The arrow shows the time of cycloheximide addition. Choriogonadotropin concentrations were measured by the poly(ethylene glycol) method, by using the latter in place of anti-(γ-globulin) antibody as a precipitant for ^{125}I-labeled antigen-antibody complexes. Poly (ethylene glycol), antiserum against choriogonadotropin-β-subunit, and other materials for RIA of choriogonadotropin were purchased from Serono Laboratories, Boston, MA, USA. (Figs. 2, 3, and 5 from Ghosh NK, Rukenstein A, Cox RP: Induction of human choriogonadotropin in HeLa-cell cultures by aliphatic monocarboxylates and inhibitors of deoxyribonucleic acid synthesis. Biochem J 166:265–274, 1977, with permission.)

tion alone does not promote HCG synthesis. For example, heptanoate (C_7) and octanoate (C_8) inhibit HeLa cell multiplication more than butyrate does, and dimethyl sulfoxide (an inducer of hemoglobin synthesis in Friend leukemia cells) is a potent inhibitor of growth, but none of these compounds significantly induce HCG production. These findings, together with the data on the kinetics of induction (Fig. 2), suggest that cell cycle events may be important in the modulation of ectopic hormone synthesis in HeLa cells. One possibility is that butyrate and other inducers of HCG synthesis may act by focusing the cell populations at a particular site in the cell cycle where this genetic locus is available for transcription.

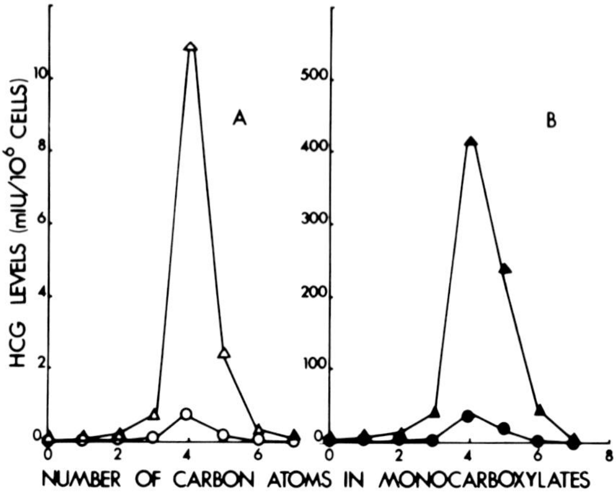

Fig. 3. HCG induction by aliphatic monocarboxylates of different chain length. HCG was measured by RIA using antiserum directed against the β-chain. A) Intracellular HCG concentrations induced by 1 mM (○) and 5 mM (△) monocarboxylates; B) extracellular concentrations of HCG secreted into media in response to 1 mM and 5 mM monocarboxylates.

INDUCTION OF HCG IN SYNCHRONOUS HeLa CELL CULTURES

The extended lag phase of 20–30 hours after adding butyrate to asynchronous HeLa cell cultures before an increase in HCG production is observed, supports the view that cell cycle events may be involved in the induction process. Figure 4 compares the effects of adding sodium butyrate to asynchronous HeLa cell cultures (cells distributed in all phases of the cell cycle) and to HeLa cell cultures synchronized by a double thymidine block [22]. At time zero the synchronized cells were released from the thymidine block. At this time the cell population was focused at the beginning of S phase. Twelve hours after release, when cells were in late G_2 or M phases, 5 mM butyrate was added to half of the replicate synchronized cultures (see Fig. 4, solid triangles). The remainder served as controls (solid circles). At the same time butyrate was added to replicate asynchronous cultures (open triangles), with HeLa cultures without butyrate as controls (open circles). HCG production during the first 10 hours of butyrate exposure appears slightly greater in synchronized cultures than in the asynchronous (Fig. 4). However, the striking finding is the marked acceleration of the induction process after this time in the synchronized cell population treated with butyrate. Parallel experiments exploring the effect of adding butyrate immediately after release from double thymidine block showed no acceleration in the induction process relative to random cultures. This and the data in Figure 4 indicate that 12 hours after release from thymidine synchronization, cells may be entering a phase of the cell cycle (G_1) required for HCG induction. These studies suggest that cell cycle location may be important in determining the availability of the HCG loci for transcription.

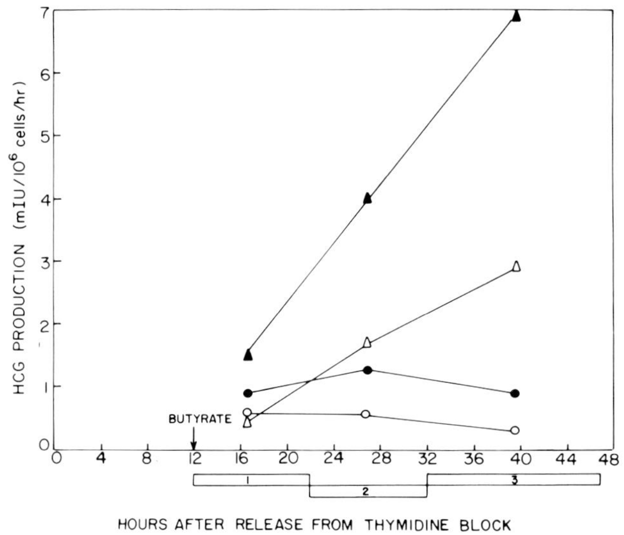

Fig. 4. Induction of HCG synthesis by butyrate in synchronous and asynchronous HeLa cultures. Replicate cultures of HeLa cells were synchronized by double thymidine block. At zero time the thymidine was removed and cells were grown for 12 hours in medium without inhibitor. At that time 5 mM butyrate was added to half the cultures, the remainder served as control. Replicate asynchronous cultures were fed with fresh medium at time zero and butyrate 5 mM was added 12 hours later to half the cultures. The remainder served as controls. The hormone collection periods are indicated by the numbered boxes below the abscissa. Synchronous control (no additions) ●——●; synchronous butyrate-treated (t = 12) ▲——▲; asynchronous control (no additions) ○——○; asynchronous butyrate-treated (t = 12) △——△.

CELL CYCLE ANALYSIS OF SODIUM BUTYRATE In HeLa CULTURES

The investigation of the effects of sodium butyrate on cell cycle events was carried out using both dynamic studies with a variety of thymidine labeling and mitotic arrest techniques, as well as static cell cycle analytic methods, such as flow microfluorometry [8]. Butyrate was compared to a well-characterized inhibitor, hydroxyurea, by the above methods. Forty-eight hours of exposure to sodium butyrate or hydroxyurea was chosen since kinetic studies of HCG induction in asynchronous HeLa cells had indicated that this is the time that hormone synthesis rates are 20- to 50-fold greater than control. Cells in early G_1, G_2, or M phase at the time of addition of either butyrate or hydroxyurea were not arrested at early time points, but by 48 hours they accumulated at a location characteristic for each drug: the G_1-S phase boundary for butyrate and early S phase for hydroxyurea. Both inhibitors prevented cells originally in S phase from reaching mitosis. S cells exposed to hydroxyurea were killed by 48 hours, but those grown with 5 mM butyrate progressed to G_2 phase where they became irreversibly arrested although not removed from the monolayer. Flow microfluorometry was used to determine the position of individual cells in the cell cycle. This technique shows the distribution of DNA content of individual cells by measuring the fluorescence emitted after laser stimulation of nuclei stained with the DNA-binding agent propidium iodide [23]. Asynchronous control cell population showed a major peak in G_1, a shoulder of cells distributed through the S phase, and a second smaller peak in G_2. Hydroxyurea-inhibited cells had accumulated in early S phase, indicating that initiation of DNA synthesis occurred but that progression through the S phase was markedly inhibited in agreement with prior work on this inhibitor [24]. Cells grown with 5 mM butyrate behaved in a different manner. At 48 hours the proportion of G_1 cells was increased and there was a marked decrease in S phase cells, but the G_2 peak was increased relative to control [8]. Although both hydroxyurea and sodium butyrate are effective inhibitors of DNA synthesis in HeLa cells [5, 25], and both decrease cell proliferation to a similar extent [8], they produce different cell cycle distributions as shown by flow microfluorometry analysis. Further studies using progression-dependent methods of cell cycle analysis showed that following release from inhibition by either sodium butyrate or hydroxyurea, the cell population initiates DNA synthesis and progresses as a synchronous population through S and G_2 phases entering mitosis approximately 12–14 hours after release from inhibition [8]. The G_2 population in butyrate-treated cultures is irreversibly inhibited and does not reenter the cell cycle. Thus, both butyrate and hydroxyurea block cell cycle progression of HeLa cell cultures and focus the majority of the population near the G_1-S boundary This similarity in cell cycle position suggests that if cell cycle-dependent events are involved in mediating glycopeptide hormone synthesis, hydroxyurea should also increase HCG production. Figure 5 shows that hydroxyurea does increase HCG synthesis by HeLa cultures. Moreover, the concentrations of hydroxyurea that were ineffective by themselves in promoting HCG production are potentiated by sodium butyrate [5]. The increased HCG induction seen when inducers are added together (Fig. 5) appears to by synergistic. This is confirmed by the data shown in Table 1. In this experiment concentrations of hydroxyurea alone, butyrate alone, and both drugs together that inhibited cell multiplication to approximately the same extent were studied with respect to the level of induction of HCG. As shown in Table 1 sodium butyrate is more effective as an inducer than hydroxyurea. However when both drugs are used together, the production of HCG is markedly increased suggesting complementary interactions of these agents. Two other inhibitors of DNA synthesis, methotrexate and 1-β-D-arabinofuranosylcytosine, that also focus cell populations at the G_1-S boundary, also mediate increased HCG synthesis in HeLa cell cultures [5]. In contrast, conditions of cell culture such as serum deprivation and isoleucine-deficient medium focus HeLa cells in *early* G_1 but do not mediate increased HCG synthesis [26]. HeLa cells collected in M phase by colcemide show a slight increase in the intracellular HCG level but a concordant decrease in extracellular hormone level [27]. This finding suggests

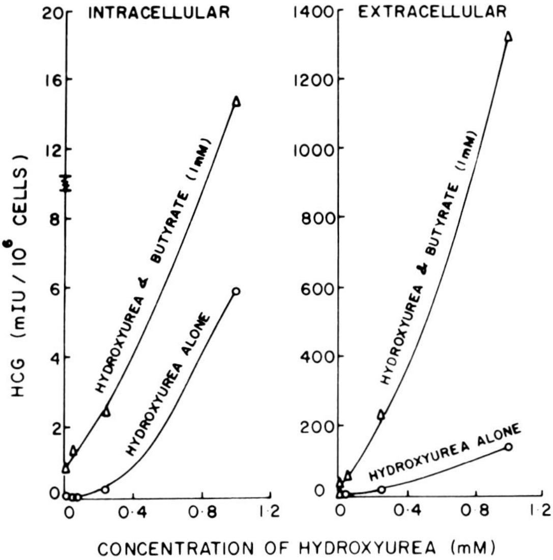

Fig. 5. Induction of HCG by hydroxyurea and its synergism with sodium butyrate. HCG was measured by RIA using antiserum directed against the β-subunit. Cells grown with different concentrations of hydroxyurea for 96 hours (○); cells grown with different concentrations of hydroxyurea and 1 mM sodium butyrate for 96 hours (△).

TABLE 1. Synergism of Butyrate and Hydroxyurea in Mediating HCG Synthesis in HeLa Cells*

Additions to medium	Percent inhibition of cell multiplication	HCG production *mIU* / 10^6 cells
None (control)	–	13.8
Hydroxyurea 0.6 mM	87.2	122.2
Butyrate 2.0 mM	84.8	482.3
Hydroxyurea 0.5 mM and Butyrate 1.0 mM	90.6	707.5

*Cultures were grown for 72 hours in medium. Methods for assaying HCG using antiserum against the β-subunit have been described [4, 5].

that microtubular integrity is needed for hormone secretion but that hormone production is not altered in cells arrested in the M phase of the cell cycle [27]. Thus, the findings presented implicate the late G_1-early S sites as being the critical phases of the cell cycle for increased production of HCG.

Lieblich and his associates at the NIH independently have found that several HeLa cell clonal lines secrete free α-chain for glycopeptide hormones [28]. Therefore, HeLa cells exhibit an unbalanced synthesis of α- and β-chains of glycopeptide hormones. Tumors that ectopically synthesize glycopeptide tropic hormones often show a loss of regulatory constraints with respect to balancing α- and β-chain synthesis [29]. Moreover in tumors and in HeLa cells the post-translational processing of α-chains may be defective since the apparent molecular weight of the α–chain is slightly larger than the normal subunit [28].

In conjunction with Dr. Lieblich and his associates we have investigated the effects of sodium butyrate in several HeLa clones. These lines secrete relatively large amounts of free α-chain and small amounts of complete HCG constitutively. When grown with sodium butyrate both α-chain and complete HCG production were markedly increased [30]. An HCG-producing cell line derived from a primary carcinoma of the lung also demonstrated marked butyrate stimulation of hormone production indicating the potential of this reagent in the study of biosynthetic mechanisms.

EFFECT OF BUTYRATE ON SYNTHESIS OF OTHER GLYCOPEPTIDE HORMONES BY HeLa CELLS

Tumors derived from a variety of tissues ectopically produce many different peptide hormones and fetal proteins depending upon the tissue of origin and the degree of differentiation [31]. A notable exception is the synthesis of pituitary glycopeptide hormones (FSH and LH) by *nonpituitary* tumors. Only one patient has been reported in which a bronchogenic carcinoma produced FSH and LH [32]. Investigation of the possible induction of these glycopeptides by butyrate in HeLa cells led to the unexpected finding that both FSH and LH synthesis were markedly stimulated. These findings necessitated a careful validation of the RIAs in view of the known production of α-subunits and HCG by HeLa cells. Two different antisera were used to measure FSH levels; one was prepared against highly purified human pituitary β-subunit of FSH and the other against the complete hormone. The anti-β-FSH serum was quite sensitive and highly specific with less than 1% cross-reactivity with HCG (see legend to Table 2). The second antiserum prepared against intact human pituitary FSH was less sensitive than the antiserum against the β-subunit but it also was highly specific (see legend to Table 2). Table 2 shows that 2 well-characterized clonal lines of HeLa cells, $HeLa_{65}$ and $HeLa_{71}$ [33], produce different constitutive levels of FSH. Similar differences between HeLa sublines have been observed with alkaline phosphatase activity [34], α-chain [28, 30], and HCG [4, 5] synthesis, and may reflect functional alterations related to the well-known karyotypic differences between these sublines. Growth of HeLa cells with 1 mM and 5 mM sodium butyrate causes a marked increase in FSH production, as shown in Table 2. Hydroxyurea also increases FSH synthesis [6].

The production of a putative pituitary hormone, FSH, by a human cervical tumor cell in culture is unexpected. We have recently found FSH-immunoreactive material in perfusates of human placenta [35, 36]. It seems likely that placenta may synthesize glycopeptide tropic hormones that previously have been assumed to be exclusively of pituitary origin.

Measurement of LH production by RIA is complicated by considerable cross-reaction between HCG and antisera against LH. Recently, antiserum against the β-subunit of LH has been prepared that has the following cross-reactivities: LH 100%; HCG < 1%; FSH 1.5%; and TSH 5%. Using this antiserum $HeLa_{65}$ cells were found to produce constitutively 1.6 mIU/10^6 cells per day. When grown for 72 hours in medium with 5 mM sodium butyrate the levels of LH were increased to 71.2 mIU/10^6 cells per day [7].

Hydroxyurea also mediated an increase in LH synthesis in HeLa cells. The production of a second putative pituitary hormone by HeLa cells and the enhanced synthesis induced by butyrate and hydroxyurea provides evidence for the coordinate effects of these compounds. TSH and human placental lactogen (HPL) could not be detected by RIAs of medium from these HeLa sublines nor could the synthesis of these glycopeptide hormones by induced by growth with sodium butyrate or hydroxyurea.

SPECULATION ON THE MECHANISM OF BUTYRATE-MEDIATED MODULATION OF GENE EXPRESSION

HeLa cells grown in medium with sodium butyrate show both morphologic and biosynthetic alterations. Cells develop ultrastructural characteristics of squamous cells with the formation of tonofilaments and desmosomes. Accompanying this morphologic "differentiation" HeLa cells synthesize increased amounts of glycopeptide hormones (HCG, FSH, and LH) and show an increase in the activity of the fetal form of alkaline phosphatase [18], 5′-nucleotidase [9], and sialyl transferase 1 [37]. The coordinate action of sodium butyrate in mediating these diverse effects suggests that this compound is affecting the availability of many genetic loci for transcription. The mechanism(s) of these effects is not known. Riggs and associates have shown that HeLa cells grown with butyrate have a rapid increase in acetylation of histones particularly the H3 and H4 subgroups [38]. The increased acetylation of histones is apparently due to inhibition of the enzyme histone deacetylase by sodium butyrate [39]. Modification of histones by acetylation would be expected to affect chromatin folding and tertiary structure; this might be associated with increased availability of certain genetic loci for transcription.

Our findings have demonstrated that several other drugs which inhibit DNA synthesis and focus cell populations at the G_1-S transition point of the cell cycle are capable of inducing glycopeptide hormone synthesis and enhancing activity

TABLE 2. Enhancement of FSH Production by Butyrate in HeLa Cells

Subline	β-Subunit of FSH antiserum: FSH (ng) secreted* by 10^6 cells			Complete FSH antiserum: FSH (mIU)† secreted* by 10^6 cells		
	Mean	Range	Proportional increase	Mean	Range	Proportional increase
$HeLa_{65}$, control	2.9	0.3–4.8	1.0	1.7	1.3–2.1	1.0
$HeLa_{65}$, 1 mM butyrate	151.7	106.1–235.8	52.0	6.0	5.2–6.7	3.5
$HeLa_{65}$, 5 mM butyrate	1,007.6	590.9–1,590.9	347.0	51.0	47.7–54.5	30.0
$HeLa_{71}$, control	116.6	65.9–204.5	1.0	2.7	2.5–2.8	1.0
$HeLa_{71}$, 1 mM butyrate	731.7	609.8–975.6	6.0	16.0	14.6–17.1	6.0
$HeLa_{71}$, 5 mM butyrate	17,555.5	9,333.3–28,333.3	151.0	313.0	293.3–333.3	116.0

*As measured in medium.

†1 mIU is equivalent to 35 ng of LER 907 FSH standard from the NIH.

Table 2 is reproduced from Nature 259:416–417, 1976, with permission [4].

$HeLa_{65}$ and $HeLa_{71}$ cells were cultured with and without sodium butyrate for 68 hours in Waymouth's medium with 10% fetal calf serum and antibiotics (penicillin 30 μg; streptomycin 50 μg, and kanamycin 30 μg ml^{-1}). The methods of subculturing, harvesting, and preparing cells for assays were as described before. The media and ultrasonicates of cells were tested for FSH by RIA using ^{125}I- FSH as the tracer antigen. Radiolabeled iodinated FSH was prepared by the chloramine-T method and purified on polyacrylamide gel. To minimize cross-reactions with other closely related glycopolypeptides, one antiserum was raised in rabbits against the β-subunit of FSH extracted and purified from fresh frozen human pituitary glands (from Diagnostic Biochem, London, Ontario, Canada). The anti-β FSH serum had the following cross-reactivities: FSH 100%; HCG < 1%; LH < 5%, TSH < 2%, and growth hormone (GH) < 1%. A second antiserum was prepared against highly purified complete human pituitary FSH (Institute of Bioendocrinology, Montreal). Antiserum against intact pituitary FSH had the following cross-reactivities: FSH 100%; TSH < 2%; LH, HCG, and GH < 0.1%. Radioactive antigen-antibody complexes were isolated by double-antibody precipitation technique using as the second precipitant antibody, an anti-rabbit γ-globulin prepared in goats with antiserum against the β-subunit and an anti-rabbit γ-globulin prepared in sheep with antiserum against complete FSH. Radiolabeled precipitate was collected by centrifugation at 6,000 g at 2°C and counted in a Beckman Biogamma II spectrometer. The percentage of binding of radioactive ^{125}I-FSH by antiserum against the β-subunit of FSH was plotted against pg concentrations of purified human pituitary FSH as the standard on logit-log graph paper. The limit of sensitivity of the assay was 50 pg. The percentage binding of radioactive ^{125}I-FSH by antiserum against complete FSH was plotted against mIU of Second International Reference Preparation of human menopausal urine gonadotropin (2nd IRP HMG) as the standard. The limit of sensitivity of the assay was 0.16 mIU. Concentrations in unknown samples were determined either from the linear standard logit-log plots or from sigmoid calibration curves on semilogarithmic scales. Apparent differences in concentrations of FSH as measured by the 2 antisera are probably the result of differences in the standards used and the higher sensitivity of the RIA with β-FSH antiserum. The results presented in this table are means of duplicate assays on 3 separate experiments carried out at different times. A standard of authentic FSH at 7 different dilutions and a sample of human serum with a known concentration of FSH were assayed concurrently with unknown samples to ensure accuracy and reproducibility of the technique. As measured by RIA, TSH and human of the fetal form of alkaline phosphatase. Inhibition in other locations in the cell cycle, such as early G_1 (isoleucine-deficient medium or serum deprivation) or M phase (colcemide), does not affect hormone production. This suggests that cell cycle events associated with the G_1 -S boundary may play an important role in mediating increased transcription of certain loci.

Pederson and Robbins [40, 41] reported marked physiochemical changes in chromatin accompanying progress of cells through G_1 to the region of the G_1 -S phase boundary, as revealed by increased accessibility to actinomycin binding or DNAase digestion. Moser and associates have developed a method to measure chromatin condensation in interphase nuclei by the binding of the fluorescent dye quinacrine dihydrochloride [42]. Cells in early G_1 phase, known to contain condensed chromatin, stain very brightly. Later in G_1, as the cells approach the G_1 -S boundary, there is considerably less staining. Fusion of interphase cells with mitotic cells causes the chromatin of the interphase cell to condense into visible strands [43]. The pattern of chromatin condensation from nuclei of late G_1 -early S phase cells is the most extended. Therefore drugs or conditions of culture that arrest the cell population at the G_1-S boundary may functionally increase transcription of selected regions of the genome. Slight differences in the site of block and perhaps in the kind of nuclear protein modification may have complementary effects. Such speculation is supported by the synergism observed in HCG induction when HeLa cells are grown with both butyrate and hydroxyurea (Table 1). Induction of glycopeptide hormone synthesis in HeLa cells indicates that cell cycle-related alterations in chromatin structure may contribute to the accessibility of genetic loci for transcription and thereby play a role in determining the biosynthetic characteristics of cells.

SUMMARY

HeLa cells can be induced to undergo morphologic and biosynthetic "differentiation" by growth in medium with sodium butyrate and certain other inhibitors of DNA synthesis. Modulations of cell phenotype include development of desmosomes and tonofilaments and production of several glycopeptide trophic hormones (HCG, FSH, and LH). Mediators of these effects focus the cell population at the G_1-S phase transition point.

REFERENCES

1. Gey GO, Coffman WD, Kubicek MT: Tissue culture studies of the proliferative capacity of cervical carcinoma and normal epithelium. (Abstract) Cancer Res 12:264–265, 1962.
2. Elson NA, Cox RP: Production of fetal-like alkaline phosphatase by HeLa cells. Biochem Genet 3:549–561, 1969.
3. Ghosh NK, Cox RP: Immunological characterization of oncofetal alkaline phosphatases from human placenta and $HeLa_{71}$ cells. Enzyme 20:35–45, 1975.
4. Ghosh NK, Cox RP: Production of human chorionic gonadotropin in HeLa cell cultures. Nature 259:416–417, 1976.

5. Ghosh NK, Rukenstein A, Cox RP: Induction of human choriogonadotropin in HeLa-cell cultures by aliphatic monocarboxylates and inhibitors of deoxyribonucleic acid synthesis. Biochem J 166:265–274, 1977.
6. Ghosh NK, Cox RP: Induction of human follicle-stimulating hormone in HeLa cells by sodium butyrate. Nature 267:435–437, 1977.
7. Ghosh D, Cox RP, Ghosh NK: Induction of ectopic luteinizing hormone (LH) production in HeLa cell cultures by inhibitors of DNA synthesis. (Abstract) Clin Res 25:666A, 1977.
8. Fallon RJ, Cox RP: Cell cycle analysis of sodium butyrate and hydroxyurea, inducers of ectopic hormone production in HeLa cells. J Cell Physiol (In press).
9. Deutsch SI, Silvers DN, Cox RP, Griffin MJ, Ghosh NK: Ultrastructural and enzymic modulation of HeLa cells induced by sodium butyrate and the effects of cytochalasin B and colcemid. J Cell Sci 21:391–406, 1976.
10. Jones HW Jr, McKusick VA, Harper PS, Wuu K-D: The HeLa cell and a reappraisal of its origin. Obstet Gynecol 38:945–949, 1971.
11. Robson EB, Harris H: Genetics of the alkaline phosphatase polymorphism of the human placenta. Nature 207:1257–1259, 1965.
12. Richter GW: Comparison of ferritins from neoplastic and non-neoplastic human cells. Nature 207:616–618, 1965.
13. Drysdale JW, Singer RM: Carcinofetal human isoferritins in placenta and HeLa cells. Cancer Res 34:3352–3354, 1974.
14. Gliksman R, Ghosh NK, Cox RP: Comparison of aldolase isozymes in placenta, HeLa cells, and human fibroblast cultures. Enzyme 22:416–419, 1977.
15. Jenkins DM, Acres MG, Peters J, Riley J: Human chorionic gonadotropin and the fetal allograft. Am J Obstet Gynecol 114:13–15, 1972.
16. Adcock EW III, Teasdale F, August CS, Cox S, Meschia G, Battaglia FC, Naughton MA: Human chorionic gonadotropin: Its possible role in maternal lymphocyte suppression. Science 181:845–847, 1973.
17. Griffin MJ, Price GH, Bazzell KL, Cox RP, Ghosh NK: A study of adenosine 3′:5′-cyclic monophosphate, sodium butyrate and cortisol as inducers of HeLa alkaline phosphatase. Arch Biochem Biophys 164:619–623, 1974.
18. Deutsch SI, Ghosh NK, Cox RP: Increased alkaline phosphatase activity in HeLa cells mediated by aliphatic monocarboxylates and inhibitors of DNA synthesis. Biochim Biophys Acta 499:382–391, 1977.
19. Rosen SW, Weintraub BD, Vaitukaitis JL, Sussman HH, Hershman JM, Muggia FM: Placental proteins and their subunits as tumor markers. Ann Intern Med 82:71–83, 1975.
20. Pierce JG: The subunits of pituitary thyrotropin – Their relationship to other glycoprotein hormones. Endocrinology 89:1331–1344, 1971.
21. Vaitukaitis JL, Braunstein GD, Ross GT: A radioimmunoassay which specifically measures human chorionic gonadotropin in the presence of human luteinizing hormone. Am J Obstet Gynecol 113:751–758, 1972.
22. Xeros N: Deoxyriboside control and synchronization of mitosis. Nature, 194:682–683, 1962.
23. Krishan A: Rapid flow cytofluorometric analysis of mammalian cell cycle by propidium iodine staining. J Cell Biol 66:188–193, 1975.
24. Walters RA, Tobey RA, Hildebrand CE: Hydroxyurea does not prevent synchronized G_1 Chinese hamster cells from entering the DNA synthetic period. Biochem Biophys Res Commun 69:212–217, 1976.
25. Hagopian HK, Riggs MG, Swartz LA, Ingram VM: Effect of n-butyrate on DNA synthesis in chick fibroblasts and HeLa cells. Cell 12:855–860, 1977.
26. Fallon RJ, Cox RP: Manuscript in preparation.

27. Fallon RJ, Ghosh NK, Cox RP: Calcium-mediated regulation of intracellular human chorionic gonadotropin in $HeLa_{65}$ cell cultures. In Wasserman RH, Corradino RA, Carafoli E, Kretsinger RH, MacLennan DH, Siegel FL (eds): "Calcium-Binding Proteins and Calcium Function." New York: Elsevier North-Holland, 1977, pp 495–497.
28. Lieblich JM, Weintraub BD, Rosen SW, Chou JY, Robinson JC: HeLa cells secrete α subunit of glycoprotein tropic hormones. Nature 260:530–532, 1976.
29. Rosen SW, Weintraub BD: Ectopic production of the isolated alpha subunit of the glycoprotein hormones. N Engl J Med 290:1441–1447, 1974.
30. Lieblich JM, Weintraub BD, Rosen SW, Ghosh NK, Cox RP: Secretion of hCG-α subunit HCG by Hela strains. Nature 265:746, 1977
31. Odell WD, Wolfsen A: Ectopic hormone secretion by tumors. In Becker FF (ed): "Cancer." New York: Plenum Press, 1975, vol 3, pp 81–97.
32. Faiman C, Colwell JA, Ryan RJ, Hershman JM, Shields TW: Gonadotropin secretion from a bronchogenic carcinoma. Demonstration by radioimmunoassay. N Engl J Med 277:1395–1399, 1967.
33. Bottomley RH, Trainer AL, Griffin MJ: Enzymatic and chromosomal characterization of HeLa variants. J Cell Biol 41:806–815, 1969.
34. Cox RP, MacLeod CM: Alkaline phosphatase content and the effects of prednisolone on mammalian cells in culture. J Gen Physiol 45:439–485, 1962.
35. Ghosh NK, Jansen V, Cox RP, Dancis J: Synthesis of follicle stimulating hormone by perfused human placenta. (Abstract) Clin Res 25:658A, 1977.
36. Dancis J, Ghosh NK, Jansen V, Schneider H, Fallon RJ, Cox RP: Secretory proteins in the perfused human placenta. Biol Neonate 35:188–193, 1979.
37. Fishman PH, Simmons JL, Brady RO, Freese E: Induction of glycolipid biosynthesis by sodium butyrate in HeLa cells. Biochem Biophys Res Commun 59:292–299, 1974.
38. Riggs MG, Whittaker RG, Neumann JR, Ingram VM: n-Butyrate causes histone modification in HeLa and Friend erythroleukaemia cells. Nature 268:462–464, 1977.
39. Candido EP, Reeves R, Davie JR: Sodium butyrate inhibits histone deacetylation in cultured cells. Cell 14:105–113, 1978.
40. Pederson T, Robbins E: Chromatin structure and the cell division cycle. Actinomycin binding in synchronized HeLa cells. J Cell Biol 55:322–327, 1972.
41. Pederson T: Chromatin structure and the cell cycle. Proc Natl Acad Sci USA 69:2224–2228, 1972.
42. Moser GC, Müller H, Robbins E: Differential nuclear fluorescence during the cell cycle. Exp Cell Res 91:73–78, 1975.
43. Johnson RT, Rao PN: Mammalian cell fusion: Induction of premature chromosome condensation in interphase nuclei. Nature 226:717–722, 1970.

The Use of the Athymic Nude Mouse for Growth of Human Tumors: Some Current Problems*

Seung-il Shin, PhD

The hairless and athymic mouse mutant "nude" is congenitally deficient in thymus-dependent cellular immunity and is unable to reject foreign tissue grafts. The nude mouse has therefore emerged as a very useful experimental tool for the growth of human tumors for laboratory investigation. However, certain highly malignant carcinomas from humans and other species fail to form growing tumors when implanted in nude mice. Evidence from several recent experiments indicates that this failure may be due to the existence in the athymic mouse of a strong thymus-independent graft resistance mechanism selectively directed against certain tumor types. By artificially suppressing this residual immunity, it may become possible to transplant the human tumors that have so far proven to be nontransplantable in nude mice.

ESTABLISHMENT OF CELL LINES FROM EXPERIMENTAL TUMORS

A detailed biochemical and genetic analysis of differentiated properties that characterize each tissue in a complex multicellular organism such as man can be greatly simplified through cell culture techniques, by which a pure population of the appropriate cell type can be maintained in a functionally differentiated state in long-term cultures. Even though the growth of normal human fibroblasts in culture can routinely be done, the growth of normal epithelial cells that continue to express the differentiated functional phenotypes is still difficult. Traditionally, investigators turned to the relatively easier task of culturing cells from experimental tumors with the relevant functional properties.

*Supported by a research grant from the National Cancer Institute (CA21054), a Genetics Center Grant to Albert Einstein College of Medicine (GM19100), and a Faculty Research Award from the American Cancer Society.

Birth Defects: Original Article Series, Volume XVI, Number 2, pages 145–153

The most notable advance in this direction was achieved by Sato and his collaborators during the early 1960s [1, 2]. Earlier work by Biskind and Biskind [3], Iglesias [4], and Furth [5] had shown that specific and sustained growth stimuli in vivo led to hypertrophy, and frequently to neoplastic transformation, of the target tissues. If such neoplastic transformation is induced in inbred laboratory animals, the tumors that arise will usually give rise to transplantable lines expressing the functional phenotypes of the tissue of origin [5]. Most epithelial cells, whether from induced experimental animal tumors or from human carcinomas, grow poorly when introduced into cell culture, and are eventually overgrown by the the stromal fibroblasts [6]. Sato and his group solved this problem through the use of repeated serial selections, first for increased culture survival in vitro and then for neoplastic growth in vivo upon reimplantation of the culture-selected cells into the host animal [1]. In this manner, many hormone-secreting or hormone-responsive cell lines were established from transplantable endocrine tumor lines of experimental animals [2, 7, 8].

However, Sato's animal-to-culture passage technique could not be applied to human carcinomas because human tumor cells could not be transplanted into experimental animals for selection in vivo, a critical step required for the elimination of the fibroblasts that usually contaminate tumor cell cultures. In order to circumvent the immunologic rejection of human tumors by experimental animals, some early workers attempted to maintain the tumors by transplantation in certain protected sites, such as hamster cheek pouch [9, 10], that are inaccessible to the host-immune mechanism, or in artificially immunosuppressed animals [11, 12]. These attempts were only partially successful.

TRANSPLANTATION OF HUMAN TUMORS IN NUDE MICE

In 1969, Rygaard and Povlsen [13] reported that malignant human tumors could be transplanted serially in the newly described athymic mouse mutant called "nude." This hairless mouse mutant was originally discovered in 1962 by Grist and studied extensively by Flanagan [14], but the fact that the nude mouse was congenitally devoid of a fully developed thymus gland and hence deficient in one of the most important immunologic defense mechanisms available to the mouse was not known until 1968 [15]. Rygaard then systematically developed the nude mouse as an experimental tool by introducing germ-free breeding techniques to prevent the microbial infection and premature death of the nude mice that was prevalent up to that time [16]. Other investigators quickly extended the initial success of Rygaard and Povlsen by demonstrating that the nude mouse is truly incapable of rejecting skin grafts from any species (including, for example, amphibian, avian, and human skin grafts) [17], and that many different types of human cancers can be grown as solid tumors by subcutaneous implantation in nude mice [18, 19].

By the mid 1970s, the optimism generated by the success of these early experiments prompted the suggestion that it should be possible to grow most human tumors, regardless of the tissue type and degree of malignancy, by transplantation in the nude mouse. Results of the initial studies that followed have been reviewed in a number of recent publications [20–25]. It became apparent through these studies that many human tumors, most notably melanomas of the skin and carcinomas of the colon, grew relatively easily as subcutaneous implants in nude mice. In contrast, certain other tumors, such as carcinomas of the breast and the prostate, and leukemias, were extremely difficult to establish as tumor lines [25]. In one experimental series, Reid and co-workers [26, 27] reported that, from more than 120 human prostate carcinoma specimens implanted in nude mice, only a few gave rise to growing tumors in the heterologous host, and that eventually only a single serially transplantable line could be isolated. In another series, Epstein and colleagues [28] reported that human leukemic cells would proliferate in nude mice only if injected intracranially. While these two may constitute the extreme examples, it is evident now that the nude mouse does not accept all human tumor grafts.

EVIDENCE FOR TUMOR GRAFT REJECTION IN NUDE MICE

Since the athymic nude mouse is demonstrably deficient in functional thymus-dependent lymphocytes (T cells) [29, 30] – the major immunologic component responsible for heterograft rejection and cell-mediated tumor immunity in the vertebrate animal – why do some highly malignant human tumors fail to grow in this host? Recent experimental evidence from several laboratories suggests that it may be due to the presence of a thymus-independent immunologic mechanism in the athymic mouse.

Working with the human prostate carcinomas, which can normally be transplanted in nude mice with less than 1% success rate, Reid and her collaborators [27], found that pretreatment of the recipient nude mice with either an antiserum prepared against mouse lymphocytes (ALS) or a sublethal cobalt irradiation of 600 rads can significantly increase the graft acceptance rate. Similarly, Giovanella and co-workers [31] reported that the growth incidence of human breast carcinomas implanted in nude mice improved when the mice were treated at the same time with ALS.

In my own laboratory, we have studied the behavior of highly malignant heterologous (allogeneic and xenogeneic) tumor cells after subcutaneous implantation in nude mice. We had observed earlier that even the highly malignant cells such as HeLa and mouse A9, which formed rapidly growing lethal tumors in nude mice with as few as 30 cells injected, never metastasized to distant sites [32, 33]. The failure of these cells to metastasize proved not to be due to the inability of the tumor cells to enter the circulation. Taking advantage of the fact that A9 cells are mutants of the mouse L cells, selected for resistance to 8-azaguanine [34], we were able to demonstrate that nude mice bearing a growing A9 tumor at a localized subcutaneous site but free of detectable metastatic nodules nevertheless contained large numbers of viable tumor cells in the major draining lymph nodes, in the spleen and lung, and in the blood withdrawn from the heart [35]. Tumor cells recovered from these sites were not only able to grow in cell culture medium containing the cytotoxic drug, but were also able to induce growing tumors when inoculated into fresh nude mice at a subcutaneous site. In addition, treatment of the A9 recipients with 2 X-irradiations at 500 rads each, 10 days before and 10 days after the implantation, or with rabbit antiserum prepared against the spleen cells from nude mice, resulted in extensive metastasis of the A9 cells in the lung [36].

In another experiment, we implanted a series of rat mammary tumors in nude mice to study the role of T-cell deficiency in tumor growth and metastasis. These rat mammary tumors were originally induced in Wistar/Fu rats by chemical carcinogens, and selected on the basis of transplantability and metastasizing properties by Kim and his colleagues [37–39]. One group of the tumors was able to induce tumors in 100% of syngeneic recipients but never metastasized spontaneously, while a second group had comparable transplantability and growth rate and in addition metastasized regularly to distant organs [39]. When these 2 contrasting groups of rat mammary tumors were transplanted into nude mice, a most unexpected result was obtained [40, 41]. The relevant data from this experiment are summarized in Table 1.

The rat mammary tumors that are highly metastatic in the natural host (eg SMT-2A and TMT-081, Table 1) often failed to induce tumors in the nude mouse, and even when tumors did develop, they showed extensive necrosis. In many instances, the tumors that started to grow in nude mice regressed completely; in no case was evidence of distant metastasis found in the nude mouse [40]. On the other hand, the nonmetastasizing rat tumors (eg MT-W9B and MT-100) showed nearly 100% acceptance in male nude mice and grew to large nonnecrotic tumors composed of well-differentiated epithelial cells typical of the mammary gland. Furthermore, these tumors formed microscopic metastatic colonies in the lung of the nude mouse [40].

Once again, evidence suggests that the failure of the metastasizing rat tumors to metastasize in the athymic mouse host may be due to a cell-mediated immunity directed against the heterologous tumor cells. In nude mice chronically immunosuppressed with a rabbit antiserum against mouse lymph node cells, the graft acceptance rate for the metastasizing rat tumors was increased to nearly 100% in males (from, for instance, the 23.5% for SMT-2A, Table 1), and more significantly, the rat tumors were now able to metastasize through the lymphatics [42].

The results of our experiments reviewed above are most consistent with the view that, even in the absence of thymus-derived lymphocytes, the nude mouse has the ability to recognize and reject certain types of highly malignant heterologous tumors, and that this thymus-independent mechanism is mediated through a

TABLE 1. Relative Transplantability of Metastasizing and Nonmetastasizing Rat Mammary Adenocarcinomas in Athymic Nude Mice

Tumor strain*	Female: No. takes/No. grafted (%)	Female: Latency, days† Mean (extremes)	Male: No. takes/No. grafted (%)	Male: Latency, days Mean (extremes)	Largest tumor (mm)	Necrosis (%)
Highly metastasizing						
SMT-2A	3/24 (12.5)	33 (31–37)	4/17 (23.5)	27 (21–30)	10	80–90
TMT-081	3/16 (18.8)	22 (21–32)	11/20 (55.0)	36 (27–43)	10	80–90
Weakly metastasizing						
STMT-058	4/4	15 (15–26)	5/5	15 (15–26)	30	20–30
STMT-29	3/3	10	12/12	6	25	20–30
Nonmetastasizing						
MT-W9B	7/10 (70.0)	26 (15–33)	15/17 (88.2)	21 (12–37)	40	0
MT-100	7/9 (77.8)	17 (11–21)	11/11 (100.0)	30 (24–41)	50	0
DMBA-1 (Fischer)	5/5 (100.0)	30	3/3 (100.0)	8	40	5–10
13762 (Fischer)	3/3 (100.0)	9(6–16)	5/5 (100.0)	7(6–8)	40	5–10

*All mammary tumors except the last 2 are in the highly inbred strain of W/Fu rats.
†Days before the tumor graft became palpable (about 3 mm in average diameter).

radiation-sensitive population of cells (lymphocytes?) that can be selectively eliminated with an antiserum directed against the total lymph node cells in the nude mouse. Whether this cell population includes the macrophages and/or the natural killer cells, and what, if any, constitutes the target cell specificities recognized by this mechanism, are yet to be clarified.

The naturally occurring cytotoxic lymphocytes, called natural killer (NK) cells, are a class of thymus-independent cells that may play an important role in immune surveillance against tumor cells in vivo [43]. NK cell activity is enhanced in the nude mouse compared to the phenotypically normal littermates [44, 45], and may provide a nonspecific immunologic mechanism by which nude mice could suppress the growth of certain tumor cells. HeLa, a human epithelial cell line derived from malignant cervical carcinoma, and BHK-21, a Syrian hamster fibroblast cell line established from a normal newborn kidney explant [46], are both highly tumorigenic in nude mice. However, when either of these cell lines is persistently infected with one of a number of RNA viruses (mumps, measles, a strain of influenza A virus, or vesicular stomatitis virus), resulting in a virus carrier state in which the cells harbor the viral genetic material but do not produce viral particles, the cells are no longer tumorigenic in nude mice [47]. Virus-producing subclones isolated from such nonproducer cells are again tumorigenic, indicating that the failure of the nonproducer cells to form tumors in nude mice is not due to a concomitant selection of nonmalignant variants [47]. More recent evidence from Reid and co-workers indicates that the persistently infected HeLa or BHK-21 cells are good inducers of the NK activity and are also more susceptible to its lytic action in vitro, compared to the tumorigenic parental cells not infected with virus [48]. Furthermore, injection of the nontumorigenic, persistently infected cells in nude mice after the mice are first irradiated with a cobalt source to suppress the residual immunity leads to the growth of the cells as tumors [48]. These results again point to the existence in the nude mouse of a very effective host-suppressive mechanism, directed against certain potentially tumorigenic cells, which is independent of the T cell functions.

CONCLUDING REMARKS

From the foregoing discussion of recent experimental data, we can conclude that the athymic nude mouse is not as innocent immunologically as it was originally believed. Indeed, the thymus-independent immunity seen in the nude mouse against the metastasizing rat mammary tumors appears to be at least as effective as the thymus-dependent tumor immunity seen in normal, immune-competent animals against highly antigenic experimental tumors.

The conclusion that the athymic nude mouse can selectively suppress the growth of certain malignant tumors naturally leads us to the next relevant question: Is it possible to grow, in artificially immunosuppressed nude mice, the types of human carcinomas that have so far resisted transplantation in untreated nude mice? The answer to this important question must be at least partially yes. The long-term maintenance of X-irradiated or ALS-treated nude mice is technically even more demanding as well as more expensive, and therefore a systematic large scale use of such mice will be difficult to carry out in most research laboratories. However, the nude mouse is the most effective living incubator of human tumor cells at the present time, and the use of immunosuppressed nude mice is likely to improve the usefulness of this animal even further.

ACKNOWLEDGMENTS

I would like to thank Dr. Lola Reid for helpful discussions and for the permission to quote unpublished results for the preparation of this paper.

REFERENCES

1. Buonassisi V, Sato G, Cohen AI: Hormone-producing cultures of adrenal and pituitary tumor origin. Proc Natl Acad Sci USA 48:1184–1190, 1962.
2. Yasumura Y, Tashjian AH Jr, Sato GH: Establishment of four functional, clonal strains of animal cells in culture. Science 154:1186–1189, 1966.
3. Biskind MS, Biskind GS: Development of tumors in the rat ovary after transplantation into the spleen. Proc Soc Exp Biol Med 55:176–179, 1944.
4. Iglesias R: Hormones and tumors. In Proc 2nd Int Cong Endocrinol, Excerpta Med. ICS 83:1072–1084, 1965.
5. Furth J: Pituitary cybernetics and neoplasia. Harvey Lect 63:47–71, 1967.
6. Sato G, Zaroff L, Mills SE: Tissue culture populations and their relation to the tissue of origin. Proc Natl Acad Sci USA 46:963–972, 1960.
7. Shin S: Studies on interstitial cells in tissue culture: Steroid biosynthesis in monolayers of mouse testicular interstitial cells. Endocrinology 81:440–448, 1967.
8. Augusti-Tocco G, Sato G: Establishment of functional clonal lines of neurons from mouse neuroblastoma. Proc Natl Acad Sci USA 64:311–315, 1969.
9. Hertz R: Choriocarcinoma of women maintained in serial passage in hamster and rat. Proc Soc Exp Biol Med 102:77–81, 1959.
10. Yohn DS, Hammon WM, Atchison RW, Casto BC: Serial heterotransplantation of human adenocarcinoma #1 in the cheek pouch of unconditioned adult Syrian hamsters. Cancer Res 22:443–448, 1962.
11. Toolan HW: Growth of human tumors in cortisone-treated laboratory animals: The possibility of obtaining permanently transplantable human tumors. Cancer Res 13:389–394, 1953.
12. Berenbaum MC, Sheard CE, Reittie JR, Bundick RW: The growth of human tumours in immunosuppressed mice and their response to chemotherapy. Br J Cancer 30:13–32, 1974.
13. Rygaard J, Povlsen CO: Heterotransplantation of a human malignant tumor to "nude" mice. Acta Pathol Microbiol Scand 77:758–760, 1969.
14. Flanagan SP: 'Nude', a new hairless gene with pleiotropic effects in the mouse. Genet Res 8:295–309, 1966.
15. Pantelouris EM: Absence of thymus in a mouse mutant. Nature 217:370–371, 1968.
16. Rygaard J: "Thymus and Self: Immunobiology of the Mouse Mutant Nude." New York: John Wiley & Sons, 1973.

17. Manning DD, Reed ND, Shaffer CF: Maintenance of skin xenografts of widely divergent phylogenetic origin on congenitally athymic (nude) mice. J Exp Med 138:488–494, 1973.
18. Giovanella BC, Yim SO, Stehlin JS, Williams LJ Jr: Brief communication: Development of invasive tumors in the "nude" mouse after injection of cultured human melanoma cells. J Natl Cancer Inst 48:1531–1533, 1972.
19. Sordat B, Fritsché R, Mach JP, Carrel S, Ozzello L, Cerottini JC: Morphological and functional evaluation of human solid tumours serially transplanted into nude mice. In "Proc 1st Int Workshop on Nude Mice (1973)." Stuttgart: Gustav Fischer Verlag, 1974, pp 269–278.
20. Giovanella BC, Fogh J: Present and future trends in investigations with the nude mouse as a recipient of human tumor transplants. In Fogh J, Giovanella BC (eds): "The Nude Mouse in Experimental and Clinical Research." New York: Academic Press, 1978, pp 282–312.
21. Schmidt M, Good RA: Transplantation of human cancers to nude mice and effects of thymus grafts. J Natl Cancer Inst 55:81–87, 1975.
22. Shimosato Y, Kameya T, Nagia K, Hirohashi S, Koide T, Hayashi H, Nomura T: Transplantation of human tumors in nude mice. J Natl Cancer Inst 56:1251–1260, 1976.
23. Shin S, Reid LC, Colburn PC, Kadish AS, Fleischer N: Development of transplantable functional endocrine tumor lines in nude mice. In "Proc 2nd Int Workshop on Nude Mice (1976)." Stuttgart: Gustav Fischer Verlag, 1977, pp 375–393.
24. Reid LM, Holland J, Jones C, Wolf B, Niwayama G, Williams R, Kaplan NO, Sato G: Some of the variables affecting the success of transplantation of human tumors into the athymic nude mouse. In Houchens D, Ovejera A (eds): "Proc Symp on the Use of Athymic (Nude) Mice." Stuttgart: Gustav Fischer Verlag, 1978, pp 107–121.
25. Reid LCM, Shin S: Transplantation of heterologous endocrine tumor cells in nude mice. Supra #20, pp 313–351.
26. Reid L, Leav I, Merk F, Albert J, Geller J: Androgen-dependent human prostatic carcinoma tumor line in nude mice. (Abstract) Proc Am Assoc Cancer Res 19:151, 1978.
27. Reid L, Merk F, Leav I, Russell P: Androgen-dependent human prostatic carcinoma tumor line in nude mice. (Abstract) Proc Am Assoc Cancer Res 19:151, 1978.
27. Reid L, Merk F, Leav I, Russell P: Androgen-dependent human prostatic tumor line and culture system. (Submitted for publication).
28. Epstein AL, Herman MM, Kim H, Dorfman RF, Kaplan HS: Biology of the human malignant lymphomas. Cancer 37:2158–2176, 1976.
29. Kindred B: Immunological unresponsiveness of genetically thymusless (nude) mice. Eur J Immunol 1:59–61, 1971.
30. Lefkovits I: In vitro complementation experiments with nude mice. Eur J Immunol 3:397–401, 1973.
31. Giovanella BC, Stehlin JS, Lee SS, Shepard R, Williams LJ: Heterotransplantation of human breast carcinomas in "nude" thymus deficient mice. (Abstract) Proc Am Assoc Cancer Res 17:124, 1976.
32. Freedman VH, Shin S: Cellular tumorigenicity in nude mice: Correlation with cell growth in semi-solid medium. Cell 3:355–359, 1974.
33. Shin S, Freedman VH: Neoplastic growth of animal cells in nude mice. Supra #23, pp 337–349.
34. Littlefield JW: Three degrees of guanylic acid-inosinic acid pyrophosphorylase deficiency in mouse fibroblasts. Nature 203:1142–1144, 1964.
35. Klein AS, Simon R, Kim U, Shin S: Host control of metastatic spread of allogeneic tumor cells in the nude mouse. (In preparation).
36. Klein AS, Kim U, Shin S: Regulation of tumor metastasis in nude mice. (Abstract) J Cell Biol 79:90a, 1978.

37. Kim U: Metastasizing mammary carcinomas in rats: Induction and study of their immunogenicity. Science 167:72–74, 1970.
38. Kim U, Depowski MJ: Progression from hormone dependence to autonomy in mammary tumors as an in vivo manifestation of sequential clonal selection. Cancer Res 35:2068–2077, 1975.
39. Kim U: Pathogenesis of spontaneously metastasizing mammary carcinomas in rats, GANN Monogr. Cancer Res 20:73–81, 1977.
40. Freedman VH, Kim U, Shin S: Metastasis of xenogeneic and allogeneic tumors in nude mice. (In preparation).
41. Freedman VH, Shin S, Kim U: Reversal of metastatic behavior of rat mammary tumors in athymic nude mice. (Abstract) In Proc XIV Int Cong Genetics, Moscow, 1978, pt II, p 428.
42. Klein AS, Freedman VH, Kim U, Shin S: Induction of metastatic spread of xenogeneic or allogeneic malignant tumors in athymic nude mice by immunosuppression. (In preparation).
43. Kiessling R, Klein E, Wigzell H: "Natural" killer cells in the mouse. I. Cytotoxic cells with specificity for mouse moloney leukemia cells. Specificity and distribution according to genotype. Eur J Immunol 5:112–117, 1975.
44. Kiessling R, Klein E, Pross H, Wigzell H: "Natural" killer cells in the mouse. II. Cytotoxic cells with specificity for mouse moloney leukemia cells. Characteristics of the killer cell. Eur J Immunol 5:117–121, 1975.
45. Herberman RB, Nunn ME, Lavrin DH: Natural cytotoxic reactivity of mouse lymphoid cells against syngeneic and allogeneic tumors. I. Distribution of reactivity and specificity. Int J Cancer 16:216–229, 1975.
46. Stoker M, Macpherson I: Syrian hamster fibroblast cell line BHK 21 and its derivatives. Nature 203:1355–1357, 1964.
47. Reid LM, Jones CL, Holland J: Virus carrier state suppresses tumorigenicity of tumor cells in nude mice. J Gen Virol 42:609–614, 1979.
48. Minato N, Bloom B, Jones C, Holland J, Reid L: Mechanism of rejection of virus persistently infected tumor cells by athymic nude mice. J Exp Med 149:1117–1133, 1979.

Epithelial Cell Cultures From Amniotic Fluid for Prenatal Diagnosis*

Paul J. Benke, MD, PhD

Cultivation of human amniotic fluid yields mixed cultures of fibroblasts and epithelial cells. Amniotic fluid fibroblasts are easier to grow than epithelial cells; generally predominate in the tissue culture dish, particularly after subculture; and have been utilized in the prenatal diagnosis of a wide variety of chromosomal and metabolic disorders. Amniotic fluid epithelial cells are not technically suitable for prenatal cytogenetic study. A prenatal diagnosis of a genetic or metabolic disorder utilizing amniotic fluid epithelial cells has not yet been accomplished. However, epithelial cells have many properties that can be distinguished from fibroblasts. Epithelial cells, not fibroblasts, have histidase activity [1]; tyrosine aminotransferase activity [2], glucuronidase activity for some substrates [3], D-amino acid oxidase activity [4], and other properties described below. It is likely that one or more unique properties of epithelial cells will be applied to prenatal diagnostic studies in the near future.

CULTIVATION OF EPITHELIAL CELLS FROM AMNIOTIC FLUID

Epithelial cells are generally easily grown from amniotic fluid cultures. Some samples, however, do not yield growth of epithelial cells. Fibroblasts take over the culture with time, particularly after subculture, unless special precautions are taken. The single most important factor in the growth of amniotic fluid cultures is the utilization of fresh, nontoxic fetal calf serum (FCS). We obtain FCS from a local slaughterhouse, filter it, and pretest each batch for epithelial cell toxicity. Two to 3 cc's of amniotic fluid samples are incubated with F12 media and enough FCS so that the final FCS concentration is 25–30%. After 4–6 days, the medium is aspirated, and 15% FCS and F12 medium is added to the culture dish. In our experience, fibroblastic cells are grown from 99% of all amniotic fluid samples, and epithelial cells from a large majority of them.

*Supported by the Hayward Foundation.

Birth Defects: Original Article Series, Volume XVI, Number 2, pages 155–159

One or more special procedures are required to facilitate the growth of epithelial cells as the predominant cell type. Undertrypsinization, as employed for different epithelial cell-fibroblast mixtures [5, 6], is useful to rid the culture of most of the fibroblast cells. *Cis*-alloproline [7] and mercurial compounds [8] are differentially toxic to fibroblast cells in mixed epithelial cell-fibroblast cultures. D-valine medias [4] may be useful in retarding fibroblastic growth, but this compound also slows the growth of normal epithelial cells. Fibroblast-specific antibodies in the presence of complement may also rid the culture of fibroblasts [9]. We have found that amniotic epithelial cells, like other epithelial cells [10], depend upon growth factors from fibroblasts or 3T3 cells for growth. Epidermal growth factor may potentially substitute for this requirement.

POTENTIAL APPLICATION OF AMNIOTIC EPITHELIAL CELLS TO THE DIAGNOSIS OF GENETIC DEFECTS

Enzyme Disorders

A large number of metabolic parameters are not present in fibroblasts. In an attempt to establish that some may be in epithelial cells, we have studied ornithine transcarbamoylase activity by published methods [11] and glyconeogenesis by the measurement of pyruvate-^{14}C incorporation into glucose. These metabolic functions could not be observed in the 10–15 mg of cellular material found in 2 P-100 tissue culture dishes. In an attempt to determine whether a study of phenylalanine hydroxylase activity would be fruitful, we grew human liver epithelial cells in a medium with low tyrosine and high phenylalanine as previously described [12]. Growth of epithelial cells under these conditions could not be observed, suggesting that there was not enough phenylalanine hydroxylase activity to allow these cells to grow on phenylalanine when tyrosine levels were low.

Recently it has been suggested that glucose-6-phosphatase activity is present in liver epithelial cells [13]. This suggests that a prenatal diagnosis of glycogen storage disease type I is feasible if amniotic fluid epithelial cells have the enzyme. However, the enzyme assay employed for glucose-6-phosphatase was colorimetric. In our experiments with amniotic fluid epithelial cells, the assay could not be scaled down to less than 2 full P-100 Petri dishes. This would not allow a prenatal diagnosis for this disorder unless a more sensitive assay for the enzyme is utilized.

Disorders of Secretion

Epithelial cells are secretory cells and genetic mutations in secretion may be expressed in epithelial cells. Although an important disorder of secretory glands, cystic fibrosis, might be expressed in epithelial cells, this has not been demonstrated, and glycoprotein secretion in epithelial cells of the intestine appears to be normal [14].

Alpha-1-Antitrypsin Deficiency

This disorder is a common genetic variant in man. It is associated with cholestatic liver disease in children [15] and early onset of emphysema in adults. The disorder is primarily that of an inability to secrete alpha-1-antitrypsin from liver [16]. Determination of pi phenotypic allele has been successful in human hepatic cell cultures [17]. If the pi phenotype can be measured in other epithelial cell types, such as amniotic fluid epithelial cells, it may be possible to identify the phenotype ZZ which carries more serious implications.

Factor VIII antigen. Factor VIII antigen, important in normal blood coagulation, is synthesized and secreted by vascular endothelial cells [18]. Synthesis of Factor VIII antigen has not yet been shown in amniotic fluid epithelial cells. However, hemophilia, an X-linked disorder, which is associated with defective Factor VIII activity, has normal Factor VIII antigen [18], and detection in amniotic fluid epithelial cells might not lead to a prenatal diagnostic test for hemophilia. Von Willebrand disease, a dominantly inherited, milder disorder of hemostasis, usually has decreased Factor VIII antigen [19], and is potentially studied prenatally.

Disorders of Membrane Response

Epithelial cells have different membrane proteins and membrane receptors than fibroblasts. These properties might be exploited for prenatal diagnosis. Membrane receptors and microtubules of epithelial cells are involved in the site of action of vasopressin [20]. If similar properties are found in amniotic fluid epithelial cells, a prenatal diagnosis of vasopressin-resistant diabetes insipidus could be made. A secretory component of epithelial cells is a surface receptor for polymeric immunoglobulins [21]. If a mutation of this property leads to defective B-T cell communication and immunodeficiency disease, and this was found in amniotic fluid epithelial cells, a prenatal diagnosis could be attempted.

Disorders of Connective Tissue and Collagen

Fibroblasts and epithelial cells differ in the collagen and proteins that they produce. Preliminary studies of the collagen production of amniotic fluid epithelial cells have appeared [22, 23]. A wide variety of disorders, including Ehlers-Danlos syndrome, Marfan syndrome, and osteogenesis imperfecta, are probably disorders of collagen metabolism. It is possible that amniotic fluid epithelial cells might be useful in prenatal diagnosis of these conditions if a defect cannot be found in amniotic fluid fibroblasts. Much remains to be done in the basic biochemistry of these disorders before this can be attempted.

Miscellaneous Disorders

Various parameters of cell-cell contact and epithelial cell function in vivo might be applied to the in vitro study of genetic disorders. For example, defects in pigmented epithelial cells of the eye may be causally related to retinal dystrophy and a form of genetic retinitis pigmentosa-like disease [24]. Retinal epithelial cells control other cell functions in the eye [25]. If these functions of epithelial cells can be further defined, it might be applied to prenatal diagnosis.

Disorders expressed in epithelial cells from various parts of the body are potentially studied in amniotic fluid epithelial cells because various epithelial cells grown in cell culture express a large number of differentiation markers in common [26], including enzymes and structural proteins. It has been suggested that lack of a distinctive phenotype of epithelial cells from various sources is due to external modulation or to dedifferentiation in culture [26]. Of course, if genetic information could be surmised from information found in amniotic fluid fibroblast DNA, as has recently been found for sickle cell disease [27], there would be no need to cultivate epithelial cells. Restriction enzyme technology, however, is potentially applied to a small number of disorders. Since epithelial cells have properties that fibroblasts do not, the application of epithelial cells for genetic studies and prenatal genetic disorders is a fruitful area of research.

SUMMARY

A prenatal diagnosis of a metabolic disorder has not yet been achieved utilizing human amniotic fluid epithelial cells. For this to be accomplished, a unique property must first be expressed in normal epithelial cells distinct from a gene function found in fibroblasts. Then, a mutation must be identified which can be quantitated in amniotic fluid epithelial cells. There appears to be the potential to study genetic disorders.

REFERENCES

1. Melancom SB, Lee SY, Nadler HL: Histidase activity in cultivated human amniotic fluid cells. Science 173:627–628, 1971.
2. Bonney RJ, Becker JE, Walker PR, Potter VR: Primary monolayer cultures of adult rat liver parenchymal cells suitable for study of the regulation of enzyme synthesis. In Vitro 9:399–413, 1974.
3. Rugstad HE, Dybing E: Glucuronidation in cultures of human skin epithelial cells. Eur J Clin Invest 5:133–137, 1975.
4. Gilbert SF, Migeon BR: Renal enzymes in kidney cells selected by D-valine medium. J Cell Physiol 92:161–168, 1977.
5. Flaxman BA, Lutzner MA, Scott EJV: Cell maturation and tissue organization in epithelial outgrowth from skin and buccal mucosa in vitro. J Invest Dermatol 49:322–332, 1967.
6. Owens RB, Smith HS, Nelson-Rees WA, Springer EL: Epithelial cell cultures from normal and cancerous human tissues. J Natl Cancer Inst 56:843–846, 1976.
7. Kao WW, Prockop DJ: Proline analogue removes fibroblasts from cultured mixed cell populations. Nature 266:63–64, 1977.
8. Braaten JT, Lee MJ, Schenk A, Mintz DH: Removal of fibroblastoid cells from primary monolayer cultures of rat neonatal endocrine pancreas by sodium ethylmercurithiosalicylate. Biochem Biophys Res Commun 61:476–482, 1974.

9. King ES, Fisher TN, Fisher E Jr: A new procedure for the destruction of human prostatic fibroblasts in explant outgrowths of cultures of mixed cell types. IRCS. J Med Sci 4:433–434, 1976.
10. Rheinwald JG, Green H: Epidermal growth factor and the multiplication of cultured human epidermal keratinocytes. Nature 265:421–424, 1977.
11. Ceriotti G, Gazzaniga A: A sensitive method for serum ornithine carbamyltransferase determination. Clin Chim Acta 14:57–62, 1966.
12. Choo KH, Cotton RGH, Danks DM: Phenylalanine hydroxylation and tyrosine requirement of cultured cells. Exp Cell Res 101:370–382, 1976.
13. Negishi H, Benke PJ: Epithelial cells and von Gierke's disease. Pediatr Res 11:936–939, 1977.
14. Neutra MR, Trier JS: Rectal mucosa in cystic fibrosis. Gastroenterology 75:701–710, 1978.
15. Lieberman J, Mittman C, Gordon HW: Alpha-1-antitrypsin in the livers of patients with emphysema. Science 175:63–65, 1972.
16. Freier EF, Sharp H, Bridges RA: Alpha-1-antitrypsin deficiency associated with familial liver disease. (Abstract) Clin Chem 14:782–783, 1968.
17. Gautier M, Martin JP, Polini G: In vitro synthesis of alpha-1-antitrypsin in long-term monolayer human liver cell cultures. Biomedicine 27:116–119, 1977.
18. Jaffe EA: Endothelial cells and the biology of Factor VIII. N Engl J Med 296:377–383, 1977.
19. Hoyer LW: Von Willebrand's disease. Prog Hemostatis Thromb 3:231–287, 1976.
20. Reaven E, Maffly R, Taylor A: Evidence for involvement of microtubules in the action of vasopressin in toad urinary bladder. III. Morphological studies on the content and distribution of microtubules in bladder epithelial cells. J Membr Biol 40:251–267, 1978.
21. Crago SS, Kulhavy R, Prince SJ, Mestecky J: Secretory component of epithelial cells is a surface receptor for polymeric immunoglobulins. J Exp Med 147:1832–1837, 1978.
22. Priest RE, Priest JH, Moinuddin JF, Keyser AJ: Differentiation in human amniotic fluid cell cultures. I. Collagen production. J Med Genet 14:157–162, 1977.
23. Megaw JM, Priest JH, Priest RE, Johnson LD: Differentiation in human amniotic fluid cell cultures. II. Secretion of an epithelial basement membrane glycoprotein. J Med Genet 14:162–167, 1977.
24. Mullen RJ, LaVail MM: Inherited retinal dystrophy: Primary defect in pigment epithelium determined with experimental rat chimeras. Science 192:799–801, 1976.
25. Parkinson EK, Edwards JG: Non-reciprocal contact inhibition of locomotion of chick embryonic choroid fibroblasts by pigmented retina epithelial cells. J Cell Sci 33:103–120, 1978.
26. Sun TT, Green H: Cultured epithelial cells of cornea, conjunctiva and skin: Absence of marked intrinsic divergence of their differentiated states. Nature 269:489–493, 1977.
27. Marx JL: Restriction enzymes: Prenatal diagnosis of genetic disease. Science 202:1068–1069, 1978.

Application of Monolayer Culture Techniques to the Study of Human Epithelium

William H.J. Douglas, PhD and Louis Terracio, PhD

During the last several years culture techniques have been developed that permit differentiated cells, derived from normal tissues, to retain specialized characteristics while undergoing a useful number of replicative cycles in vitro. This was first accomplished by the application of differentiated cell culture techniques to enzymatically dispersed suspensions of chick embryo skeletal muscle [1], and subsequently extended to cartilage [2], pigmented retina [3], thyroid [4], liver [5], pituitary [6, 7], keratinocytes [8], vascular endothelial cells [9], vascular smooth muscle [10], and other cell types.

In all of these reports, cells have been isolated that retain a differentiated phenotype in culture; thus meeting the basic requirement for cells to be used for in vitro experimentation. The successful culture of differentiated cells relies upon the ability to separate the desired cell type (eg epithelial cells) from the heterogeneous population of cells present in the intact organ. For the most part, adequate cell separation must occur prior to maintenance in culture, if the epithelial cells are going to survive for prolonged periods of time and permit useful experimentation in vitro. The need to separate these various cell types prior to culture is due to the fact that fibroblasts and other stromal cells generally have shorter generation times in culture than do epithelial cells [11]. This difference in replication rates results in the fibroblasts rapidly becoming the dominant cell type unless the various cell types are adequately separated and the epithelial population can grow in the absence of fibroblasts.

The basic techniques of primary culture form the foundation of current methods for the isolation and culture of specific epithelial cell types. However, the diversity of functional cell types present in any one organ, make it necessary for the cell culturist to draw upon a broad spectrum of techniques in order to design a procedure that will yield an enriched population of a specific Cell type. Most cell culture systems utilizing human epithelium start by dissociating the epithelial tissue using

Birth Defects: Original Article Series, Volume XVI, Number 2, pages 161–165

enzymatic or nonenzymatic procedures to yield a suspension of viable cells of mixed origin. The cell type of interest is then isolated using physical cell separation methods or in vitro enrichment techniques.

PHYSICAL CELL SEPARATION METHODS

The most commonly used physical methods take advantage of differences in cell size and density to separate the epithelial cells from stromal elements. These techniques include: velocity sedimentation in isokinetic and isopycnic gradients [12, 13]; sedimentation at unit gravity in gradients [14], and centrifugal elutriation [15, 16].

Velocity sedimentation in an isokinetic gradient separates cells primarily based on differences in cell size. A cell suspension is placed on a continuous Ficoll gradient in culture media and centrifuged. The gradient balances the increasing centrifugal force encountered by the sedimenting cells against the increasing viscous drag of the gradient medium. Thus, cells of distinctly different size come to rest at various levels in the gradient and are separated.

Velocity sedimentation in an isopycnic gradient, separates cells based primarily on differences in cell density. Cell density is a function of the chemical composition of the cell rather than its size. Since most cells are composed of basically the same components, there is only a slight variation in the proportion of the components and therefore only a narrow range of cell densities. However, cells with different nucleus-to-cytoplasm ratios, or a high content of lipid or secretory granules usually have a sufficiently different density and can be separated. When cells are centrifuged in a density gradient, they rise or sink until they reach an area in the gradient that corresponds to their buoyant density. Thus, cells with different densities come to rest at different levels in the gradient and are separated.

Sedimentation at unit gravity in an isokinetic gradient is based on the same principles as velocity sedimentation in an isokinetic gradient except that it uses the force of gravity to separate cells instead of the increased forces generated by the centrifuge rotor. Cells of different sizes settle out in narrow bands in the gradient and are then easily separated.

Centrifugal elutriation separates cells of different sizes and densities by counterstreaming the cells, suspended in culture medium, against the centrifugal force generated by a specialized rotor in a centrifuge. A monodisperse cell suspension is pumped through the special centrifuge rotor against a set centrifugal force generated by the rotor. When the counterstream force generated by the flow of culture medium being pumped through the rotor is less than or equal to the centrifugal force of the rotor, the cells remain in the rotor. When the flow is increased, its force becomes greater than that of the rotor and small cells are washed from the rotor and collected. As the flow rate is increased larger cells are removed from the rotor and collected. This technique allows for the separation of a variety of cell types with little damage to the cells.

IN VITRO ENRICHMENT TECHNIQUES

The in vitro enrichment techniques are based upon the fact that cell function and origin can affect the rate of attachment to culture vessels [17, 18]. Thus by varying the cell culture substrate [19, 20, 21], the environmental conditions (pH, serum concentration, etc [22]), and the time allotted for attachment in sequential platings, a pure population of the desired cell type can be obtained. The resultant cell populations are highly enriched for epithelial cells and can be used directly for the study of normal epithelial cell development, function, and metabolism in vitro, or they can be further "purified" by other culture techniques. When grown in primary culture, these enriched cell populations may show signs of residual fibroblast contamination. The residual fibroblasts can be removed by periodic treatment of the culture with low concentrations of enzymes [23, 24, 25] or chelating agents [25, 26]. Since epithelial cells adhere to the culture substrate more firmly than do fibroblasts, short exposures to the enzymes or chelators will remove the fibroblasts with little or no effect on the epithelial cells. Using this procedure, pure cultures of epithelial cells devoid of fibroblast contamination can be obtained [24, 25].

The procedures described above result in enriched primary cultures of epithelial cells. Although cultures obtained from these enriched populations have proven to be useful for the majority of in vitro experiments, they may contain more than one cell type and thus be unacceptable for certain specialized procedures that require a homogeneous population of cells. To produce such a population, single cells are isolated from enriched cultures and propagated separately to form pure cultures. These populations in which all the individuals cells are descendants of a single cell are called clones. Although cloning is tedious and time consuming, it has several unique advantages: 1) since a clonal population is derived from a single cell, overgrowth by contaminating stromal cells is completely eliminated; 2) several cell lines can be isolated from the same specimen, each with maximal epigenetic purity; 3) clonal growth of cells at low population densities avoids rapid depletion of essential components from the medium and thus allows for closer control of cell nutrition.

All of these techniques can and have been employed with human epithelial cells to yield a variety of purified epithelial cell systems. These systems provide an opportunity to study differentiated cells in a highly controlled environment, free from the complicating cellular and hormonal environment found in vivo.

REFERENCES

1. Konigsberg IR: Clonal analysis of myogenesis. Science 140: 1273–1284, 1963.
2. Coon HG: Clonal stability and phenotypic expression of chick cartilage cells in vitro. Proc Natl Acad Sci USA 55:66–73, 1966.

3. Cahn RD, Cahn MB: Heritability of cellular differentiation: Clonal growth and expression of differentiation in retinal pigment cells in vitro. Proc Natl Acad Sci USA 55:106–114, 1966.
4. Spooner BS: The expression of differentiation by chick embryo thyroid in cell culture. I. Functional and fine structural stability in mass and clonal culture. J Cell Physiol 75:33–48, 1970.
5. Kaighn ME, Prince AM: Production of albumin and other serum proteins by clonal cultures of normal human liver. Proc Natl Acad Sci USA 68:2396–2400, 1971.
6. Tashjian AH Jr, Yasumura Y, Levine L, Sato GH, Parker ML: Establishment of clonal strains of rat pituitary tumor cells that secrete growth hormone. Endocrinology 82: 342–352, 1968.
7. Tashjian AH Jr, Bancroft FC, Levine L: Production of both prolactin and growth hormone by clonal strains of rat pituitary tumor cells: Differential effects of hydrocortisone and tissue extracts. J Cell Biol 47:61–70, 1970.
8. Sun T-T, Green H: Differentiation of the epidermal keratinocyte in cell culture: Formation of the cornified envelope. Cell 9:511–521, 1976.
9. Gimbrone MA Jr, Cotran RS, Folkman J: Human vascular endothelial cells in culture. J Cell Biol 60:673–684, 1974.
10. Gimbrone MA Jr, Cotran RS: Human vascular smooth muscle in culture. Lab Invest 33:16–27, 1975.
11. Douglas WHJ, Kaighn ME: Clonal isolation of differentiated rat lung cells. In Vitro 10:230–237, 1974.
12. Dow SH, Pretlow TG II: Separation of cells exhibiting acid phosphatase activity from disaggregated hamster prostate cells in an isokinetic gradient of Ficoll in tissue culture medium. J Natl Cancer Inst 54:147–150, 1975.
13. Pretlow TG II, Luberoff DE: A new method for separating lymphocytes and granulocytes from human peripheral blood using programmed gradient sedimentation in an isokinetic gradient. Immunology 24:85–92, 1973.
14. Hymer WC, Evans WH, Kraicer J, Mastro A, Davis J, Griswold E: Enrichment of cell types from the rat adenohypophysis by sedimentation at unit gravity. Endocrinology 92:275–287, 1973.
15. Lindahl PE: On counter streaming centrifugation in the separation of cells and cell fragments. Biochim Biophys Acta 21:411–415, 1956.
16. Mason RJ, Williams MC, Greenleaf RD, Clements JA: Isolation and properties of type II alveolar cells from rat lung. Am Rev Respir Dis 115:1015–1026, 1977.
17. Williams GM, Weisburger EK, Weisburger JH: Isolation and long-term cell culture of epithelial-like cells from rat liver. Exp Cell Res 69:106–112, 1971.
18. Kasten FH: Rat myocardial cells in vitro: Mitosis and differentiated properties. In Vitro 8(3):128–149, 1972.
19. Harris A: Behavior of cultured cells on substrata of variable adhesiveness. Exp Cell Res 77:285–297, 1973.
20. Grinnell F: Studies on the mechanisms of cell attachment to a substratum: Evidence for three biochemically distinct processes. Arch Biochem Biophys 160:304–310, 1974.
21. Martin GR, Rubin H: Effects of cell adhesion to the substratum on the growth of chick embryo fibroblasts. Exp Cell Res 85:319–333, 1974,
22. Takeichi M, Okada TS: Rolls of magnesium and calcium ions in cell-to-substrate adhesion. Exp Cell Res 74:51–60, 1972.
23. Owens RB, Smith HS, Hackett AJ: Epithelial cell cultures from normal glandular tissue of mice. J Natl Cancer Inst 53:261–269, 1974.

24. Lasfargues EY, Moore DH: A method for the continuous cultivation of mammary epithelium. In Vitro 7:21–25, 1971.
25. White MT, Hu ASL, Hamamoto ST, Nandi S: In vitro analysis of proliferating epithelial cell populations from the mouse mammary gland: Fibroblast-free growth and serial passage. In Vitro 14:271–281, 1978.
26. Lechner JF, Narayan KS, Ohnuki Y, Babcock MS, Jones LW, Kaighn ME: Replicative epithelial cell cultures from normal human prostate gland. J Natl Cancer Inst 60:797–801, 1978.

PART II:
Possibilities, Feasibility, Future of Studying Human Birth Defects Expressed in Epithelium in Tissue Systems

In Vitro Growth and Characterization of Human Skin Cells

Aaron E. Freeman, PhD

Skin cells have been cultivated in vitro by trypsinization procedures [1–5], plasma clot method [6–11], floating explant method [12–14], on organ culture grids [15,16], and in hanging drops [17–21]. A variety of substrates including glass [1, 6–8, 10, 11], plastic [2,5,9–11], gelatin [22], fibrin [6], cellophane [23], paper [24], collagen [25], cellulose sponge [26–28], pigskin [29,30], and irradiated feeder cells [31] have been used as supporting surfaces and substrates. Although significant studies have been made with each of these methods, the current state of the art centers on four major methods, ie classical trypsinization [1–5], growth of trypsin-collagenase digests on irradiated feeder cells [31], outgrowth of explants on plastic [2–5, 9–11], and outgrowth of explants on irradiated pigskin [29,30].

BASIC REVIEW OF METHODS

When skin is minced and trypsinized, the cell outgrowth tends to have fibroblastic morphology. There are, however, several methods for selecting cultures consisting predominantly of epithelial cells. The first of these methods involves growth and differentiation of skin explants or trypsin-collagenase digests of skin on a layer of 6000 r irradiated mouse 3T3 fibroblast feeders. In this system [31] the feeder served to accelerate the growth of epithelial cells (keratinocytes) while simultaneously retarding the growth of dermal fibroblasts which invariably contaminate primary skin cultures. Subcultures are achieved by preliminary versene (EDTA) removal of feeders and a small number of skin fibroblasts followed by complete dissociation of epithelium with trypsin-EDTA. Upon replanting on new mouse 3T3 feeders, new epithelial islands arise with approximately 1% plating efficiency. Two to four subcultures are feasible. The disadvantages of this system are the possible contamination of human cells with mouse endogenous viruses or other mouse genetic material, and interference by mouse cells of biochemical analyses

Birth Defects: Original Article Series, Volume XVI, Number 2, pages 169–173

on the donors' epithelial elements. Due to the low plating efficiency it is difficult to increase the total population of epithelial cells on subculture.

A second method for culturing skin epithelial cells is conventional explant outgrowth on tissue culture grade plastic [32]. Superior growth longevity of primary cultures is obtained in a closed or low gas exchange vessel. Open dishes, for unknown reasons, yield slower growth and premature keratinization. Foreskin or biopsy skin minced pieces are placed on a dry vessel surface and allowed to adhere for 0.5–3.0 hours without medium (dried on). Dulbecco's modified Eagle's medium (DMEM) containing 5–10% fetal bovine serum is then added. After 20–50 days incubation at 36.5°C in a humidified incubator at 10% CO_2, certain minced pieces yield exclusively fibroblast colonies and others yield true keratinizing epithelial colonies. If the original skin sample is cleaned exhaustively by scraping away most of the dermis and underlying connective tissue, 70–90% of the minced pieces will yield epithelial colonies free of fibroblasts. Each donor sample will vary with respect to the relative growth of epithelial versus fibroblastic elements. This is dependent on the amount of dermis in each minced piece and the number of minced pieces per unit area of the culture vessel.

A third method for growing skin epithelial cells is the culturing of skin explants on a substrate of sterile dead pigskin [29, 30]. In this system minced skin pieces are planted on pigskin which rest dermal side up on an organ culture-type grid. Medium is added to the level of the grid such that the mince is nourished through the pigskin. After a period of 5–9 days, epithelial cells migrate and begin to grow from the mince onto the pigskin dermis. A continuous process of replication and differentiation ensues over the following weeks as clearing of the pigskin through digestion of the dermal substrate occurs. These clear areas represent digested pigskin dermis covered with the four layers of skin found in vivo, ie basal layer (germinative layer), squamous layer, granular layer, and horny layer (keratin). Expansion of the epithelium continues until the new epithelium is confluent on the pigskin surface. Several subcultures to new pigskin substrate can be achieved by either scraping new growth from the digested pigskin, mincing and replanting onto new pigskin, or by cutting out clear areas and inverting on new pigskin. The pigskin system is especially appropriate for in vitro studies because vertical sectioning of cells growing on pigskin yield histologic sections with excellent definition.

CHARACTERIZATION OF CULTURED HUMAN SKIN CELLS

My colleagues and I began our studies of human skin cells in vitro with attempts to culture epithelium and to use the newly proliferated cells as grafts for burn patients. We have also been interested in the comparative roles of epithelial cells and fibroblasts in the metabolism of chemical carcinogens and as target cells for transforming and mutating agents produced during the metabolic processes. The results of these studies are briefly outlined herein.

1) Human skin epithelium grows as organotypic cultures on the surface of sterile dead pigskin [29, 30, 32].
2) These cultures can serve as epithelial grafts to cover third-degree burn wounds in the donor [30].
3) Human skin epithelial cells invariably have greater hydrocarbon metabolizing activity than skin fibroblasts from the same donor [33].
4) Human fibroblasts are not transformed by methylcholanthrene (MCA), but fibroblasts treated with MCA in the presence of skin epithelial cells become heteroploid after continued culture [33].
5) Human skin epithelial cells show increased levels of unscheduled DNA synthesis upon exposure to chemical carcinogens, but not on exposure to noncarcinogens [34].
6) Human fibroblasts are not mutated to ouabain resistance by MCA, but fibroblasts treated with MCA in the presence of skin epithelial cells mutate at a rate of 1×10^{-6} [35].

CONCLUSIONS

The in vitro culturing of human skin epithelial cells has progressed rapidly in the last few years and methods are now available for producing organotypic, metabolically functional primary and semicontinuous cultures. These techniques may be very valuable in the study of metabolic diseases in general and birth defects in particular because skin is the most readily available of all human organs.

REFERENCES

1. Billingham RE, Reynolds J: Transplantation studies on sheets of pure epidermal epithelium and on epidermal cell suspensions. Br J Plast Surg 5:25–36, 1952.
2. Constable H: Ultrastructure of adult epidermal cells in monolayer culture. Br J Dermatol 86:27–39, 1972.
3. Fusenig NE: Isolation and cultivation of epidermal cells from embryonic mouse skin. Naturwissenschaften 58:421, 1971.
4. Fusenig NE, Worst PKM: Mouse epidermal cell cultures. I. Isolation and cultivation of epidermal cells from adult mouse skin. J Invest Dermatol 63:187–193, 1974.
5. Yuspa SH, Morgan DL, Walker RJ, Bates RR: The growth of fetal mouse skin in cell culture and transplantation to F_1 mice. J Invest Dermatol 55:379–389, 1970.
6. Parshley MS, Simms HS: Cultivation of adult skin epithelial cells (chicken and human) in vitro. Am J Anat 86:163–189, 1950.
7. Harnden DG: A human skin culture technique used for cytological examinations. Br J Exp Pathol 41:31–37, 1960.
8. Karasek MA: In vitro culture of human skin epithelial cells. J Invest Dermatol 47:533–540, 1966.
9. Friedman-Kien AE, Morrill S, Prose PH, Liebhaber H: Culture of adult human skin: In vitro growth and keratinization of epidermal cells. Nature 212:1583–1584, 1966.

10. Flaxman BA, Lutzner MA, Van Scott EJ: Cell maturation and tissue organization in epithelial outgrowths from skin and buccal mucosa in vitro. J Invest Dermatol 49:322–332, 1967.
11. Chopra DP, Flaxman BA: Human epidermal cell cycle in vitro. Br J Dermatol 87:13–17, 1972.
12. Medawar PB: The behavior of mammalian skin epithelium under strictly anaerobic conditions. Quart J Micr Sci 88:27–37, 1947.
13. Medawar PB: The cultivation of adult mammalian skin epithelium in vitro. Quart J Micr Sci 89:187–196, 1948.
14. Bailey PJ: The metabolism of glucose in skin maintained in tissue culture. Br J Dermatol 85:264–271, 1971.
15. Hambrick GW Jr, Lamberg SI, Bloomberg R: Observations on keratinization of human skin in vitro. J Invest Dermatol 47:541–550, 1966.
16. Prose PH, Friedman-Kien AE, Neistein S: Ultrastructural studies of organ cultures of adult human skin. In vitro growth and keratinization of epidermal cells. Lab Invest 17:693–716, 1967.
17. Ulloa-Gregori O, Blocker TG Jr, Nowinski WW, Pomerat CM: The effect of ascitic fluid and of blood serum on the outgrowth of epidermal cells from the human skin in tissue culture. Tex Rep Biol Med 8:400–409, 1950.
18. Everett ET, Livingood CS, Pomerat CM, Hu F: Tissue culture studies on human skin. II. Comparative effects of certain specific contact allergens on sensitized and non-sensitized human skin. J Invest Dermatol 18:193–204, 1952.
19. Hsu TC: Tissue culture studies on human skin. III. Some cytological features of the outgrowth of epithelial cells. Tex Rep Biol Med 10:336–352, 1952.
20. Hu F, Livingood CS, Johnson P, Pomerat CM: Tissue culture studies on human skin. IV. The comparative toxic effects of antibiotics on tissue culture explants of human skin and embryonic chick spleen. J Invest Dermatol 20:357–372, 1953.
21. Matoltsy AG: Human epidermal cells in tissue culture. Transplant Bull 3:99–100, 1956.
22. Smulow JB, Rustigian R, Tye M: Cultivation in vitro of adult human skin and oral mucosa on gelatin film. Proc Soc Exp Biol Med 106:757–762, 1961.
23. Bassett CAL, Evans VJ, Campbell DH, Earle WR: Characteristics and potentials of long-term cultures of human skin. Research Report, Project NM 007 081.10.11, Naval Medical Research Institute, pp 509–528, 1955.
24. Sarkany I, Grice K, Caron GA: Organ culture of adult human skin. Br J Dermatol 77:65–76, 1965.
25. Worst PKM, Valentine EA, Fusenig NE: Formation of epidermis after reimplantation of pure primary epidermal cell cultures from perinatal mouse skin. J Natl Cancer Inst 53:1061–1064, 1974.
26. Reinertson RP: Stratum corneum formation in auto-implants and in explants of human skin. J Invest Dermatol 36:345–357, 1961.
27. Reaven EP, Cox AJ Jr: Organ culture of human skin. J Invest Dermatol 44:151–156, 1965.
28. Reaven EP, Cox AJ: Behavior of adult human skin in organ culture. II. Effects of cellophane tape stripping, temperature, oxygen tension, pH and serum. J Invest Dermatol 50:118–128, 1968.
29. Freeman AE, Igel HJ, Waldman NL, Losikoff AM: A new method for covering large surface area wounds with autografts. I. In vitro multiplication of rabbit-skin epithelial cells. Arch Surg 108:721–723, 1974.
30. Igel HJ, Freeman AE, Boeckman CR, Kleinfeld KL: A new method for covering large surface area wounds with autografts. II. Surgical application of tissue culture expanded rabbit-skin autografts. Arch Surg 108:724–729, 1974.

31. Rheinwald JG, Green H: Serial cultivation of strains of human epidermal keratinocytes: The formation of keratinizing colonies from single cells. Cell 6:331–344, 1975.
32. Lake RS, Freeman AE, Igel HJ, Pezzutti MR, Kropko ML: In vitro culture of diploid human skin epithelial cells for chemical transformation studies. In Saffiotti U, Autrup H (eds): "In Vitro Carcinogenesis. Guide to the Literature, Recent Advances and Laboratory Procedures." NCI Carcinogenesis Tech Rep Ser No 44. DHEW Publ No (NIH) 78–844, 1978, pp 283–291.
33. Freeman AE, Lake RS, Igel HJ, Gernand L, Pezzutti MR, Malone JM, Mark C, Benedict WF: Heteroploid conversion of human skin cells by methylcholanthrene. Proc Natl Acad Sci USA 74:2451–2455, 1977.
34. Lake RS, Kropko ML, Pezzutti MR, Shoemaker RH, Igel HJ: Chemical induction of unscheduled DNA synthesis in human skin epithelial cell cultures. Cancer Res 38:2091–2098, 1978
35. Curren RD, Homer CJ, Price PJ, Freeman AE: Mutagenesis of human cells by 3-methylcholanthrene. Mutat Res 60:109–113, 1979.

In Vitro Growth of Normal and Abnormal Keratinocytes*

Howard P. Baden, MD and Joseph Kubilus, PhD

Human epidermis is a multilayered tissue which undergoes constant replication as a result of cell division in the lowest basal layer. Cells ascend through the spinous layer, granular layer, and stratum corneum, from which they are finally shed. In most areas of the body this transit time is about 28 days with half the time being spent in the viable layers and half in the cornified dead stratum corneum. Cells which leave the basal layer are no longer capable of division and undergo differentiation. The stimulus for this process is not "mitotic pressure" but part of the regulatory process controlling epidermal differentiation.

The most characteristic and constant product of the epidermal cell is the fibrous protein which is organized into filaments that run through the cell and into the attachment plaques of desmosomes [1]. The filaments have a diameter of 80 Å and are organized into larger bundles. These bundles are also present in the cornified cells of the horny layer, although the protein, as discussed below, has altered physicochemical properties. Studies of bovine snout [2, 3] and perihoof epidermis [4] have shown that the protein of the malpighian (living) layer can be extracted by citrate buffer, pH 2.65, and is insoluble in the pH range of 3 to 10. Polyacrylamide gel electrophoresis (PAGE) in the presence of SDS indicates that up to 7 fibrous polypeptides are present in the fibrous protein, but that 3 polypeptides are organized into a basic α-helical fibrous protein which shows 9.8 Å equatorial and 5.14 Å meridional reflections by x-ray diffraction [5, 6]. No single polypeptide, however, is capable of forming the fibrous protein. These data indicate there are a number of keratin molecules in the cell consisting of different combinations of the fibrous polypeptides. When the protein is allowed to aggregate, dimers are formed, with 2 molecules lying side by side, and then more extensive polymerization occurs with end-to-end as well as side-to-side attachment.

*Supported by NIH grant AM-06838 and a gift from the Avon Corporation.

Birth Defects: Original Article Series, Volume XVI, Number 2, pages 175–181

In human epidermis the citrate-soluble protein consists of 4 principal fibrous polypeptides with molecular weights of 47,000, 51,000, 59,000, and 67,000 daltons, as well as 3 minor ones [7]. The fibrous proteins from different individuals show variation in the relative proportion of the different polypeptides. The solubility of the fibrous protein is similar to that observed in bovine epidermis as is the x-ray diffraction pattern. It has not as yet been demonstrated whether the arrangement of polypeptides is the same as in bovine epidermis. The fibrous protein of the stratum corneum requires denaturing solvents for solubilization and 0.1 M Tris, pH 9.0, with 8.0 M urea and 0.1 M mercaptoethanol (Tris-urea-mercaptoethanol) is an excellent one. The polypeptide composition of whole stratum corneum fibrous protein is very similar to that of the citrate-soluble protein, but disulfide cross-links are present in the former and not in the latter. Stratum corneum obtained by scraping the surface of the skin is quite different, however, showing bands of 50,000 and 62,000 daltons, indicating some posttranslational modifications of the fibrous proteins.

Another important structural component of the epidermis is keratohyalin which is synthesized in the granular layer just beneath the stratum corneum and appears as various sized granules [8]. The granules contain 2 morphologically distinct components, at least in some species [9]. The small ones (DHD) contain a histidine-rich protein. The proline- and cystine-rich protein gives rise to the cornified envelope (discussed below) [10] and the histidine-rich protein may act as a matrix material around the filaments in the stratum corneum.

As the cells of the granular layer cornify, an envelope is deposited under the plasma membrane. This cornified membrane is insoluble even in denaturing solvents as a result of ϵ - (γ - glutamyl) lysine cross-links [11]. A transglutaminase enzyme has been identified in the epidermis which produces these cross-links [12]. The envelope is rich in cystine and proline and probably consists of a number of different polypeptides [13].

Lamellar granules (MCGs) also appear in the granular layer and consist of lipids and proteins [14]. These are extruded into the intercellular space and fill it, which suggests they act as a cementing substance and contribute to the barrier function of the stratum corneum [15].

Another essential structure in the epidermis is the desmosome [16], a multi-layered structure connecting adjacent cell surfaces. As cells move in the viable epidermis the desmosomes come apart and are reformed, but it has not been established how this occurs. The desmosome is progressively modified in the stratum corneum where it is broken down as the cells are shed from the surface.

There are 2 other important enzyme markers of epidermis, histidase [17] and the arginine-to-citrulline-converting enzyme [18]. Histidase deaminates free histidine to urocanic acid which remains in the stratum corneum. It is absent in malignant tumors of the epidermis and is not found in the epidermis of mucous membranes. The other enzyme converts peptide-bound arginine to peptide-bound citrulline and is specific for certain substrates. It does not deaminate free arginine. It has only recently been described and little is known about it.

A final characteristic marker of epidermis is a lipid with a 4.15 Å meridional x-ray diffraction pattern [19]. It is a polar lipid but not saponifiable and its structure has not been elucidated.

A number of techniques for growing epidermis have been described by Freeman (this volume) but we have had the most experience with the 3T3 feeder technique described by Rheinwald and Green [20]. The 3T3 cells are killed by treatment with mitomycin C (10 μg/ml) and 140,000 cells are plated on 35-mm plastic dishes. Epidermis is separated from skin by overnight treatment with 0.25% trypsin at 4°C. The cells are suspended in Dulbecco medium with 20% fetal calf serum (FCS) and 100,000 are plated on the 3T3 cells. The primary cultures have a plating efficiency of about 0.1% but show plating efficiencies of about 10% in subsequent passages. The cells reach confluency in about 2 weeks, have a doubling time of about 24 hours, and can be passed through about 50 generations. Hydrocortisone is said to help growth and epidermal growth factor increases the number of passages but not the growth rate of the cells. The cultures show multiple layers after reaching confluency, with the upper layers appearing as flat squames. Cornified cells are shed into the medium at this time.

We have found that both citrate buffer, pH 2.65, soluble as well as Tris-urea-mercaptoethanol soluble protein can be isolated from the cultures. The percentage of Tris-urea-mercaptoethanol soluble protein increases in late cultures and is the only protein found in the shed cornified cells. The SDS PAGE patterns of citrate-soluble and Tris-urea-mercaptoethanol soluble proteins of cultured cells are identical but different than those of the epidermis from which they were derived (Fig. 1), with 2 bands apparently missing. Although there appears to be a new band, a weak band with similar mobility is seen in some samples of normal epidermis. Therefore it may be a normal component but present in much greater amount.

Cornified envelopes resistant to solubilization by 1% SDS and 1% mercapto-ethanol in 0.1 M Tris, pH 9.0, are present in cultures. ϵ - (γ - glutamyl) Lysine cross-links have been identified in the envelopes and the cross-linking enzyme is present in cell extracts.

Histidase activity is absent in cultured cells after the first medium change and is not found in cells allowed to grow for up to 45 days. The arginine-to-citrulline-converting enzyme does appear to be present. The lipid with a 4.15 Å equatorial reflection is not found in growing keratinocytes or in cells shed into the medium.

Desmosomes can be readily identified in cultured cells but MCGs have not been looked for thoroughly. Keratohyalin granules are very sparse but we have not looked for the 2 protein components.

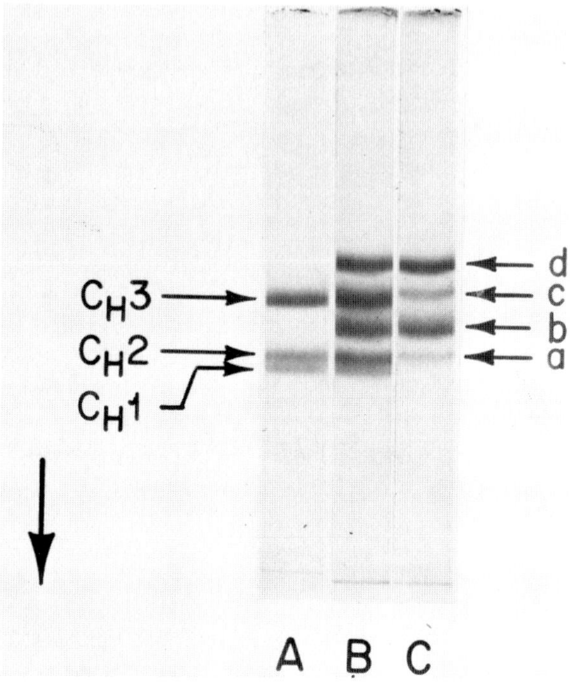

Fig. 1. SDS PAGE of fibrous proteins of cultured human keratinocytes (A) and the epidermis from which they were derived (C). "B" is coelectrophoresis of "A" and "C." A band corresponding to C_H1 is found in some samples of human epidermis. (From Kubilus J, Macdonald MJ, Baden HP: Epidermal proteins of cultured human and bovine keratinocytes. Biochim Biophys Acta, 1979, with permission.)

There are a number of genetic disorders that could be conveniently and effectively studied using tissue culture techniques. These include the various forms of ichthyosis, ichthyosis vulgaris, X-linked ichthyosis, lamellar ichthyosis, and epidermolytic hyperkeratosis [21]. These disorders have distinctive morphologic features which can readily be recognized in culture, such as thickening of the stratum corneum or ballooning of the granular layer. The report that X-linked ichthyosis occurred in families with absent steroid sulfatase [22] prompted us to look for the enzyme in individuals who were ascertained as having X-linked ichthyosis. Nine individuals in 8 families were found to be missing the enzyme in their cultured fibroblasts. One individual with ichthyosis vulgaris had normal activity as did one with lamellar ichthyosis. Epidermis was cultured from 2 affected individuals and the enzyme was found to be missing, although cultured normal keratinocytes had enzyme activity comparable to that of normal cultured fibroblasts. The epidermal cultures did not appear to grow abnormally, but the cells were only carried for 20 days and all the plates were used for enzyme assay. Finding the enzyme abnormality in affected epidermis coupled with the failure to find other tissue involved, suggests there may be a primary abnormality of sulfate metabolism in the epidermis. This enzyme is known to have a number of substrates and one may be important for cell attachment.

In both ichthyosis vulgaris and X-linked ichthyosis the primary morphologic defect appears to be retention of stratum corneum cells. Since an absence of steroid sulfatase is only found in the X-linked form, it is clear that the genetic defect must be different in these diseases. Tissue culture affords the opportunity of studying the epidermal cells in a defined environment and observing whether there is an abnormal retention of cornified cells. One difficulty with our present culture technique is that it does not permit a full expression of differentiation. For example, retention of nuclei and absence of lipids is characteristic of cultured cells but not of intact normal stratum corneum. It may be necessary to modify culture conditions to favor differentiation. One alternative is to use a different support such as dead pigskin which appears, at least at the histologic level, to produce a very complete stratum corneum [23]. Thus cells could be started on 3T3 feeders and then tested on another feeder such as dead pigskin.

In epidermolytic hyperkeratosis, abnormalities are observed in the malpighian layer with ballooning of cells at the granular level. These kinds of changes would be readily recognized by microscopy and the abnormality in the disease would easily be recognized in culture. This is also true for another disorder of keratinization, Darier disease [24], where acantholysis (premature separation of cells) and abnormally differentiated cells are a striking feature. In both these diseases the skin may not be universally involved and it would be important to compare epidermis from affected and normal skin. Here again, if the abnormality was not brought out by our usual culture system, modifications could be tried including different substrates.

A very common and important disorder of the skin which is amenable to study is psoriasis. It has been shown that epidermal hyperplasia and abnormal scale production are important features and that the relative proportion of epidermal fibrous polypeptides in affected epidermis is different than normal and unaffected epidermis (Fig. 2) [25, 26]. It has not been established that there is a primary epidermal defect and the epidermal change could be a response to some dermal abnormality such as in the vasculature or in fibroblast metabolism. We have begun studies evaluating psoriatic fibroblasts as feeder layers and have not as yet observed any difference from normal fibroblasts or 3T3 cells. Initial studies on the growth and differentiation of psoriatic epidermal cells in culture have also not shown abnormal findings. These results are still too preliminary, and further work along such lines should lead to a more complete understanding of the disease.

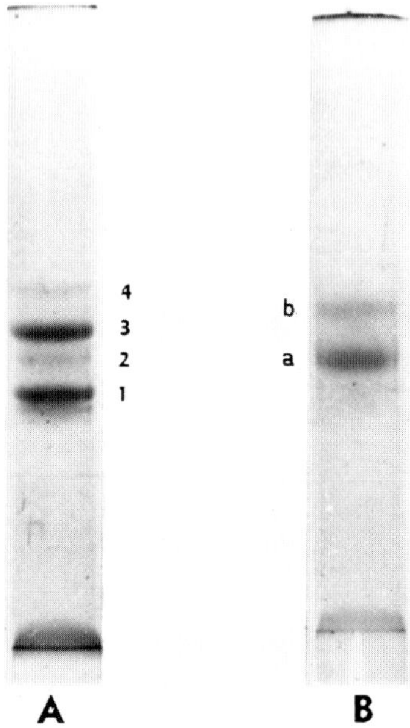

Fig. 2. SDS PAGE of fibrous proteins extracted from stratum corneum scraped from the surface of affected psoriatic skin (A) and normal skin (B). "a" and "2" have the same mobility and "b" is between "3" and "4". (From Baden HP, McGilvray N, Cheng CK, Lee LD, Kubilus J: The keratin polypeptides of psoriatic epidermis. J Invest Dermatol 70:294–297, 1978, with permission.)

CONCLUSION

Differentiation of normal epidermis involves a series of complex morphologic and biochemical changes which can now be studied in the laboratory. Tissue culture can be used to study these events and holds promise for examining genetic disorders of the epidermis where many of these pathways may be abnormal.

REFERENCES

1. Brody I: The ultrastructure of the tonofibrils in the keratinization process of normal human epidermis. J Ultrastruct Res 4:264–297, 1960.
2. Matoltsy AG: Soluble prekeratin. In Lyne AG, Short BF (eds): "Biology of the Skin and Hair Growth." New York: American Elsevier Publishing Co, 1965, pp 291–305.
3. Lee LD, Fleming BC, Waitkus RF, Baden HP: Isolation of the polypeptide chains of prekeratin. Biochim Biophys Acta 412:82–90, 1975.

4. Steinert PM, Idler WW: Polypeptide composition of bovine epidermal α-keratin. Biochem J 151:603–614, 1975.
5. Steinert PM: The mechanism of assembly of bovine epidermal keratin filaments in vitro. In Seiji M, Bernstein IA (eds): "Biochemistry of Cutaneous Epidermal Differentiation." Baltimore: University Park Press, 1977, pp 444–466.
6. Baden HP, Lee LD: The structure of epidermal keratin. Ibid pp 478–492.
7. Baden HP, Lee LD, Kubilus J: The fibrous proteins of stratum corneum. J Invest Dermatol 67:573–576, 1976.
8. Selby CC: An electron microscope study of thin sections of human skin. J Invest Dermatol 29:131–149, 1957.
9. Fukuyama K, Wier KA, Epstein WL: Dense homogeneous deposits of keratohyalin granules in newborn rat epidermis. J Ultrastruct Res 38:16–26, 1972.
10. Matoltsy AG, Matoltsy MN: Chemical nature of keratohyalin granules of the epidermis. J Cell Biol 47:593–603, 1970.
11. Sugawara K: Intermolecular cross-links in epidermal differentiation. Supra #5 pp 387–397.
12. Goldsmith LA, Baden HP, Roth SI, Colman R, Lee L, Fleming B: Vertebral epidermal transamidases. Biochim Biophys Acta 351:113–125, 1974.
13. Matoltsy AG, Matoltsy MN: The membrane protein of horny cells. J Invest Dermatol 46:127–129, 1966.
14. Odland GF: A submicroscopic granular component in human epidermis. J Invest Dermatol 34:11–15, 1960.
15. Elias PM, Goerke J, Friend DS: Mammalian epidermal barrier layer lipids: Composition and influence on structure. J Invest Dermatol 69:535–546, 1977.
16. Odland GF: The fine structure of the interrelationship of cells in human epidermis. J Biophys Biochem Cytol 4:529–538, 1958.
17. Baden HP, Pathak MA: Urocanic acid in keratinizing tissue. Biochim Biophys Acta 104:200–204, 1965.
18. Kubilus J, Baden HP: The enzymatic conversion of protein bound arginine to protein bound citrulline in epidermis. Fed Proc 37:2795, 1978.
19. Goldsmith LA, Baden HP: Uniquely oriented epidermal lipid. Nature 225:1052–1053, 1970.
20. Rheinwald JG, Green H: Serial cultivation of strains of human epidermal keratinocytes: The formation of keratinizing colonies from single cells. Cell 6:331–344, 1975.
21. Frost P, Weinstein GD: Ichthyosiform dermatoses. In Fitzpatrick TB, Arndt KA, Clark WH Jr, Eisen AZ, Van Scott EJ, Vaughan JH (eds): "Dermatology in General Medicine." New York: McGraw-Hill Co, 1971, pp 249–265.
22. Shapiro LJ, Weiss R, Webster D, France JT: X-linked ichthyosis due to steroid-sulphatase deficiency. Lancet 1:70–72, 1978.
23. Freeman AE, Igel HJ, Waldman NL, Losikoff AM: In vitro multiplication of rabbit-skin epithelial cells. Arch Surg 108:721–723, 1974.
24. White JC: A case of keratosis (ichthyosis) follicularis. J Cutan Genito-Urin Dis 7:201–209, 1889.
25. Van Scott EJ, Ekel TM: Kinetics of hyperplasia in psoriasis. Arch Dermatol 88:373–381, 1963.
26. Baden HP, McGilvray N, Cheng CK, Lee LD, Kubilus J: The keratin polypeptides of psoriatic epidermis. J Invest Dermatol 70:294-297, 1978.

The Use of Antikeratin Antibodies for the Identification of Cultured Epithelial Cells*

Tung-Tien Sun, PhD,† Thomas I. Doran, PhD, and Alda Vidrich, PhD

INTRODUCTION

Cell culture techniques have been used extensively for the study of the molecular basis of hereditary diseases. Although epithelial abnormalities are known to exist in a number of these diseases, most work has been done with fibroblasts which adapt well to culture conditions and frequently outgrow other cell types [1]. In order to facilitate the study of normal and abnormal epithelial cells in culture, a simple and specific way of identifying these cells is desirable.

Since the morphology of cultured cells can sometimes be affected drastically by alterations of culture conditions [2], examination of these cells by light microscopy does not always provide reliable information concerning their identity.

Certain characteristic subcellular structures, if they exist, can be used for the identification of cell types. For example, tonofilaments and desmosomes are found in many epithelial cells and have been frequently regarded as markers for these cells. However, the use of such morphologic markers, even at the electron microscopic level, can sometimes be misleading. Filaments with diameters similar to those of tonofilaments are present in many nonepithelial cell types. These include the neurofilaments and glial filaments of nerve cells, desmin filaments of muscle cells, and intermediate-sized filaments of fibroblasts, endothelial cells, and melanocytes [3–6]. Although there is ample evidence suggesting that tonofilaments and the above-mentioned filaments are distinct biochemically, it may

*Supported in part by grants from the National Eye Institute (EY 02472), the National Institute of Arthritis, Metabolism and Digestive Diseases (AM 25140 and AM 21358), and the American Cancer Society (IN-11p).

†Recipient of a Research Career Development Award from the National Eye Institute (EY 00125).

Birth Defects: Original Article Series, Volume XVI, Number 2, pages 183–196

be difficult to distinguish them morphologically. In addition, desmosomes are present in a number of nonepithelial, mesenchyme-derived cells such as those of cardiac muscle [7]. Thus, the demonstration of (tono) filaments and/or desmosomes in a particular cell type does not constitute a proof that the cells in question are of epithelial origin. An additional limitation in the use of electron microscopy for the identification of cultured cells is that only a small number of cells can be examined, rendering the detection and identification of minor cell types in a heterogeneous population difficult and impractical.

IMMUNOLOGIC MARKERS OF CULTURED CELLS

By definition, differentiated cell types are distinct from each other morphologically and functionally. The molecular basis of such differences may be qualitative since certain molecules may be present only in special cell types, or quantitative since certain molecules may be present in greater quantities in particular cell types, or a combination of both. Although quantitative differences are useful, specific qualitative differences provide the greatest potential usefulness for the unambiguous identification of different cell types.

The molecular marker(s) specific for a particular cell type may be isolated and used for antiserum production. With specific antibodies, cells containing relevant antigens can be identified by the immunofluorescent staining technique. The advantages of using such an approach for identifying cultured cells include: 1) Simplicity: With cells grown on glass coverslips, the staining reaction can be completed within 4–5 hours and rapid decisions concerning the subsequent manipulation of parallel cultures can be made. 2) Specificity: The staining is highly specific if proper controls are performed to ensure the immunologic nature of the reaction. The staining also yields information concerning cellular localization (eg cytoplasmic or nuclear) as well as any special organization (eg fibrous or granular) of the antigens. 3) Sensitivity: Small quantities of antigens, even if present in a single cell among a heterogeneous population, can sometimes be detected easily. 4) Versatility: Mixed as well as pure cell populations can be used as substrate for the immunofluorescent staining. Furthermore, parallel samples can be stained with antibodies prepared against different antigens and the results compared.

Recently, keratins from stratum corneum of human epidermis have been isolated and specific antisera prepared in rabbits [3, 8, 9]. With these antisera, Sun and Green [3, 8, 10] found that keratin-related filaments are present in a wide variety of epithelial cells, many of them covering the surface of internal organs. Similar conclusions have been reached by Franke and co-workers [5, 11, 12]. Antikeratin can therefore be used as an immunologic reagent for the detection and identification of these epithelial cells in culture. Experimental evidence in support of this statement will be reviewed in the following sections.

KERATIN FILAMENTS IN EPIDERMAL CELLS: GENERAL ASPECTS

Keratins are a group of water-insoluble structural proteins associated with tonofilaments of the epidermal cell and its appendages [13]. Epidermal keratins from cows [5, 11, 14–20], rats [21–24], and humans [8, 9, 25–27] have been studied extensively in recent years. In general, these keratins consist of 2–6 related polypeptide chains which can be reassembled in vitro into 80 Å filaments [9, 28, 29].

Using lethally irradiated fibroblasts as feeder cells, Rheinwald and Green [30] succeeded in the serial cultivation of human epidermal cells, thereby opening a new avenue for studying keratins in living epidermal cells. Such cells synthesize abundant water-insoluble proteins (approximately 30% of the total cellular protein) similar to keratins isolated from human (in vivo) stratum corneum in their molecular weight range (40,000–63,000), their immunologic reactivity, and their ability to reconstitute filaments in vitro. However, detailed comparison of the proteins by 2-dimensional gel electrophoresis shows that there are differences between the keratins of cultured human epidermal cells and of stratum corneum with respect to their exact molecular size, their number of components, and their charge heterogeneity. The latter is in part related to the extensive phosphorylation of some of the keratin proteins [9].

It has also been found that keratins of (dead) stratum corneum are completely crosslinked by intermolecular disulfide bonds, whereas most of the keratins of (living) cultured human epidermal cells are not. When tonofilaments of cultured epidermal cells or stratum corneum are solubilized and the filaments reconstituted under aerobic conditions, they both become completely disulfide-crosslinked and consequently become insoluble in solutions of 8 M urea or sodium dodecyl sulfate. These results suggest that the degree of disulfide-crosslinking of the keratins is determined by the oxidative state of the environment. When, as a result of terminal differentiation, cellular metabolism ceases and the reducing environment of the cytoplasm is lost, the sulfhydryl groups of the keratin proteins are oxidized and neighboring proteins in the tonofilaments become disulfide-crosslinked and stabilized [9].

IMMUNOLOGIC STUDIES OF KERATIN PROTEINS

The purification and characterization of keratin antigens from human stratum corneum have been described previously [8, 9, 31]. Sun and Green [9] isolated keratins from epidermal callus clipped from fingers and toes. This callus (which consists of a form of stratum corneum) was minced, extracted with 20 mM Tris-HCl (pH 7.4), and then extracted again with the same buffer containing 8 M urea to remove the nonkeratin proteins. The remaining keratins, stabilized by intermolecular disulfide bonds, were dissolved in 8 M urea containing β-mercaptoethanol. In SDS gel electrophoresis the solubilized keratin fraction produces 4 major and 3 minor bands, all with molecular weights between 40,000 and 63,000. The proteins can be assembled in vitro into typical 80 Å filaments [9].

Antisera against this keratin fraction were raised in rabbits [9] and their specificity for keratins established in a variety of tests. In double immunodiffusion the antisera produce precipitin bands when tested against stratum corneum keratins and against the extracts of cultured epidermal cells. No precipitin band is formed with serum proteins or extracts of fibroblasts [8]. The antisera contain antibodies against all major keratin bands and stain by indirect immunofluorescence all cellular layers of the epidermis [3].

Such antisera have been used to study the intracellular distribution and organization of the keratin proteins in cultured cells. When epithelial cells of skin and cornea are grown on coverslips and stained by indirect immunofluorescence with antikeratin, their cytoplasm stains very brightly. In those cells which are flattened, a discrete network of fibers can be observed (Fig. 1).

Even though our antisera were prepared against keratins isolated from human stratum corneum, the same antisera cross-react with keratins from rabbits [3], mice [3], and rat kangaroos [10]. Similar immunologic cross-reactivity has been described for keratins from several vertebrates [31, 32], including the amphibian [12]. Thus, the primary structure of keratin proteins seems to be conserved to a large extent during evolution.

Recently, keratins of human stratum corneum have been fractionated electrophoretically and antisera prepared against the major purified components. Rabbit antisera against the 63K and 46K keratins were prepared by Fuchs and Green [27] and those against the 65K and 55K proteins by us. Guinea pig antisera against all 4 major human proteins have also been obtained (Vidrich and Sun, in preparation).

Antisera against the 63K and 46K keratins were found to cross-react with all major human epidermal keratin subunits [27], a result consistent with the findings that different keratin subunits are structurally related [17] and contain common peptides [27]. Common antigenic determinants in various keratin subunits have also been demonstrated in keratins of the rat [22] and the cow [18].

KERATIN-RELATED FILAMENTS ARE PRESENT IN A VARIETY OF EPITHELIAL CELLS

As mentioned previously, filaments with a diameter of approximately 80 Å are present in many epithelial cells and are frequently associated with desmosomes. Although they have often been called "tonofilaments," the relationships between them and the (keratin) tonofilaments of epidermal cells were not known until recently [3, 5, 10, 11]. In experiments conducted by Sun, Shih, and

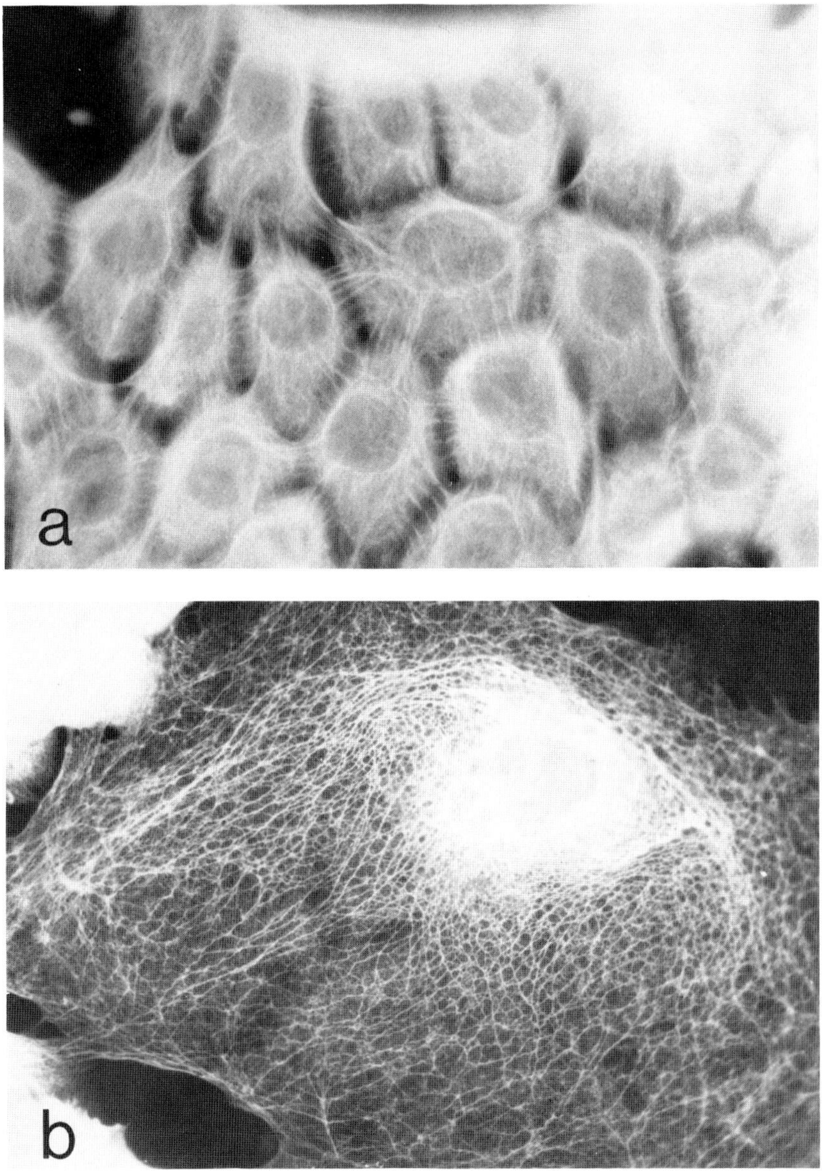

Fig. 1. Immunofluorescent staining of keratin fibers in cultured keratinocytes. a) Human epidermal cells and b) rabbit corneal epithelial cells. These cells were grown on glass coverslips, fixed with 10% formalin, made permeable with methanol, reacted with rabbit antikeratin and then with FITC-conjugated goat anti-rabbit IgG[3]. Viewed by fluorescent microscopy. (From Sun T-T, Green H: Immunofluorescent staining of keratin fibers in cultured cells. Cell 14:469–476, 1978, copyright © by The MIT Press, with permission.)

Green [10], a rabbit antiserum against human epidermal keratins has been used to detect related antigens in frozen sections of various rabbit and human tissues by indirect immunofluorescent staining. Strong staining can be observed in all stratified squamous epithelia (epidermis, cornea, tongue, esophagus, and anus), in epidermal appendages (hair follicle, sebaceous gland, ductal and myoepithelial cells of the sweat gland), and in Hassall corpuscle of the thymus, indicating that all contain abundant keratins. The antiserum also stains the cells of epithelia of the gastrointestinal tract, the urinary tract (urethra, bladder, ureter, collecting ducts of the kidney), the female genital tract (cervix, cervical glands, uterus, oviduct), and the respiratory tract (trachea, bronchi). Epithelial cells of the fine ductal systems in the pancreas and submaxillary gland also stain well. The results [10] are summarized schematically in Figure 2. This figure illustrates that, perhaps with the exception of Hassall corpuscles, all epithelial cells so far shown to contain keratins cover luminal surfaces which are contiguous with the external body integument.

Since it is difficult to demonstrate the detailed nature of the staining in frozen sections, cells from several of the internal organs, including bladder (see below), kidney, intestine, and trachea, have been grown on glass coverslips and stained with antikeratin [10]. Fibrillar networks similar to those of the cultured epidermal cells are observed in "epithelial" cells but not in "fibroblastic" cells. The fact that these fibers are resistant to cytochalasin B and colcemid suggests that they are distinct from microfilaments and microtubules [3]. Similar results have been obtained by Franke et al [5, 11, 12] in which guinea pig antisera against total and purified bovine keratins have been found to cross-react with tonofilament-like structures in a number of epithelial cells. These results show that keratins constitute a cytoskeleton in epithelial cells of diverse morphology and embryologic origin [3, 5, 8, 10–12]. The stability of keratin tonofilaments presumably confers the structural strength necessary for epithelial cells covering a free surface [10].

KERATIN FILAMENTS ARE DISTINCT FROM INTERMEDIATE-SIZED FILAMENTS OF NONEPITHELIAL CELLS

The intermediate-sized filaments of many nonepithelial cells (eg fibroblasts, nerve cells, and muscle cells) may be distinguished from each other immunologically and biochemically [4, 6, 34]. Furthermore, desmin (muscle) filaments [6] and fibroblast filaments [3, 5] seem to be unrelated to keratin filaments.

Fig. 2. A schematic drawing summarizing the distribution of keratin-containing epithelial cells, based on the results described by Sun et al [10]. Frozen sections of various tissues were stained by immunofluorescence with antikeratin and epithelial cells which stain very strongly (solid lines), strongly (cross-hatched lines), or moderately (hatched lines) are indicated.

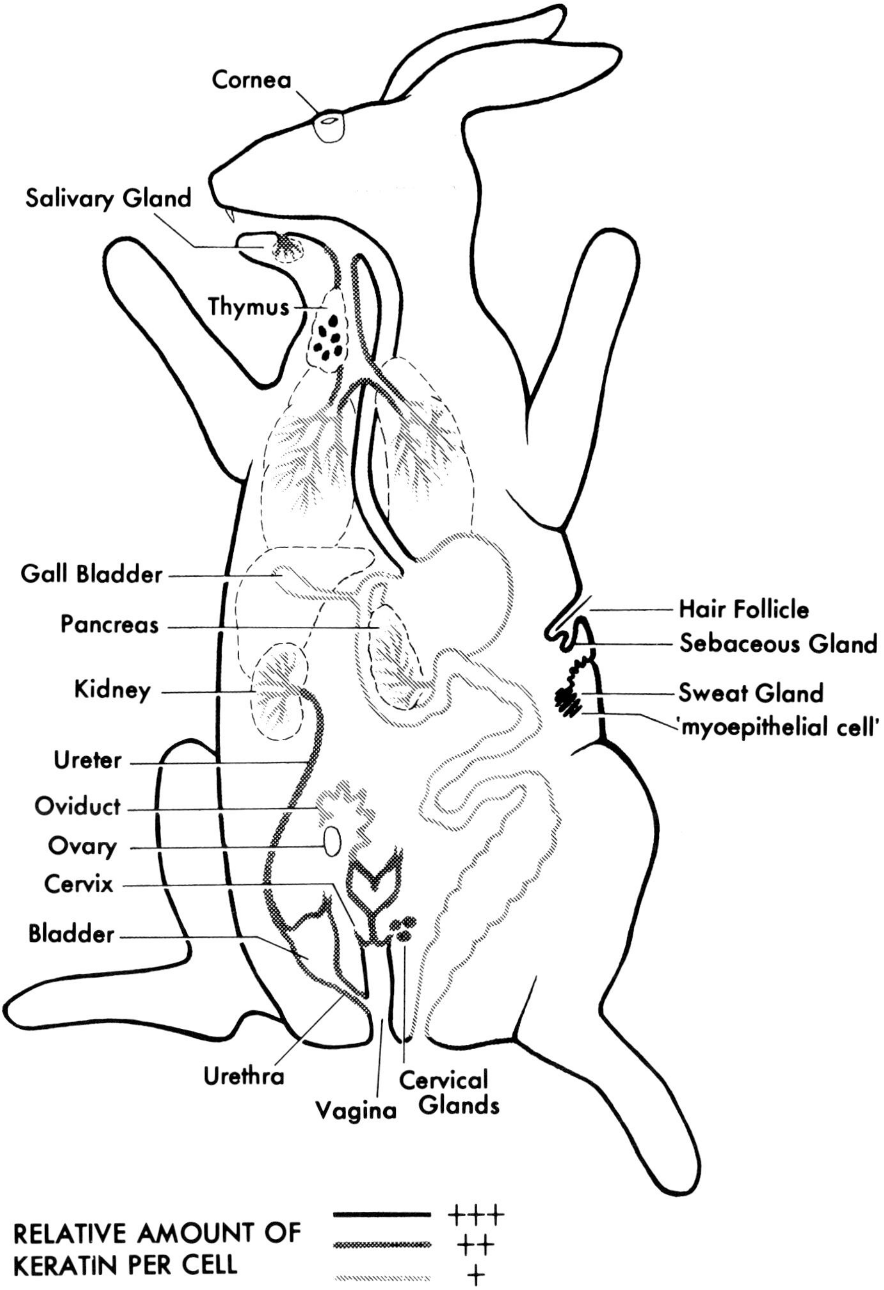
Cornea
Salivary Gland
Thymus
Gall Bladder
Pancreas
Kidney
Ureter
Oviduct
Ovary
Cervix
Bladder
Urethra
Vagina
Cervical Glands
Hair Follicle
Sebaceous Gland
Sweat Gland
'myoepithelial cell'
RELATIVE AMOUNT OF KERATIN PER CELL
+++
++
+

To investigate further the relationship between keratin and other filaments, antikeratin was used to stain frozen sections of tissues and cultured cells known to contain intermediate filaments. The finding that none of the nonepithelial cells are stained by the antisera indicates that their filament systems are immunologically distinct from keratins [3, 5, 10]. Antikeratin can therefore be used to distinguish those epithelial cells which contain tonofilaments from other cells including fibroblasts, muscle cells, nerve cells, and endothelial cells.

IDENTIFICATION OF RABBIT URINARY BLADDER EPITHELIAL CELLS IN CULTURE

As has been shown previously [10], frozen sections of bladder epithelium stained well by immunofluorescence with antikeratin (Fig. 3). Experiments involving the isolation and cultivation of rabbit bladder epithelial cells [10] (also Sun, Doran, and Bonitz, in preparation) will be briefly described here to illustrate the use of antikeratin antibodies for the identification of cultured epithelial cells.

Cells from the mucosa of the urinary bladder of freshly killed rabbit were disaggregated by brief trypsinization and then plated in Dulbecco's modified Eagle's medium containing 20% fetal bovine serum. Two major morphologic cell types were obtained in culture: one was "epithelial" in morphology and the other was "fibroblastic." The epithelial cells formed well-defined colonies (Fig. 4a) with a stratified squamous structure somewhat similar to that of cultured epidermal cells [30, 37] and corneal epithelial cells [8]. Like keratinocytes (stratified squamous epithelial cells which contain a large amount of keratins [10]), their colony initiation at low plating density depended absolutely on suitable fibroblast support. When tested with antikeratin antibodies, the cells showed strong cytoplasmic staining (Fig. 4c); flattened cells showed stained cytoplasmic networks of discrete fibers. Such results suggest that this cell type is derived from bladder epithelium.*

*Occasionally, another "epithelial" cell type appeared in culture. These cells showed "contact-inhibition" of growth and formed a cobblestone-like monolayer when confluent. Unlike keratinocytes, they grew well without the support of fibroblasts. Staining with antikeratin was weak, indicating that they did not contain keratins. Since some of these properties are consistent with those described for endothelial cells [35] and since abundant blood vessels are known to be present immediately underneath the bladder epithelium [36], it is possible that this cell type represents endothelial cells. Further investigations are in progress to identify this cell type.

Fig. 3. Immunofluorescent staining of frozen sections of rabbit bladder by antikeratin antiserum. a) Phase contrast microscopy. b) Same section as shown in (a) stained with antikeratin and viewed by fluorescent microscopy. Note the strong staining of all cellular layers of the epithelium which is barely discernible in (a), and the absence of staining in the underlying connective tissues. c) A neighboring section treated with pre-immune serum. Viewed by fluorescent microscopy.

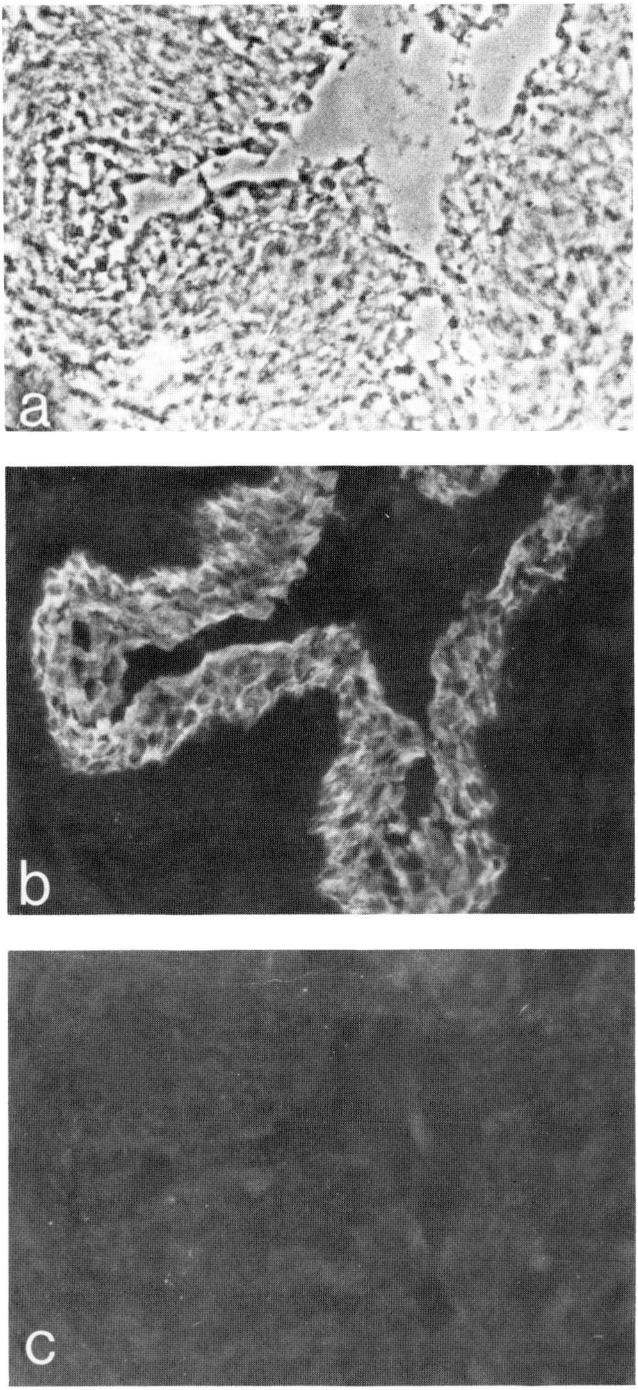
a
b
c

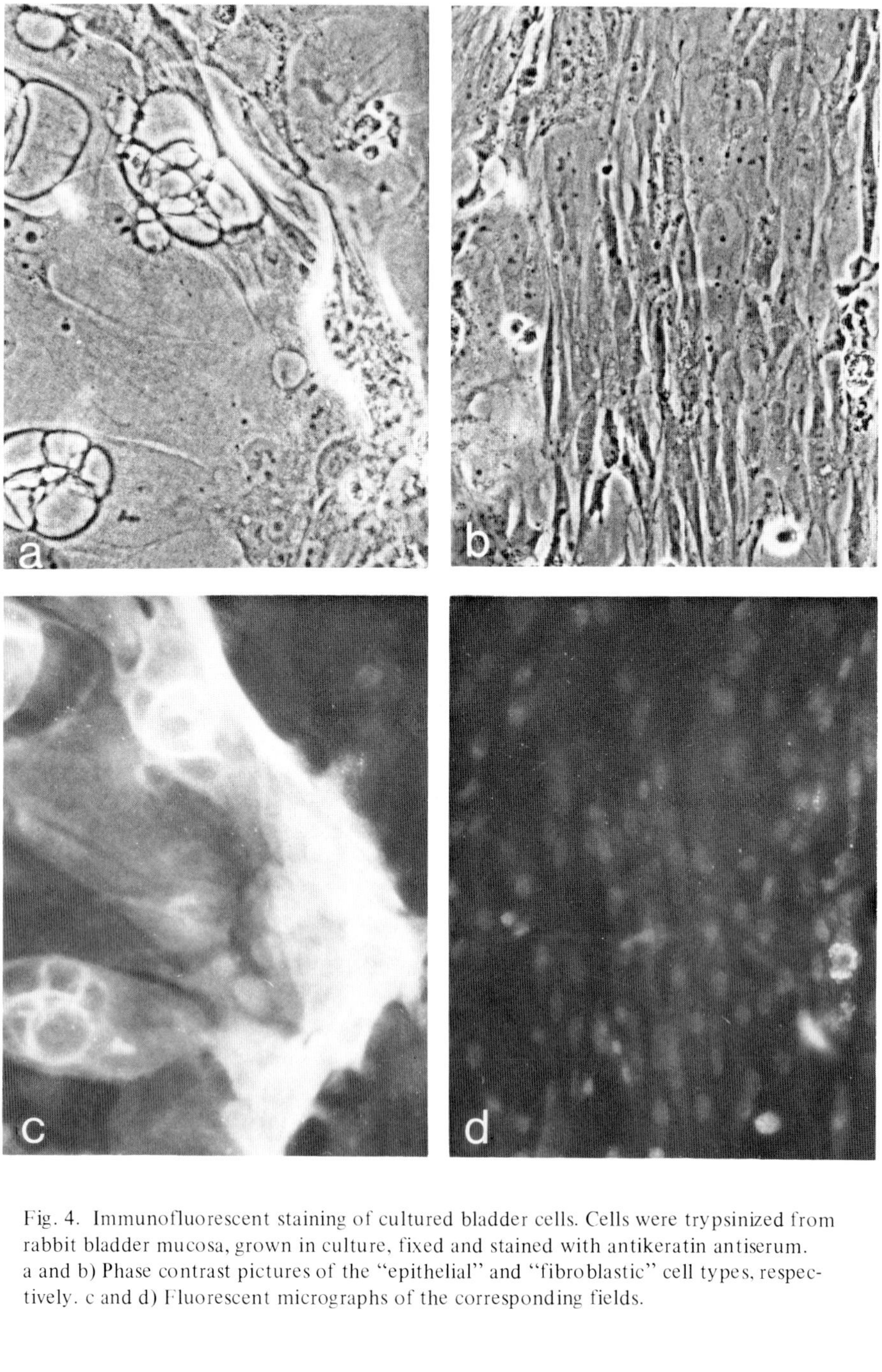

Fig. 4. Immunofluorescent staining of cultured bladder cells. Cells were trypsinized from rabbit bladder mucosa, grown in culture, fixed and stained with antikeratin antiserum. a and b) Phase contrast pictures of the "epithelial" and "fibroblastic" cell types, respectively. c and d) Fluorescent micrographs of the corresponding fields.

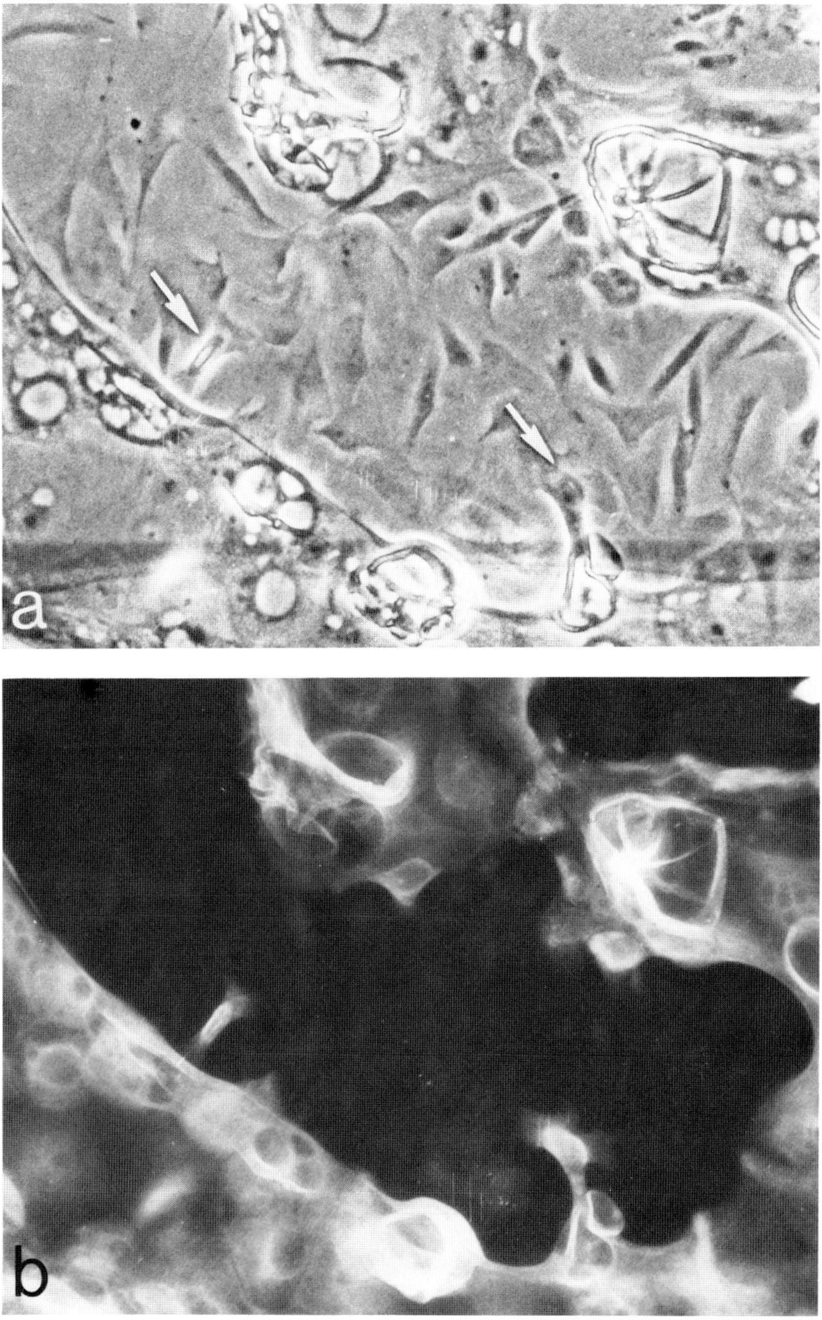

Fig. 5. Identification of single bladder epithelial cells in culture by antikeratin staining. An 11-day-old primary culture of bladder cells was fixed and stained. a) Phase contrast microscopy of a group of fibroblastic cells surrounded by epithelial cells. Arrows indicate 2 cells which are somewhat fibroblast-like. The strong staining of these 2 cells by antikeratin, however, indicates their epithelial nature. b) Fluorescent picture of the same field.

The morphology and growth properties of the other major cell type (Fig. 4b) are similar to those of fibroblasts from other sources. Consistent with such a presumptive fibroblastic nature, no staining was observed with the antikeratin antibodies (Fig. 4d) [3, 5, 10].

The sensitivity of antikeratin staining for the detection of single epithelial cells in a mixed cell population is illustrated in Figure 5 [3]. Figure 5a is the phase contrast picture of a group of rabbit bladder fibroblasts surrounded by epithelial cells, and Figure 5b is the immunofluorescent picture of the same field after antikeratin staining. Comparison of the 2 pictures (5a and b) indicates that 2 cells (arrows), morphologically similar to the surrounding fibroblasts, are strongly stained and must be bladder epithelial cells, probably migrating out from the main colony.

CONCLUSIONS

An antiserum prepared against the total keratin fraction of human stratum corneum has been shown by indirect immunofluorescence to stain a wide variety of epithelial cells [3, 10], many of them lining the surfaces of internal organs and known to contain tonofilament-like subcellular structures. The specificity of the staining reaction is supported by the observation that similar staining can be obtained with antibodies prepared against individual purified keratin subunits (Vidrich and Sun, in preparation). Furthermore, fibrillar cytoplasmic staining patterns are observed when epithelial cells derived from such organs are grown on coverslips and stained with the antiserum. Similar results have been obtained by Franke and co-workers [5, 11, 12]. Thus, tonofilaments of epidermal cells and many other epithelial cells are related immunologically.

Since connective-tissue-derived cells, including fibroblasts, endothelial cells, and muscle cells, do not contain any appreciable amount of keratins, the staining of cultured cells by antikeratin provides a simple, specific, and sensitive method for the detection and identification of epithelial cells derived from many organs.

Furthermore, the immunofluorescent staining pattern of frozen sections of the intact organs yields information concerning the in vivo origin of the cultured epithelial cells [10]. Because keratin structures have been relatively conserved during evolution, antisera prepared against human keratins can be used as a general reagent to identify cultured epithelial cells from human and from a variety of laboratory animals.

ACKNOWLEDGMENT

It is a pleasure for us to acknowledge the contribution by Dr. Howard Green of MIT in whose laboratory much of the cited earlier work was performed.

REFERENCES

1. Wigley CB: Differentiated cells in vitro. Differentiation 4:25–55, 1975.
2. Puck TT: "The Mammalian Cell as a Microorganism: Genetic and Biochemical Studies In Vitro." San Francisco: Holden-Day, 1972, p 15.
3. Sun T-T, Green H: Immunofluorescent staining of keratin fibers in cultured cells. Cell 14: 469–476, 1978.
4. Bennett GS, Fellini SA, Croop JM, Otto JJ, Bryan J, Holtzer H: Differences among 100-Å filament subunits from different cell types. Proc Natl Acad Sci USA 75:4364–4368, 1978.
5. Franke WW, Schmid E, Osborn M, Weber K: Different intermediate-sized filaments distinguished by immunofluorescence microscopy. Proc Natl Acad Sci USA 75:5034–5038, 1978.
6. Lazarides E, Balzer DR Jr: Specificity of desmin to avian and mammalian muscle cells. Cell 14:429–438, 1978.
7. Ross R, Greenlee TK Jr: Electron microscopy: Attachment sites between connective tissue cells. Science 153:997–999, 1966.
8. Sun T-T, Green H: Cultured epithelial cells of cornea, conjunctiva and skin: Absence of marked intrinsic divergence of their differentiated states. Nature 269:489–493, 1977.
9. Sun T-T, Green H: Keratin filaments of cultured human epidermal cells: Formation of intermolecular disulfide bonds during terminal differentiation. J Biol Chem 253:2053–2060, 1978.
10. Sun T-T, Shih C, Green H: Keratin cytoskeletons in epithelial cells of internal organs. Proc Natl Acad Sci USA 76:2813–2817, 1979.
11. Franke WW, Weber K, Osborn M, Schmid E, Freudenstein C: Antibody to prekeratin: Decoration of tonofilament-like arrays in various cells of epithelial character. Exp Cell Res 116:429–445, 1978.
12. Freudenstein C, Franke WW, Osborn M, Weber K: Reaction of tonofilament-like intermediate-sized filaments with antibodies raised against isolated defined polypeptides of bovine hoof prekeratin. Cell Biol Int Rep 2:591–600, 1978.
13. Matoltsy AG: What is keratin? Adv Biol Skin 9:559–569, 1969.
14. Matoltsy AG: Soluble prekeratin. In Lyne AG, Short BF (eds): "Biology of the Skin and Hair Growth." New York: American Elsevier, 1965, pp 291–305.
15. Baden HP, Gifford AM, Goldsmith LA: The precursor of the α-fibrous protein of epidermis. J Invest Dermatol 56:446–449, 1971.
16. Skerrow D, Matoltsy AG, Matoltsy MN: Isolation and characterization of the α-helical regions of epidermal prekeratin. J Biol Chem 248:4820–4826, 1973.
17. Steinert PM, Idler WW: The polypeptide composition of bovine epidermal α-keratin. Biochem J 151:603–614, 1975.
18. Lee LD, Fleming BC, Waitkus RF, Baden HP: Isolation of the polypeptide chains of prekeratin. Biochim Biophys Acta 412:82–90, 1975.
19. Baden HP, Lee LD, Kubilus J: The fibrous proteins of stratum corneum. J Invest Dermatol 67:573–576, 1976.
20. Steinert PM: Structure of the three-chain unit of the bovine epidermal keratin filament. J Mol Biol 123:49–70, 1978.
21. Tezuka T, Freedberg IM: Epidermal structural proteins. II. Isolation and purification of tonofilaments of the newborn rat. Biochim Biophys Acta 263:382–396, 1972.
22. Huang L-Y, Stern IB, Clagett JA, Chi EY: Two polypeptide chain constituents of the major protein of the cornified layer of newborn rat epidermis. Biochemistry 14:3573–3580, 1975.

23. Culbertson VB, Freedberg IM: Mammalian epidermal keratin: Isolation and characterization of the α-helical proteins from newborn rat. Biochim Biophys Acta 490:178–191, 1977.
24. Brysk MM, Gray RH, Bernstein IA: Tonofilament proteins from newborn rat epidermis: Isolation, localization, and biosynthesis of marker of epidermal differentiation. J Biol Chem 252:2127–2133, 1977.
25. Baden HP, Bonar L, Katz E: Fibrous proteins of epidermis. J Invest Dermatol 50:301–307, 1968.
26. Baden HP, Lee LD: Fibrous protein of human epidermis. J Invest Dermatol 71:148–151, 1978.
27. Fuchs E, Green H: The expression of keratin genes in epidermis and cultured epidermal cells. Cell 15:887–897, 1978.
28. Steinert PM, Gullino MI: Bovine epidermal keratin filament assembly in vitro. Biochem Biophys Res Commun 70:221–227, 1976.
29. Steinert PM, Idler WW, Zimmerman SB: Self-assembly of bovine epidermal keratin filaments in vitro. J Mol Biol 108:547–567, 1976.
30. Rheinwald JG, Green H: Serial cultivation of strains of human epidermal keratinocytes: The formation of keratinizing colonies from single cells. Cell 6:331–344, 1975.
31. Lee LD, Baden HP, Kubilus J, Fleming BF: Immunology of epidermal fibrous proteins. J Invest Dermatol 67:521–525, 1976.
32. Inoue N, Fukuyama K, Epstein WL: Immunochemical studies of proteins in epidermal cornified cells of human and newborn rat. Biochim Biophys Acta 439:95–106, 1976.
33. Osborn M, Franke WW, Weber K: Visualization of a system of filaments 7–10 nm thick in cultured cells of an epithelioid line (Pt K2) by immunofluorescence microscopy. Proc Natl Acad Sci USA 74:2490–2494, 1977.
34. Davison PF, Hong B-S, Cooke P: Classes of distinguishable 10nm cytoplasmic filaments. Exp Cell Res 109:471–474, 1977.
35. Schwartz SM: Selection and characterization of bovine aortic endothelial cells. In Vitro 14:966–980, 1978.
36. Hicks RM: The mammalian urinary bladder: An accommodating organ. Biol Rev 50: 215–246, 1975.
37. Sun T-T, Green H: Differentiation of the epidermal keratinocyte in cell culture: Formation of cornified envelope. Cell 9:511–521, 1976.

Disorders Affecting Cellular Communications in Oral Tissues: Gap Junctions

Carl J. Witkop, Jr., DDS, MS

The availability of reproducible, dependable cultures of oral epithelial cells would not only provide the technical avenue to answering important questions of normative development of oral structures so ably described in this volume by Dr. Slavkin, but also would provide the key to our understanding numerous defects involving the teeth and oral structures. There are 2 general major questions, among others, that techniques for culture of epithelial cells could address: the first concerns whether the defect in question is intrinsic to the epithelial cell or whether it involves the cellular environment. The second concerns involvement of cell-to-cell communicative systems in the genesis of certain defects. I will give a few examples of oral diseases in which the first question is possibly involved and devote the major portion of this paper to disorders where there is some evidence for involvement of cell-to-cell communications.

INTRINSIC CELL DEFECTS

Odontodysplasia is a developmental defect of teeth usually limited to adjacent teeth in a segment of the jaw [1]. Radiographically, the affected teeth have a "ghost" appearance with little demarcation on radiographs between enamel and dentin (Fig. 1). The teeth are hypoplastic, having only a thin layer of enamel and dentin, calcifications in the dental pulp, abnormalities in the structure of enamel and dentin [2], and degenerative changes in the ameloblasts and odontoblasts. The cause is unknown. The condition is not inherited, as all reported patients

Birth Defects: Original Article Series, Volume XVI, Number 2, pages 197–209

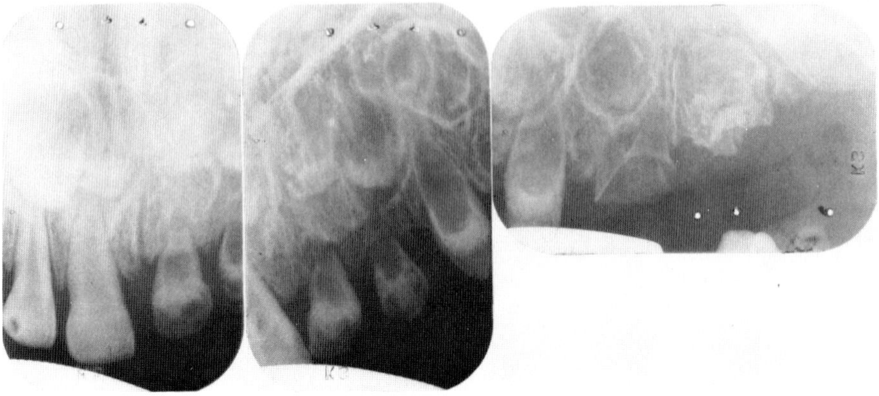

Fig. 1. Radiograph of the maxillary left arch of a patient with odontodysplasia. Note the ghost appearance of both the primary and the unerupted permanent teeth of the entire left quadrant. It is not known if the defect is intrinsic to the odontogenic cells, or if the defect resides in the environment of the developing dental organ.

have occurred as isolated cases [3]. A specific etiology for the disorder has not been established. Among those suggested are local infection, local ischemia, local trauma, irradiation, metabolic or vitamin deficiency, Rh incompatibility, hyperpyrexia, and somatic mutation [3]. Most of these suggested etiologic agents can be ruled out on the evidence of the combined cases.

Evidence suggesting that the condition results from a local vascular defect has recently been presented [3]. Cases in which abnormal teeth occurred in all 4 quadrants, separated by normal teeth, and examples in which unaffected teeth developed from the distal extension of a mesially affected dental lamina would make the somatic mutational theory highly unlikely. It is not known, however, if odontogenic cells themselves are intrinsically defective or whether local factors in environment are responsible for suppression of the developing odontogenic organ. Theoretically, if the defect is intrinsic to cells forming hard tissue, it could reside either in the ectodermally derived inner enamel epithelial cells, which normally induce the differentiation of odontoblasts from mesenchymal cells of the papilla; in the mesenchymal cells or their induced odontoblasts which, in turn, normally induce differentiation of ameloblasts in the inner enamel epithelial cells; or in the ameloblasts themselves. The ability to culture both ectodermally derived and mesodermally derived cells of the dental organ could provide the answer to the question of whether there is an intrinsic cellular defect in the odontogenic cells from patients with odontodysplasia.

Amelogenesis imperfecta is a group of inherited diseases in which only the enamel of teeth is affected without clinical evidence of defects in other structures or metabolic processes. This suggests that these diseases represent mutations at loci that are specific for the development and function of ameloblasts. Eleven different forms of amelogenesis imperfecta have been distinguished on the basis of their clinical, histologic, and genetics features [4]. These 11 different forms can be grouped by their general clinical features into hypoplastic, hypomaturation, and hypocalcified types. The enamel in the hypoplastic types does not reach normal thickness. The enamel in the hypomaturation types does not develop normal enamel rods or enamel rod sheaths, while in the hypocalcified forms there is a gross deficiency of mineralization of the enamel matrix.

Briefly, formation of normal enamel involves the formation of a protein enamel matrix, deposition of organically bound transported calcium salts in the matrix, and maturation of apatite crystals in enamel rods. Matrix is synthesized in the endoplasmic reticulum and assembled in membrane-bound secretory granules in a system of Golgi and endoplasmic reticulum. The secretory granule is released from the terminal end of the ameloblast, Tomes process, into the extracellular space [5]. The nucleation of apatite crystals begins immediately or concomitantly with matrix secretion as long, thin crystals which are oriented perpendicularly to the convex face of the secreting end of the ameloblast. The crystals enlarge in width and thickness during the maturational phase which is a slower process than the initial nucleation. Because the crystals develop perpendicularly to the cell face, the crystals at the periphery change orientation and are short, accounting for the prismatic sheath at the periphery of the enamel rod. The newly formed matrix is composed of enamel protein, the enamlins or amelogens. During calcification and maturation, 90% of the original protein is lost [6]. Further, the organic content of the prismatic sheath is higher than that of the rod portion. It is postulated that 2 distinct steps account for these findings. Nucleation of apatite progresses first in the center of the enamel rod and then progresses to the area of the rod sheath. There is enzymatic hydrolysis of the matrix, and at the periphery an enzymatic resorption of these peptides back into the ameloblast.

The different types of amelogenesis imperfecta are compatible with this postulated normative formation of enamel. The autosomal dominantly inherited forms of hypoplastic amelogenesis imperfecta reflect defects in ameloblastic differentiation, viability, and production of matrix, and probably involve defects in structural proteins. The hypocalcified forms most likely reflect defects in the transport and deposition of calcium salts into the matrix as the histologic and histochemical properties of the matrix resemble normal embryonic matrix. The autosomal recessive pigmented amelogenesis imperfecta most likely represents a defect in the enzyme responsible for the hydrolysis of the initial matrix or esotropic gel. Histologically, the enamel of this type of amelogenesis imperfecta contains deposits of esotropic gel in both the rods and the rod sheaths [4]. The X-linked hypomaturation type of amelogenesis imperfecta contains pools of esotropic gel in the rod sheaths, compatible with a defect in the postulated enzyme responsible for resorption of the hydrolyzed gel back into the ameloblast [4].

The ability to develop cultures of ameloblasts isolated from these defects would provide the source of sufficient tissue to investigate these problems. These mutations affecting formation of human enamel could then be fully used to delineate the steps in the genetic control of normative as well as defective amelogenesis.

PROBLEMS OF CELL-CELL COMMUNICATION

Gap Junctions

Developmental biologists have long recognized the importance of cellular interactions in the developmental process [7, 8]. In the last decade, attention was focused upon the gap junction as one putative mechanism for the direct exchange from cell to cell of small molecules of up to approximately 1,000 daltons [9] that may be important in normal development [10, 11]. Gap junctions provide the avenue for the direct exchange of small molecules isolated from the intercellular space. Gap junctions are found throughout the metazoa [12, 13] in embryonic and adult tissues [8], and in most epithelial tissue [14]. Gap junctions form between cells in tissue culture [15], between differentiated cells [16], and between cells of different species [17]. They are found in high density in tissues that function under anoxic and avascular conditions, where glycolysis plays a major role in energy metabolism, such as in the lens [18, 19] and cornea [20].

The exact mechanism whereby gap junctions form is not known [9]; however, the experiments of Rose and Loewenstein [21] showed that after damage to a cell in which gap junctions become uncoupled, new junctions form within 30 minutes. The regulation of uncoupling of gap junctions is a function of the level of intracellular calcium. Holes experimentally punched in cells permit the entrance of extracellular fluid containing high levels of ionic calcium, which results in immediate uncoupling of the damaged cell from adjacent noninjured cells.

Goodenough and co-workers [18, 22] have isolated gap junction protein that maintains its morphologic integrity by electron microscopy and consists of one major protein, connexin, which consists of 2 chains of amino acid units with a molecular weight of 18,000 daltons. They have shown that, depending upon the method of isolation, the isolated gap junction protein appears as pentalamellar strands as seen in the intact cell or multistrand aggregates. The x-ray diffractive studies indicate that the intercellular connecting "pipes" consist of 6 dumbbell-shaped protein subunits that form the wall of the "pipe" that spans the cell membrane with a central channel of about 20 Å in diameter.

Garant [23] has demonstrated that the developing enamel organ is particularly rich in gap junctions. The ectodermally derived cells of the enamel organ consist of the ameloblasts, the stratum intermedium, the stellate reticulum, and the outer enamel epithelium. The mesodermally derived cells consist of the odontoblasts and their adjacent papillary cells from which the former are derived. He found that extensive gap junctions occur between cells of different types as well as cells of the same type. Not only were gap junctions found between ameloblasts and cells of the stratum intermedium, and stellate and outer enamel epithelial cells, but also between papillary cells and ameloblasts. Barnett and Szabo [24] found gap junctions present in all layers of gingival keratinizing epithelium except the stratum corneum and proposed that they play a role in the synchronous differentiation of normal human gingival keratinizing epithelium.

Gap junctions in amelogenesis. Evidence that gap junctions may play a role in formation of enamel comes from studies on X-linked hypomaturation amelogenesis imperfecta [25, 26]. Hemizygous males have a mottled yellow-white enamel which histologically shows defects in the enamel rod sheaths with accumulations of pink staining (H & E and Masson's trichrome) material within these voids resembling the esotropic gel of the initial protein matrix produced by Tomes processes. It is postulated that this defect is a result of the functional absence of the enzyme that resorbs the hydrolyzed gel back into the ameloblast.

Females heterozygous for the trait show alternating vertical bands of hypomature and normal-appearing enamel. The bands are not symmetric on homologous teeth in the right and left sides of the dental arches, but are randomly distributed; an occasional tooth may show a predominance of hypomature or normal enamel. As the enamel organ develops, daughter cells are added at the edge of the cup-shaped enamel organ as it proliferates into the underlying mesenchyme similar to a cookie-cutter proceeding into dough. Thus, any clonal lines of ameloblasts containing either a normal active X-chromosome or an X-chromosome with the abnormal gene which develop from the inner enamel epithelium are arranged in a vertical fashion. The subsequent enamel formed by these cells then becomes a visual representation of vertical clones of 2 different gene products. Figure 2 shows the scanning electron photomicrographic appearance of a hypomature band of enamel with surrounding normal enamel from a tooth of a heterozygous woman.

Analysis by electron probe of the mineral content of the enamel of hemizygous males showed that the percent of calcium by weight of the defective enamel was approximately 28%, while that of enamel from normal males was approximately 36%. It was expected that a probe of the normal and hypomature bands of enamel of heterozygous females would show 2 distinct patterns: normal enamel containing 36% calcium and the abnormal bands containing 28% calcium. However, analysis by electron probe of the enamel of the heterozygous female did not yield the expected results. An analysis by electron probe (Fig. 3) of a 250-μm section shown by the bar in Figure 2 demonstrated that the normal-appearing enamel had a calcium content (36%) similar to that of enamel from a normal male. However, as the probe proceeded into the area of hypomature enamel, there was a gradual decrease rather than an abrupt change in the calcium content, and even at the center of the band the calcium content did not drop to the level of that shown by the enamel from her hemizygous son (28%). It was only when the bands. of hypomature enamel involved most of the teeth that this value was approached. It should be noted that similar evidence for a partial correction of the defective enamel of heterozygous women occurs in the X-linked hypoplastic form of amelogenesis imperfecta.

It is postulated that the enzyme or a product of the normal cells is passed to the defective cells in the hypomaturation type partially correcting the cellular defect. The distance that the electron probe moved and still encountered enamel with a higher than expected calcium content argues in favor of a mechanism-like gap junction being involved in the partial correction of the defect. Tissue culture experiments would be invaluable in resolving this issue as well as in providing a tool for the isolation of the correcting factor, which could possibly lead to a treatment of this disorder.

Gap junction disease of the mucosa. Hereditary mucoepithelial dysplasia is a recently described disorder which appears to be a disease of gap junction and desmosomal formation [27, 28]. This autosomal dominantly inherited disorder affects all orificial mucosa. The mouth, pharynx, nose, anus, vagina, conjuctiva, and urethra are firey red due to a thin noncornifying or nonkeratinizing mucosal epithelium. In infancy the patients develop nystagmus, photophobia, keratoconjunctivitis, vascularization of the cornea, and chronic rhinorrhea. At 6–7 years of age, cataracts of the lenses develop, leading to blindness by 9–11 years of age. The patients develop a follicular keratosis of unexposed skin. Nonscarring alopecia accompanies

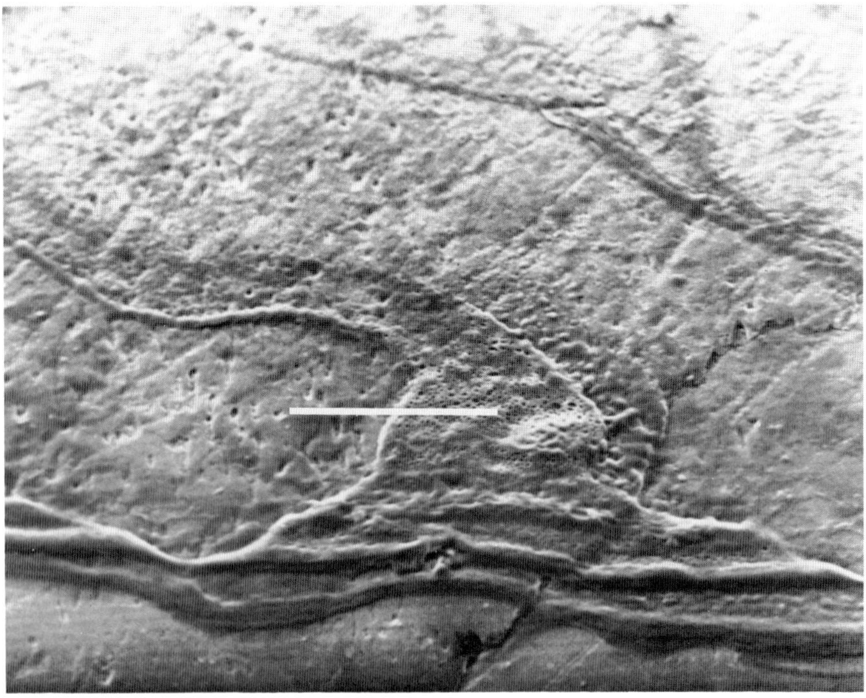

Fig. 2. Scanning electron microscopic appearance of the enamel surface of a tooth of a woman heterozygous for X-linked hypomaturation amelogenesis imperfecta. The vertical band in the center is hypomature enamel while the surrounding enamel is clinically normal. The white line approximates the scan path of the electron probe, the results of which are shown in Fig. 3. (Courtesy of Dr. John J. Sauk, Jr.)

repeated bouts of pneumonia which are associated with frequent episodes of diarrhea, melena, hematuria, and bladder or urethral obstruction. As adults, patients experience numerous bouts of spontaneous pneumothorax, develop fibrocystic lung disease, and die of cor pulmonale. Women have had repeated abnormal vaginal and cervical Papanicolaou smears, conizations, and cryotherapy for prolonged cervical metaplasia following delivery.

Histologically, the mucosa shows a decrease in thickness of the epithelial cell layer, vacuolization and "dyshesion" of cells, dense staining folded nuclei, a lack of cornification or keratinization (palate and gingivae), and small round dyskeratotic cells. Cytologically, the mucosal cells show lack of maturation, anisocytosis,

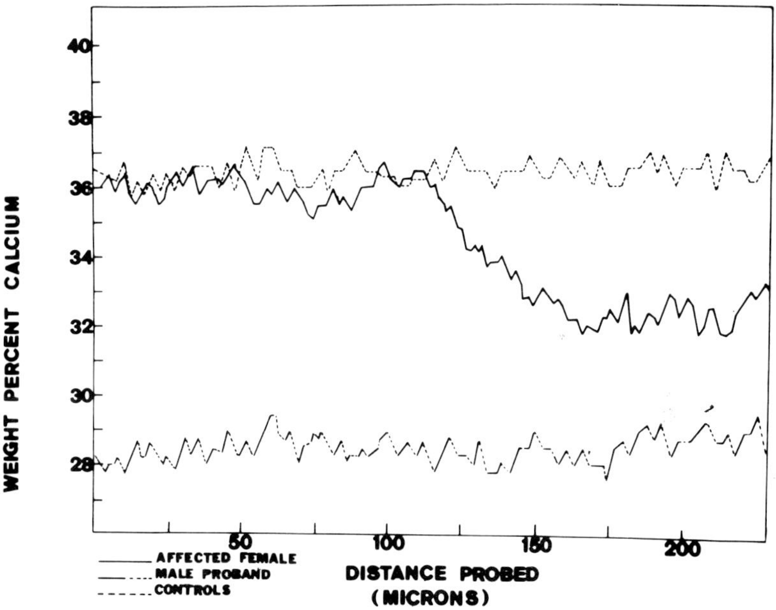

Fig. 3. Scanning electron probe microanalysis of the weight percent calcium content of enamel from a normal male control (– – –), a male hemizygous for hypomaturation amelogenesis imperfecta (– - - -), and a female heterozygous for the defect (—). The latter scan path is shown in Figure 2. Note that when the probe passed over clinically normal enamel, the calcium content was like that of the enamel of the normal male. However, instead of an abrupt drop to the level of the values of the affected male, there is a gradual decrease over approximately 60 μm. Note also that the probe values do not reach the approximately 28% calcium level of her affected son. (From Sauk JJ Jr et al: Electron optic microanalysis of two gene products in enamel of females heterozygous for X-linked hypomaturation amelogenesis imperfecta. Am J Hum Genet 24:267–276, © 1972 by the American Society of Human Genetics, published by The University of Chicago Press, with permission.)

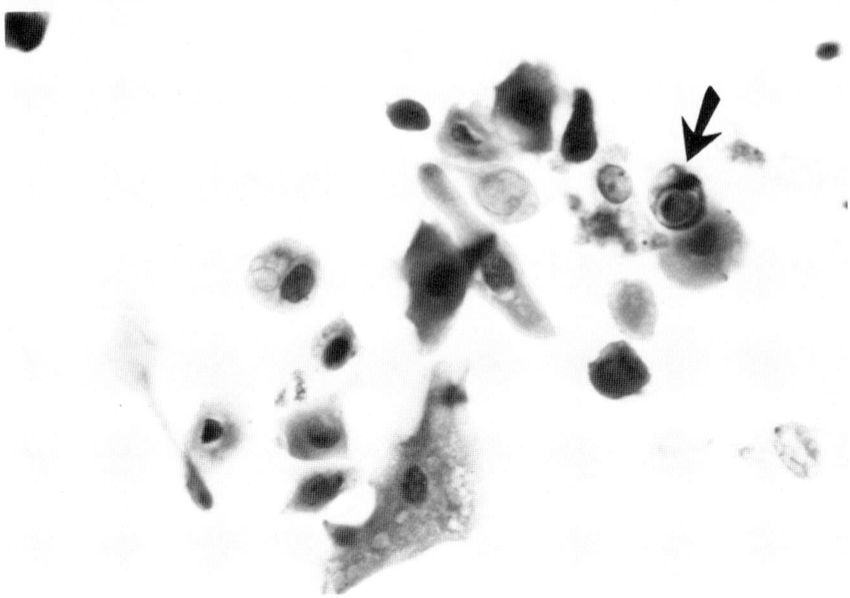

Fig. 4. Exfoliated epithelial cells from the hard palate of a woman affected with hereditary mucoepithelial dysplasia. Note the lack of maturation of cells which normally would be all anuclear keratinized cells. Anisocytosis, poikilocytosis, cytoplasmic vacuoles, and strand-shaped cytoplasmic inclusions characterize this disorder. A dyskeratotic cell is present (↑) (Papanicoleau stain, ×480).

poikilocytosis, large paranuclear vacuoles, strand-shaped inclusions in the cytoplasm, and small round dyskeratotic cells (Fig. 4). Cytologic abnormalities have been observed in oral, nasal, vaginal, and bladder epithelial cells. Ultrastructural features inlcude a paucity of desmosomal attachments, accumulation of amorphous material in intercellular spaces, desmosomes poor in tonofilaments, large paranuclear vacuoles, paranuclear accumulations of bundles of large wheat-sheaf-like fibers and long strands of pentalamellar material (Fig. 5). This latter material develops as ribosomally bound strands in the paranuclear cytoplasm and has the appearance and dimensions of gap junction protein (Fig. 6). The pentalamellar bands aggregate into multilamellar bands (Fig. 7) similar to the stacking of gap junction protein isolated in vitro as shown by Goodenough [29] (Fig. 8). We interpret these findings to indicate that this is a disease of desmosome and gap junction formation in which the material for these structures is formed but does not occupy the normal gap junction and desmosomal sites on the cell surface, and remains trapped within the cytoplasm.

This disorder raises several important questions, some of which we are attempting to answer by the culture of the abnormal epithelium isolated from bladder cells. As a first step, we would like to isolate sufficient material to see if it indeed

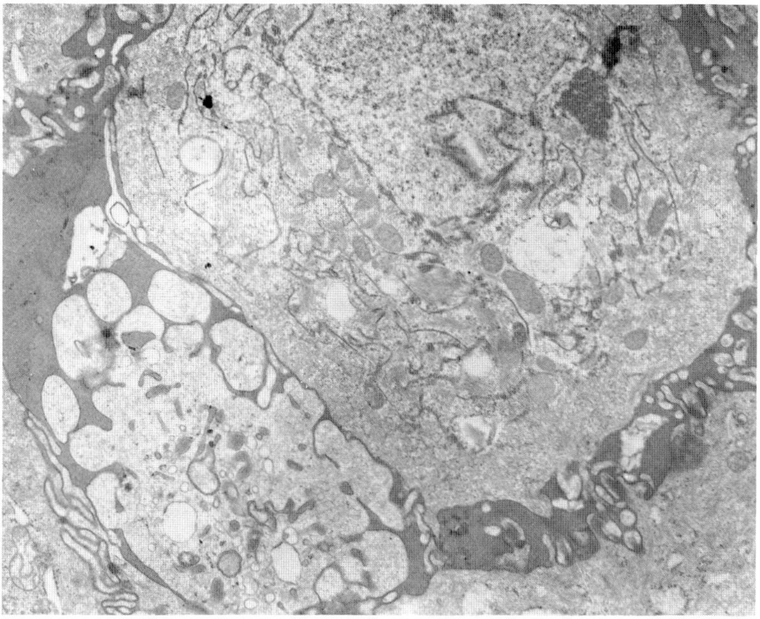

Fig. 5. Cell from the palate of a patient with hereditary mucoepithelial dysplasia showing accumulation of moderately electron dense amorphous intercellular material, a paucity of desmosomes, accumulations of included material in the perinuclear cytoplasm and strand-shaped material in the cytoplasm (×10,000).

is connexin. If so, then this disorder may elucidate how and where gap junction material is formed. There are also several important clinical observations which may be addressed. Clinical evidence suggests that the condition primarily involves epithelia. We have no evidence of malfunction in other tissues where gap junctions have been observed such as liver, smooth muscle, and neurons. Is it possible that junctions at these sites are somehow different from epithelial junctions?

It has been noted that elevations in intracellular calcium cause disconnection of gap junctions [9, 21]. It is interesting that the lesions become intensified after contact with substances containing high amounts of calcium such as milk, toothpaste, and calcium carbonate dusting powders. We are investigating ciliary action in respiratory mucosa because of the chronic rhinorrhea and respiratory problems in these patients. With even slight manipulation, these patients have massive mucosal glandular secretion. Simply by everting the eyelids a copious outpouring from the the Meibomian glands can be observed. We have been unable to bronchoscope these patients because of the massive mucosal secretion induced by this procedure. Barnett and Szabo [24] postulated that a function of gap junctions was to coordinate the development of cornification or keratinization in oral epithelia. The clinical,

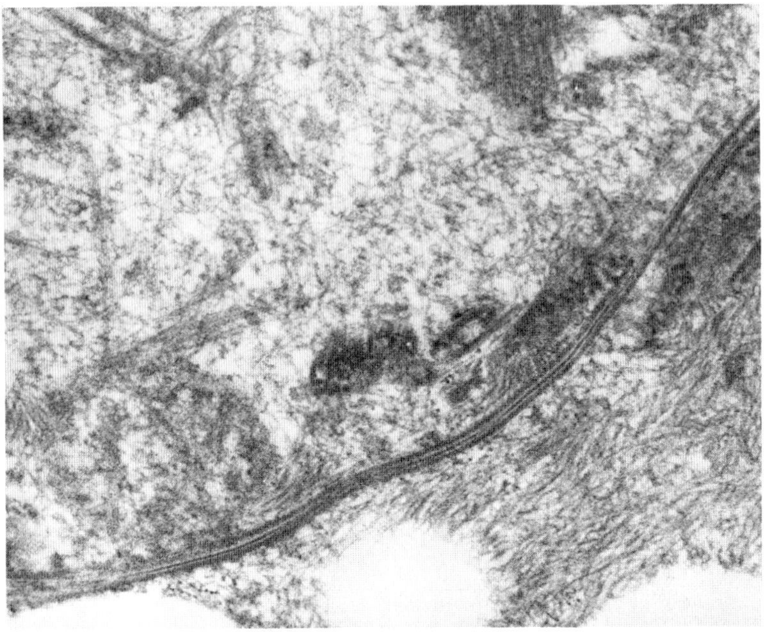

Fig. 6. Strand-shaped material in the cytoplasm has a pentalamellar configuration and dimensions similar to those of gap junction material (×72,000).

histologic, cytologic, and ultrastructural findings in this disease strongly suggest that lack of cellular maturation in all mucosal surfaces is related to the lack of intercellular communication.

Of special importance is the development of cataracts in these patients. Theoretically, as this is a dominantly inherited trait, the normal gene should be coding for normal structural protein. Thus, these patients would be expected to have some normal connections. The fact that they do not have congenital cataracts, but develop them in childhood, suggests that the lens functions normally for a time but then develops a premature cataract. As the lens depends to a great extent on gap junctions, a defect in these connections may be involved in this disease.

It was observed that the exposed tanned skin of patients lacked the follicular lesion seen on untanned, unexposed skin. Two patients received 3 minimal erythemal doses of ultraviolet light to the unexposed skin. Following this procedure, the skin lesions disappeared but reappeared after 6 weeks. We would like to examine the effect of ultraviolet light on cultured cells from this disorder.

Finally, if cells from this disorder were to be successfully cultured, they could possibly provide a mutant cell line lacking gap junctions which could be used as a tool in experiments involving cell-to-cell cooperation.

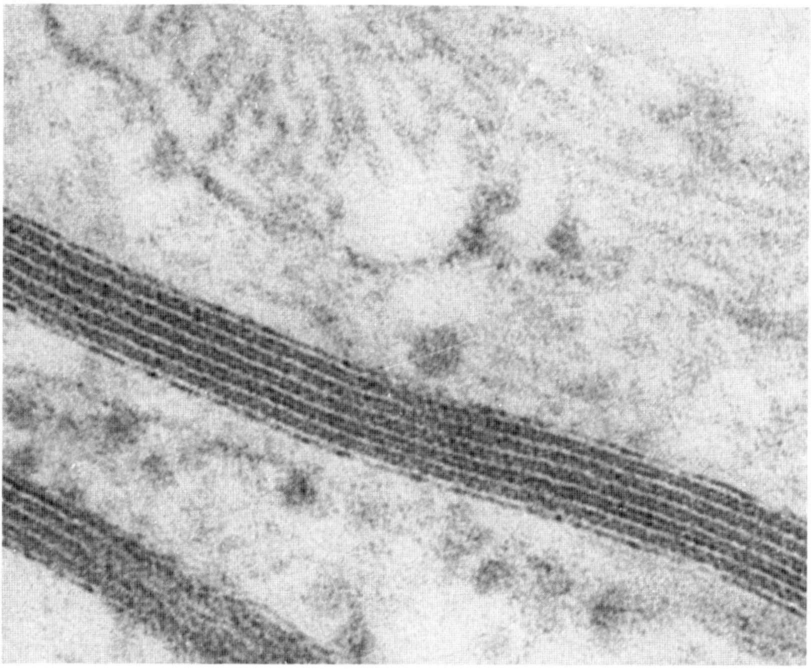

Fig. 7. Aggregates of individual strands are found within the cellular cytoplasm and resemble the stacked aggregates of gap junction protein isolated in vitro as shown in Fig. 8.

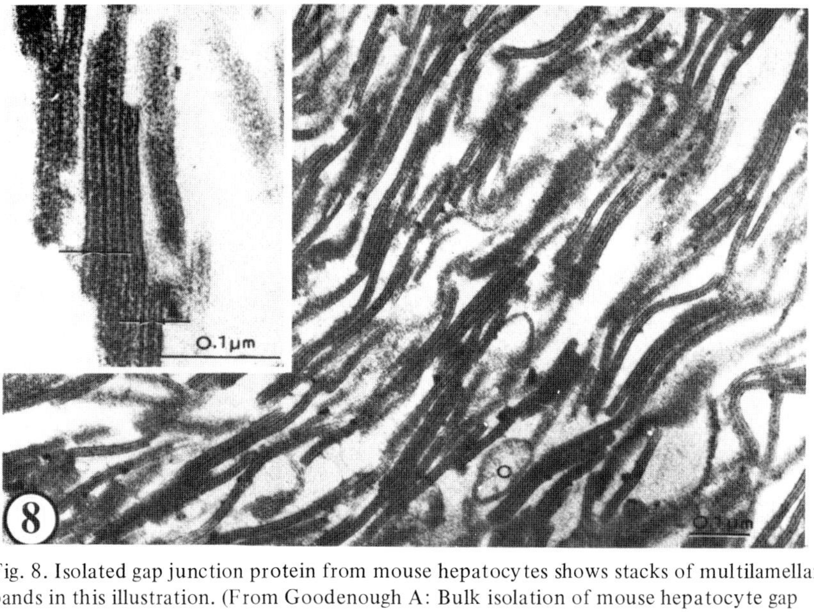

Fig. 8. Isolated gap junction protein from mouse hepatocytes shows stacks of multilamellar bands in this illustration. (From Goodenough A: Bulk isolation of mouse hepatocyte gap junctions. J Cell Biol 61:557–563, 1974, with permission.)

SUMMARY

There are numerous defects of teeth and oral tissues in which important questions concerning the pathogenesis of these disorders could be investigated in epithelial cell cultures. Cell cultures can be invaluable in such conditions as odontodysplasia and amelogenesis imperfecta in determining whether the basic defect is intrinsic to the epithelial cell or resides in the cell's environment. Problems in cell-cell communications particularly as they might involve gap junctions in normal as well as pathologic amelogenesis can be investigated in cultured cells. Evidence for a possible role of gap junctions in amelogenesis comes from a study by electron probe of enamel of women heterozygous for X-linked hypomaturation amelogenesis imperfecta who have 2 distinct types of enamel representing the clonal cell products of different genes on the 2 X chromosomes. Autosomal dominantly inherited mucoepithelial dysplasia, a disease involving all orificial mucosa with cataracts, spontaneous pneumothorax, and death from cor pulmonale, appears to be a disease of formation of desmosomes and gap junctions. The lack of keratinization, the development of cataracts, and the defects in ciliary action possibly result from lack of cellular communication in this disorder.

REFERENCES

1. Rushton MA: Odontodysplasia: "Ghost teeth." Br Dent J 119:109–113, 1965.
2. Gardner DG: The dentinal changes in regional odontodysplasia. Oral Surg 38:887–897, 1974.
3. Walton JL, Witkop CJ Jr, Walker PO: Odontodysplasia. Report of three cases with vascular nevi overlying the adjacent skin of the face. Oral Surg 46:676–684, 1978.
4. Witkop CJ Jr, Sauk JJ Jr: Heritable defects of enamel. In Stewart RE, Prescott GH (eds): "Oral Facial Genetics." St. Louis: CV Mosby, 1976, pp 151–226.
5. Reith EJ, Butcher EO: Microanatomy and histochemistry of amelogenesis. In Miles AEW (ed): "Structural and Chemical Organization of Teeth." New York: Academic Press, 1967, vol 1, pp 371–397.
6. Glimcher MJ: Studies of embryonic and mature dental enamel; the "enamelins." In "Chemistry and Physiology of Enamel, University of Michigan Symposium." Ann Arbor: University of Michigan Press, 1971, pp 2–4.
7. Cox RP (ed): "Cell Communication." New York: John Wiley & Sons, 1974.
8. Sheridan JD: Low-resistance junctions: Some functional considerations. In Moscona AA (ed): "The Cell Surface in Development." New York: John Wiley & Sons, 1974, pp 187–206.
9. Staehelin LA, Hull BE: Junctions between living cells. Sci Am 238:141–152, 1978.
10. Furshpan EJ, Potter DD: Low-resistance junctions between cells in embryos and tissue culture. In Moscona AA, Monroy A (eds): "Current Topics in Developmental Biology." New York: Academic Press, 1968, vol 3, pp 95–127.
11. Loewenstein WR: Emergence of order in tissues and organs. Communication through cell junctions: Implications in growth control and differentiation. Dev Biol 2(Suppl):151–183, 1968.
12. Satir P, Gilula NB: The fine structure of membranes and intercellular communication in insects. Annu Rev Entomol 18:143–166, 1973.
13. McNutt NS, Weinstein RS: Membrane ultrastructure at mammalian intercellular junctions. Prog Biophys Mol Biol 26:45–101, 1973.

14. Friend DS, Gilula NB: Variations in tight and gap junctions in mammalian tissues. J Cell Biol 53:758–776, 1972.
15. Gilula NB, Reeves OR, Steinbach A: Metabolic coupling, ionic coupling and cell contacts. Nature 235:262–265, 1972.
16. Johnson RG, Herman WS, Preus DM: Homocellular and heterocellular gap junctions in *Limulus:* A thin-section and freeze-fracture study. J Ultrastruc Res 43:298–312, 1973.
17. Michalke W, Loewenstein WR: Communication between cells of different type. Nature 232:121–122, 1971.
18. Goodenough DA, Paul DL, Culbert KE: Correlative gap junction ultrastructure. In Lerner RA, Bergsma D (eds): "The Molecular Basis of Cell-Cell Interaction." New York: Alan R Liss for The National Foundation-March of Dimes, BD:OAS XIV(2):83–97, 1978.
19. Philipson BT, Hanninen L, Balazs EA: Cell contacts in human and bovine lenses. Exp Eye Res 21:205–219, 1975.
20. Kreutziger GO: Lateral membrane morphology and gap junction structure in rabbit corneal endothelium. Exp Eye Res 23:285–293, 1976.
21. Rose B, Loewenstein WR: Permeability of cell junction depends on local cytoplasmic calcium activity. Nature 254:250–252, 1975.
22. Caspar DLD, Goodenough DA, Makowski L, Phillips WC: Gap junction structures. I. Correlated electron microscopy and x-ray diffraction. J Cell Biol 74:605–628, 1977.
23. Garant PR: The demonstration of complex gap junctions between the cells of the enamel organ with lanthanum nitrate. J Ultrastruct Res 40:333–348, 1972.
24. Barnett ML, Szabo G: Gap junctions in human gingival keratinized epithelium. J Periodont Res 8:111–126, 1973.
25. Witkop CJ Jr: Partial expression of sex-linked recessive amelogenesis imperfecta in females compatible with the Lyon hypothesis. Oral Surg 23:174–182, 1967.
26. Sauk JJ Jr, Lyon HW, Witkop CJ Jr: Electron optic microanalysis of two gene products in enamel of females heterozygous for X-linked hypomaturation amelogenesis imperfecta. Am J Hum Genet 24:267–276, 1972.
27. Witkop CJ Jr, White JG, King RA, Dahl MV, Young WG, Sauk JJ Jr: Hereditary mucoepithelial dysplasia. Am J Hum Genet 31:414–427, 1979.
28. Witkop CJ Jr, White JG, Sauk JJ Jr, King RA: Clinical, histologic, cytologic, and ultrastructural characteristics of the oral lesions from hereditary mucoepithelial dysplasia. A disease of gap junction and desmosome formation. Oral Surg 46:645–657, 1978.
29. Goodenough DA: Bulk isolation of mouse hepatocyte gap junctions. J Cell Biol 61:557–563, 1974.

Tooth Epithelial Differentiation In Vitro and Congenital Craniofacial Malformation*

Harold C. Slavkin, DDS, Marie Yamada, DDS, PhD, Pablo Bringas, Jr., BS, and Martin Grodin, BS, MA

INTRODUCTION

"Experiments of Nature" have been reported to disfigure the human face, cranium, and intraoral structures since Man's recorded history. Abnormal morphogenesis and function of the human craniofacial complex represents one of the most common of congenital malformations, afflicting 1 out of every 600 live-births [1]. These congenital malformations include cleft lip and/or palate, hemifacial microsomia, orbital hypertelorism, inner and middle ear malformations, tongue malformations, anencephaly, craniostenosis, dentinogenesis and amelogenesis imperfecta, numerous aberrations in tooth morphogenesis, and, in later years, malocclusion of the dentition [1]. In considering causation of these craniofacial malformations, both genetic determinants (or "predisposition") and environmental factors have been demonstrated, although the precise etiology for most of these birth defects remain as yet unknown.

Normal development of the tongue, lips, jaws, palate, teeth, and pharynx involve transformation of the 1st and 2nd branchial arches into discernible structures [1, 2]. The most sensitive period for the induction of congenital craniofacial malformations lies between the initiation and developmental expression of branchial arch morphogenesis (ca 19 days in Man and 7.5–8.0 days in mouse) through the 12th week of embyogenesis in Man (through the 14th day in mouse [1–3]. In fact, organogenesis, consisting of histogenesis and cytodifferentiation, is determined during the most critical Embryonic Period of embryogenesis (Fig. 1).

*Supported by grants DE-02848 and DE-03569 from the National Institute for Dental Research, US Public Health Service.

Birth Defects: Original Article Series, Volume XVI, Number 2, pages 211–230

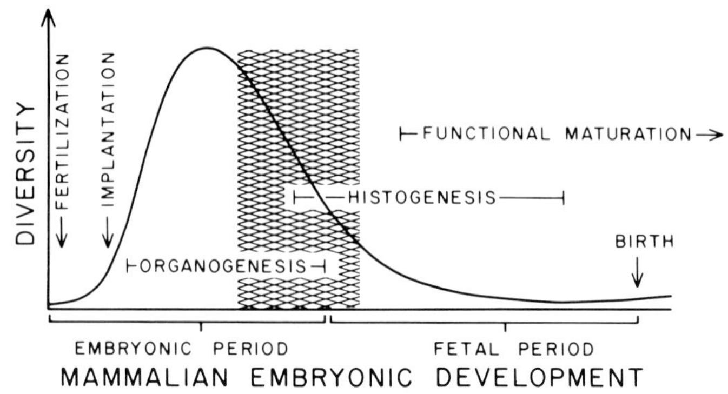

Fig. 1. During the Embryonic Period many different formations of organs occur during the ontogenesis of the human embryo. These ontogenetic differentiations are biodynamically essential changes of the appearance of the growing individual organism. Among the numerous organ systems being determined in the first few weeks following implantation, the various deciduous and permanent tooth organs (eg incisor, canine, premolar, molar) are initially determined by 40–44 days following fertilization. Tooth morphogenesis, histogenesis, and cytodifferentiation within each individual tooth organ is expressed in a gradient with respect to time and spatial position within the organism – anteroposterior morphogenetic and metabolic gradients.

The regulatory processes operating during secondary embryonic inductions, so-called epithelial-mesenchymal interactions, associated with various types of epidermal organogenesis are as yet obscure [4–9]. Examples of several extensively described epithelial-mesenchymal organ systems include salivary gland [4], kidney [10], pancreas [7], lung, limb, feather, and tooth morphogenesis [11–23]. Critical to each of these developing organ systems is the initiation or determination and maintenance of the epithelial phenotype. The objective of this discussion is to select critical issues associated with fetal tooth epithelial differentiation and to suggest their relevance to basic problems in human birth defects.

HUMAN PRENATAL TOOTH MORPHOGENESIS: GENERAL CONSIDERATIONS

Human tooth morphogenesis is initiated during the Embryonic Period of embryogenesis (ca 6th week) [1, 24–26]. Following the migration of the cranial neural crest cells into the forming maxillary and mandibular segments, derived from the 1st and 2nd branchial arches, a series of interactions between oral ectoderm and adjacent cranial neural crest-derived ectomesenchyme initiates the formation of the dental lamina and tooth morphogenesis. In Man, there are 2 different sets of teeth. Therefore, the embryonic epithelial-mesenchymal interactions, giving rise to the tooth anlagen, serve both the deciduous and the permanent sets of teeth

(Fig. 2). In Table 1 "highlights" of human tooth morphogenesis, histogenesis, cytodifferentiation, and extracellular matrix formation are presented in a comparison of embryonic or fetal age, crown-rump length, and general features of tooth development.

In all types of epidermal organogenesis (eg hair, salivary gland, skin, and tooth morphogenesis), both the embryonic and the maternal genotypes are extremely relevant to the structural and functional integrity of the resulting developing organ system. Each tooth organ in the deciduous or primary dentition, as

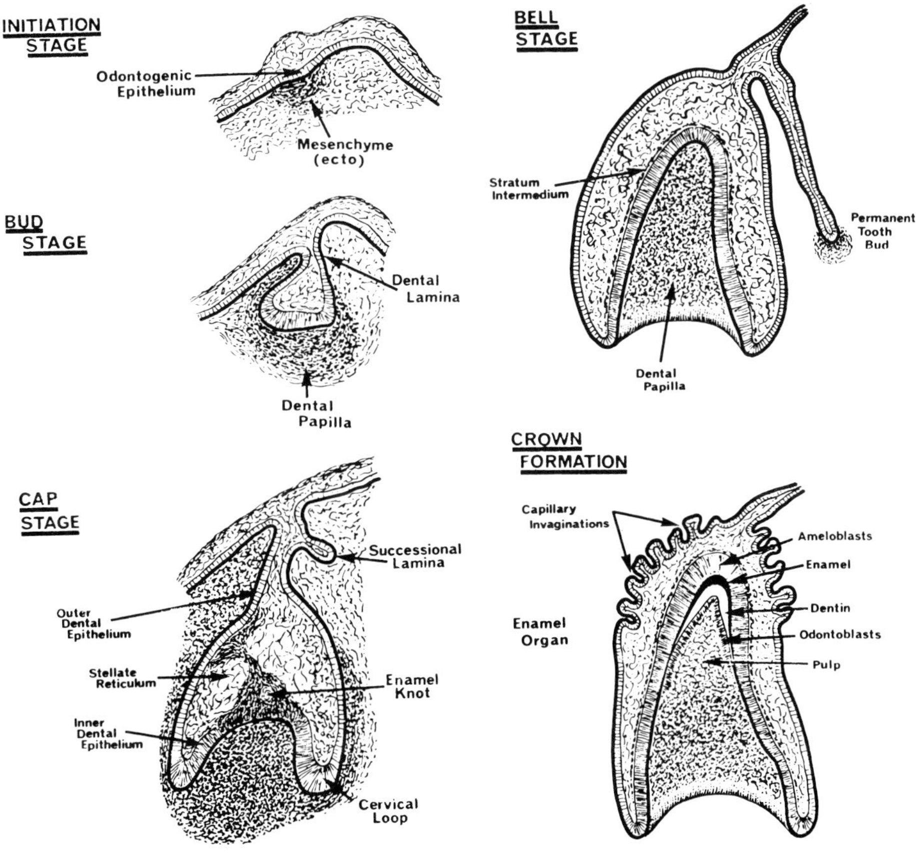

Fig. 2. The development of the human deciduous incisor tooth organ (ie initiation, bud, bell, and cap stages of morphogenesis; histogenesis; and differentiation through crown formation). Note the determination of the permanent incisor tooth analagen is clearly evident by the bell stage (after diagrams provided by Dr. Charles Smith, McGill University, Montreal, Canada).

well as in the permanent dentition, is an individual organ system; each organ has independent nerve innervation, vascularization, and lymphatic drainage [24–26]. Since tooth morphogenesis, histogenesis, cytodifferentiation, dentin and enamel extracellular matrix formation and calcification span a developmental period extending from the Embryonic Period to well beyond birth, numerous genetic as well as environmental factors are implicated in congenital malformations involving dental tissues. Obvious defects of tooth development include

TABLE I. Highlights of Human Embryonic and Fetal Tooth Development

Embryo or fetal age	Crown-rump length (mm)	Developmental characteristics
40–44 days	8–14	Oral ectodermal proliferation in prospective regions of the maxillary and mandibular deciduous 1st and 2nd incisor, canine, and molar tooth organs.
42–48 days	12–15	Dental lamina forms for the deciduous incisor, canine, and molar tooth anlagen.
50–56 days	17–22	Tooth "bud stage" of deciduous incisor, canine, and molar tooth anlagen.
70 days	40–45	Tooth "cap stage" is expressed by deciduous tooth anlagen with dental papilla mesenchyme cell condensation adjacent to the basal lamina of the enamel organ inner enamel epithelium.
14 weeks	116	Tooth "bell stage" is expressed by deciduous tooth organs with the differentiation of odontoblasts, predentin and dentin extracellular matrix formation and calcification; the permanent tooth "bud stage" is now expressed.
18 weeks	164	Dentin calcification continues in deciduous tooth organs and enamel extracellular matrix formation begins with secretory ameloblast cell differentiation in incisor, canine, and molar teeth; permanent "cap stage" is expressed.
32 weeks	302	All deciduous tooth crowns are completed with dentin and enamel extracellular matrix formation and calcification; cusps of teeth are fused; permanent molar tooth organs now show dentin calcification.
36 weeks	341	Dentin and enamel extracellular matrix formation begins in permanent 1st molar tooth organs.

adontia, malformed teeth, supernumerary teeth, dentinogenesis imperfecta (reflecting the extracellular organic matrix and/or subsequent mineralization and calcification), and amelogenesis imperfecta (Table 2).

TABLE 2. Examples of Genetic Disorders in Human Tooth Morphogenesis, Histogenesis, and Differentiation

Genetic disorder	Pattern(s) of inheritance
Nonsyndrome aberrations in number, size, and shape of teeth	
no central incisors	X-linked recessive
absent or "pegged" lateral incisors	autosomal dominant
dens invaginatus	autosomal dominant or multifactorial
hypodontia	autosomal dominant or multifactorial
microdontia	autosomal dominant or multifactorial
supernumerary teeth	autosomal dominant, X-linked recessive and/or multifactorial
Syndromes with hypodontia	
Ellis-van Crevald syndrome	autosomal recessive
Goltz syndrome	X-linked dominant
hypohidrotic ectodermal dysplasia	X-linked or autosomal recessive
Syndromes with supernumerary teeth	
cleidocranial dysplasia	autosomal dominant
Gardner syndrome	autosomal dominant
Nonsyndrome enamel matrix dysplasias	
hypoplasia	autosomal dominant
hypocalcification	autosomal dominant
hypomaturation	X-linked recessive
hypomaturation with pigmentation	autosomal recessive
Syndromes with enamel matrix dysplasias	
Aarskog syndrome	X-linked recessive
Goltz syndrome	X-linked dominant
trichodentoosseous syndrome	autosomal dominant
Nonsyndrome dentin matrix dysplasias	
dentin dysplasia – I	autosomal dominant
dentin dysplasia – II	autosomal dominant
Brandywine opalescent dentin	autosomal dominant
Syndromes with dentin matrix dysplasias	
hypophosphatasia	autosomal dominant
osteogenesis imperfecta	autosomal dominant
Nonsyndrome cementum matrix dysplasias	
multiple cementomas	autosomal dominant
idiopathic juvenile periodontitis (periodontosis)	X-linked recessive
Syndromes with cementum matrix dysplasias	
cleidocranial dysplasia	autosomal dominant
hypophosphatasia	autosomal recessive

Closer examination suggests that regulatory processes operating during epithelial-mesenchymal interactions associated with tooth morphogenesis are crucial determinants in normal development. Each tooth organ represents a high degree of developmental programming for sequential synthesis and secretion of unique extracellular matrix macromolecules derived from either cranial neural crest-derived ectomesenchyme (eg preodontoblast and odontoblast cells) or from the inner enamel epithelial cells differentiating into secretory ameloblast cells [27]. During differentiation a changing program of macromolecular synthesis and secretion characterize tooth morphogenesis. For example, the odontoblast cells synthesize preprocollagen, subsequently process this gene product to procollagen, and then secrete type I collagen and α(I) trimer collagen coincident with dentin proteoglycans [11]. Subsequently, odontoblast cells synthesize and secrete dentin phosphoproteins after the initiation of calcium hydroxyapatite crystals within matrix vesicles.

Since the dental papilla mesenchyme, including the odontoblast cells, synthesize and secrete type I collagen, various types of proteoglycans, glycosaminoglycans, and dentin phosphoproteins (constituents of the forming dentin organic extracellular matrix), one would predict that genetic diseases such as Ehlers-Danlos syndrome, osteogenesis imperfecta, achondroplasia (in which there is some controversy), and mucopolysaccharidosis IV (Morquio syndrome) will have associated tooth malformations especially related to the connective tissue elements involved in dentin and cememtum formation [28–30].

Adjacent inner enamel epithelial cells synthesize tonofilaments and also synthesize and secrete a basal lamina allegedly formed with type IV collagens [31]. A class of glycosaminoglycans is also secreted by these epithelial cells into the matrix of the basal lamina [32]. Thereafter, these preameloblast epithelial cells demonstrate a cessation in cell division, become highly elongated as tall columnar epithelial cells, acquire an extreme nuclear polarity, no longer possess a discernible basal lamina, and synthesize and secrete enamel matrix proteins (Figs. 3 and 4). As such, the secretory ameloblast cells also regulate the mineralization and calcification of calcium hydroxyapatite crystals in the forming enamel matrix. Subtle genetic and/or epigenetic factors which perturbate the flow of information within and between these heterotypic cell types are reflected in major and minor malformations of the deciduous and/or permanent dentitions. The etiology of many of these defects is as yet difficult to identify, especially within the intact organism, and necessitates combined in vivo and in vitro experimental strategies.

ISSUES REGARDING TOOTH EPITHELIAL DIFFERENTIATION

It has become axiomatic that developmental instructions for morphogenesis are related to differential gene expression leading to unique gene products, and that somatic eucaryotic cells contain identical concentrations of deoxyribonucleic acid (DNA). The timing and sequence of genetic expression reside within inherited structural genes contained within chromatin. Whereas so much information is encoded within DNA (ca 80,000 different unique structural genes in addition to the enormous number of repetitive genes for transfer ribonucleic acid [tRNA] and ribosomal ribonucleic acid [rRNA]), it is also evident that subtle

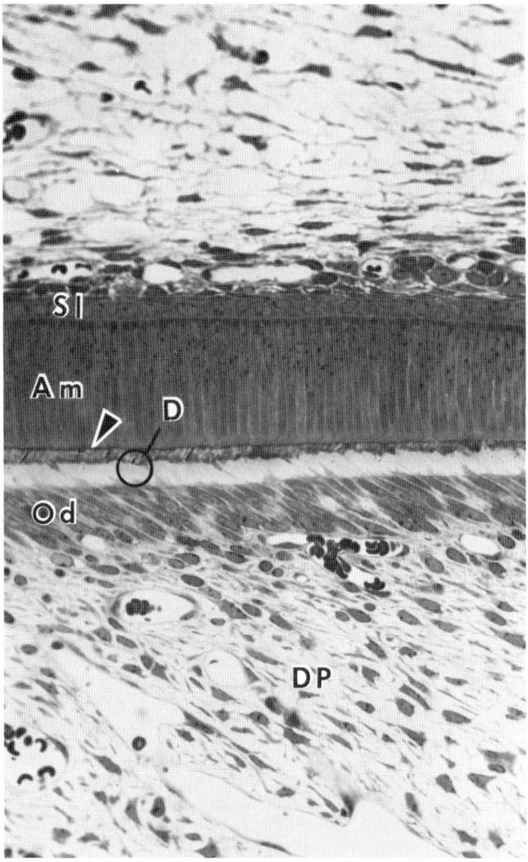

Fig. 3. General histologic characteristics of mammalian dentinogenesis and amelogenesis. Oral ectodermally derived inner enamel epithelium has differentiated into nondividing, highly elongated, and polarized secretory ameloblasts (Am) producing enamel extracellular matrix (arrow). Cranial neural crest-derived ectomesenchyme has formed the dental papilla (DP) and those cells at the periphery have differentiated into nondividing, highly elongated, and polarized secretory odontoblasts (Od) producing dentin extracellular matrix (D). The secretory ameloblast cells within the epithelium remain avascular. Note the sheet of epithelial cells, stratum intermedium (SI), interposed between vasculature and ameloblasts. Vascular elements are readily apparent adjacent to the mesenchymal odontoblast cells.

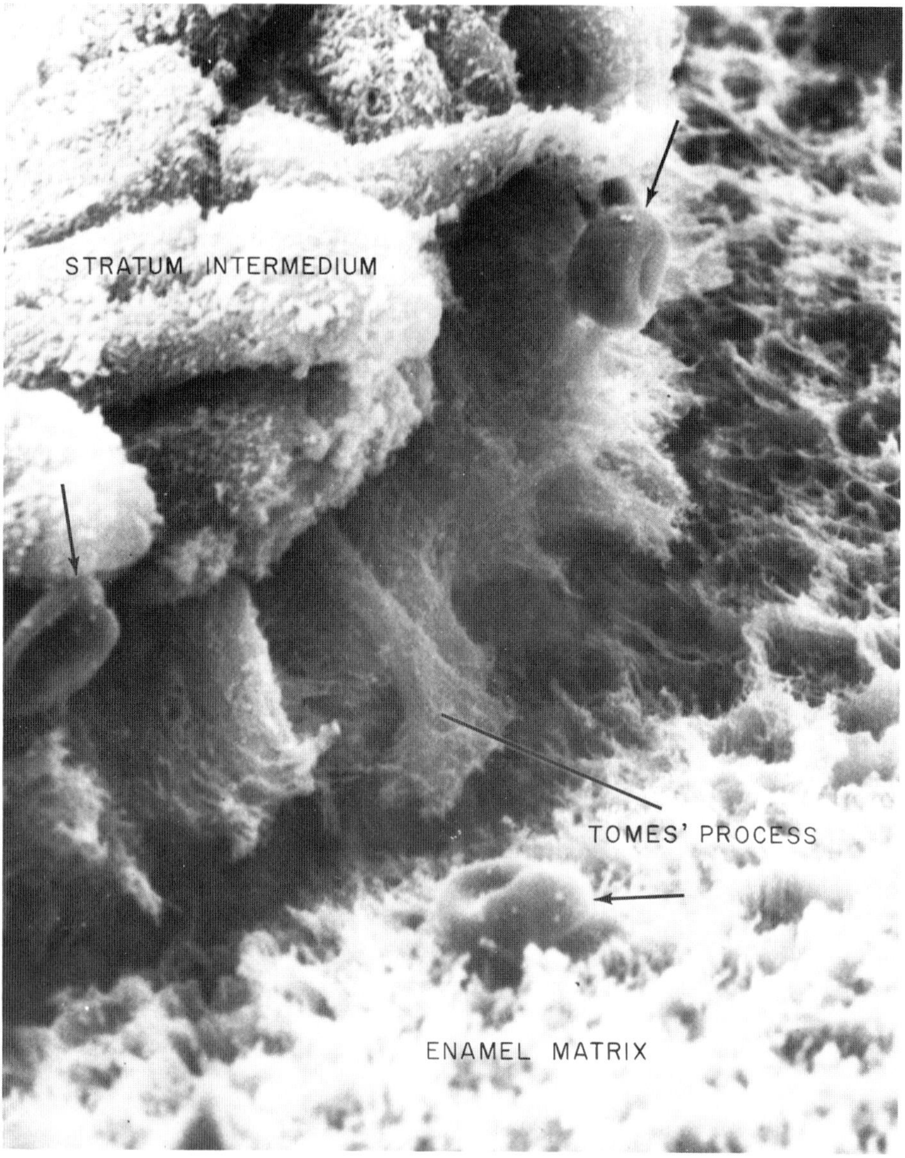

Fig. 4. Scanning electron microscopy provides topographic observations of secretory ameloblast cell processes (ie Tomes processes) during the secretion of fetal enamel extracellular matrix constituents (eg enamel polypeptides, glycosaminoglycans, calcium ions). During the laboratory preparation of this specimen, red blood cells (arrows) have been displaced from the vasculature adjacent to the stratum intermedium. In vivo, nutrients for the ameloblasts must diffuse through the stratum intermedium.

perturbations outside of chromatin, so-called extrachromosomal or epigenetic, serve to regulate timing, sequencing, and duration of differential gene expression. This theme repeats itself throughout eucaryotic cell differentiation, histogenesis, and morphogenesis (Fig. 5).

One very interesting question regarding the nature of epithelial-mesenchymal interactions during tooth morphogenesis is the issue of *determination* [23, 32]. When are these heterotypic interactions determined? When have specific RNA polymerases initiated the transcription of unique sequences of DNA leading to biochemical markers for differentiation? When do inner enamel epithelial cells initiate the transcription of cell surface-specific glycoproteins, preprocollagens, glycosylating enzymes, phosphokinases, preproenamel proteins, or alkaline phosphatases? When do preodontoblast cells initiate preprocollagen synthesis? When does the induction for dentin phosphoprotein, glycosyl transferase, or proteoglycans occur? How are molecular determinants regulated?

These questions survey various molecular *responses* that individual cells make as a consequence of both epithelial-mesenchymal interactions and pattern information during tooth morphogenesis. How are these responses initiated? How do epigenetic processes mediate the amplification or suppression of gene expression? That heterotypic tissue interactions are required for these various

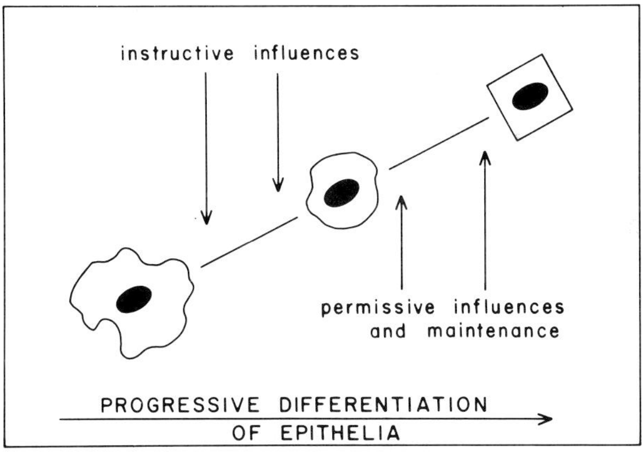

Fig. 5. During embryogenesis both *instructive* and *permissive or maintenance* influences are required for progressive epithelial differentiation. Instructive or "inductive" influences may include 1) direct cell-cell contacts between mesenchyme and adjacent epithelial cells, 2) specific interactions between the epithelial cells and constituents of the forming extracellular matrix (eg collagens, proteoglycans, glycosaminoglycans, anions, cations), 3) diffusion of "chemical signals" from adjacent cells (so-called "short-range" intercellular communications), or 4) diffusion from other parts of the organism (eg long-range diffusion of growth-promoting humoral factors such as insulin, thyroxine, glucocorticosteroids, somatomedin, epidermal growth factor, nerve growth factor, mesenchymal growth factor, etc). Permissive or maintenance factors suggest those nutritional requirements essential to maintain already determined epithelial phenotype.

types of gene expression appears today to be unequivocal. What is not clear is whether these epithelial-mesenchymal interactions are causally related to the determination of differential gene expression associated with differentiation, or whether these same intercellular interactions serve to regulate predetermined events; events determined prior to the histologic identification of inner enamel epithelium within the tooth anlagen.

Determination of epithelial tissue might be envisioned to begin with induction of unique and diverse mRNAs. The popular paradigm for induction has been to consider "on" (derepression) and "off" (repression) controls of gene activation and expression. Unique structural genes, such as collagen, myosin, actin, keratin, and enamel protein, are either "on" or "off." Epithelial-mesenchymal interactions could provide a mechanism to selectively activate previously inactive and unique structural genes in the inner enamel epithelium. An alternative concept is to consider that all unique structural genes are essentially activated in the epithelium and appropriate hnRNAs (heterogeneous nuclear RNAs) are synthesized earlier in embyronic development. In this concept potential mRNA (messenger RNA) transcripts are physically available for translation prior to epithelial-mesenchymal interactions, yet require "activation" as a direct consequence of heterologous tissue-tissue interactions. Determination at the gene level of biologic organization has already occurred. Subsequently, *differentiating* inner enamel epithelial cells become increasingly restricted as a consequence of a net loss in their capacity to express gene products and cessation of cell division. Differentiation is a nonreversible process. Nondividing cells, such as ameloblasts, synthesize phenotypically characteristic enamel protein gene products as their terminal expression of diversity. Aberrations in *rates* of production and absolute *concentration* of gene product produced results in various forms of amelogenesis imperfecta, including hypoplasia, hypomineralization, and hypocalcification.

IN VITRO TOOTH EPITHELIAL DIFFERENTIATION

The experimental protocol used in numerous investigations of epidermal organ systems has attempted to study developmental processes in vitro, independent from cumbersome interpretations often required when evaluating in vivo experimentation. Discrete fetal organs or organ primordia are cultured in an "artificial" environment. The sequences of differentiation, histogenesis, and morphogenesis are monitored using histologic criteria. The "defined" artificial environment (such as the chick chorioallantoic membrane [CAM], subcutaneous grafts, anterior chamber of the eye, or "semi-defined" organ culture conditions employing fetal serum and chick embryonic extract supplementation) contain ubiquitous growth factors of unknown concentration or identity. If intact fetal organ explants develop into more complex structures and shapes, can isolated epithelial or mesenchymal tissues differentiate, express characteristic histogenesis, and even generate form? Both tissues appear to be required in recombination in order to achieve "normal" morphogenesis [4]. Can these heterologous tissues be separated in juxtaposition to a filter and continue to differentiate, express histogenesis and morphogenesis in an artificial environment?

Available data suggest that epithelial-mesenchymal interactions require direct intercellular cell-cell contact between heterologous tissues for some duration in order to accommodate subsequent differentiation, histogenesis, and morphogenesis [10, 32–34]. The data are equivocal but highly suggestive [10]. If cells cannot penetrate through interposed Millipore or Nucleopore filters (usually 0.45 μm pore size and 25 μm in thickness), subsequent stages of differentiation, histogenesis and morphogenesis are inhibited [15–17, 21, 35].

Experimental embryologic studies have clearly shown that both epithelial and mesenchymal tissues in association are required for tooth development [11]. Of special interest have been the elegant studies of Kollar and his collaborators showing that 16-day fetal molar tooth mesenchyme is a potent "inducer" of tooth morphogenesis in responding non-tooth, oral epithelium or in non-oral epithelium such as the foot pad epidermis [22, 36, 37]. Further, Kollar and Baird provided studies which indicate that tooth organ form is dependent upon the dental papilla mesenchyme [37]. A large number of other studies, especially those from Ruch's group in Strasbourg [12, 13], Koch in North Carolina [21, 35] and ourselves in Los Angeles [9, 11, 27], have demonstrated that mesenchymal specificity is crucial in tooth morphogenesis as well as in many other epithelial-mesenchymal interacting systems [4, 7, 8, 10, 38]. These studies, and many others, have significantly affected the rationale within this field of development by providing rather extensive examples of mesenchymal influences upon epithelial cytodifferentiation and morphogenesis in many different organ systems. In fact, several papers have used "mesenchymal-epithelial interactions" to describe their intellectual bias regarding this question.

Of course, as you might imagine, investigators have also indicated that the ectodermally derived epithelium is "inductive" of mesenchymal differentiation, histogenesis, and morphogenesis. Using comparable types of heterotypic and heterochronic tissue recombinants in vitro, these investigations have indicated that ectodermally derived epithelium induced a responding mesenchyme to differentiate and express various morphogenetic characteristics [23, 31]. One major difference between the "mesenchyme induction" and "epithelium induction" studies has been in terms of temporal factors [11]. During early development associated with dental lamina formation and early stages of tooth morphogenesis, epithelial tissues (ie inner enamel epithelium) appear to synthesize and secrete several types of collagen *prior to* the synthesis and secretion of collagen within adjacent mesenchymal cells (Figs. 6–8) [29, 39].

An interesting comparison can be made between tooth morphogenesis and primary corneal stroma morphogenesis [8, 40–42]. During avian eye morphogenesis, corneal ectodermally derived epithelial cells synthesize and secrete basal lamina collagens. A "template" of type I corneal collagen is formed which serves as the primary matrix for the subsequent formation of the corneal stroma [41]. No mesenchymal cells are physically present at this stage of morphogenesis [40]. Subsequently, invading mesenchymal cells align themselves adjacent to the epithelial-secreted collagen matrix and then the mesenchymal cells begin to

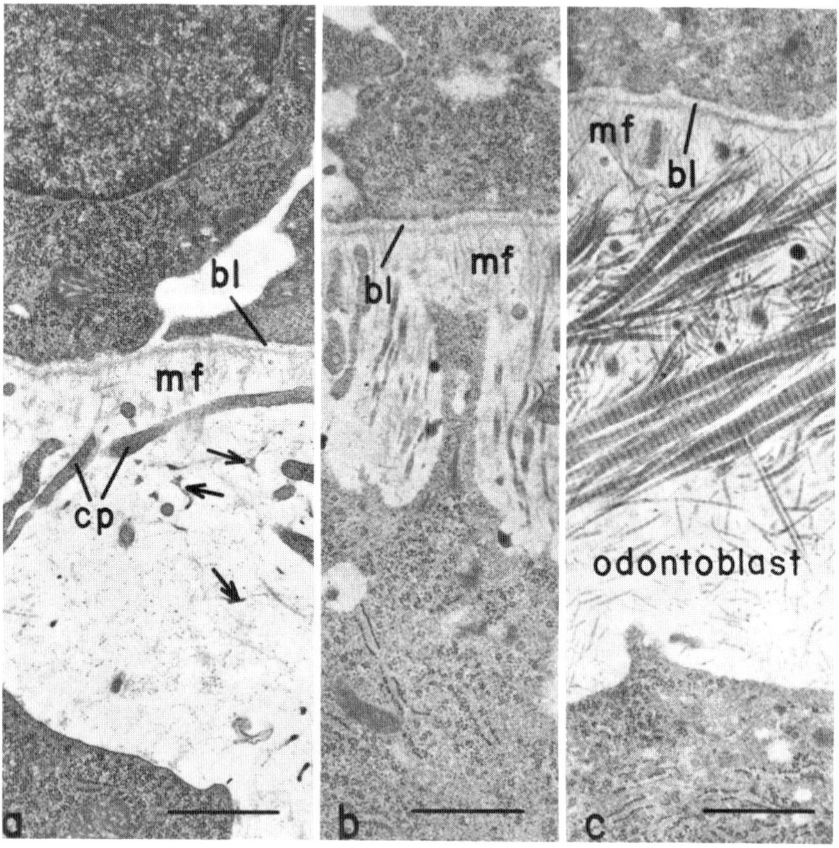

Fig. 6. A sequential series of electron photomicrographs of comparable magnification (bar line = 0.5 μm) illustrating the differentiative changes at the interface during embryonic tooth epithelial-mesenchymal interactions. a) Inner enamel epithelial cells secrete a basal lamina (bl) (allegedly type IV collagen and sulphated glycosaminoglycans) and microfilaments (mf) which may represent yet another type of collagen; arrows, proteoglycan-like material known to positively stain with Ruthenium Red; cp, mesenchymal cell processes. b) The ectomesenchyme cells have differentiated into preodontoblast cells extending long cell processes towards the undersurface of the inner enamel epithelial cells. c) The preodontoblast cells have differentiated into nondividing, elongated, and polarized odontoblast cells which synthesize and secrete type I collagen, proteoglycans, and dentin phosphoproteins at least 48 hours before epithelial cells differentiate into secretory ameloblasts. These observations illustrate both in vivo and in vitro tooth development, albeit somewhat slower in vitro.

synthesize and secrete corneal collagen which is spatially and phenotypically complementary with that previously made by the ectodermally derived epithelium. It is further interesting to note that after the mesenchymal cells begin to secrete corneal collagen, the adjacent epithelial cells no longer synthesize and secrete collagen [38]. These observations suggest a significant reciprocal set of heterotypic tissue interactions mediated by gene products present in the extracellular matrix interface [8]. Comparable temporal events appear to occur during tooth morphogenesis [30, 34, 39].

EPITHELIAL OR MESENCHYMAL INDUCTION?

Grobstein critically discussed the "state of the art" regarding epithelial-mesenchymal interactions related to organogenesis, and concluded that *reciprocal and interdependent* heterotypic tissue interactions were a prerequisite to epidermal

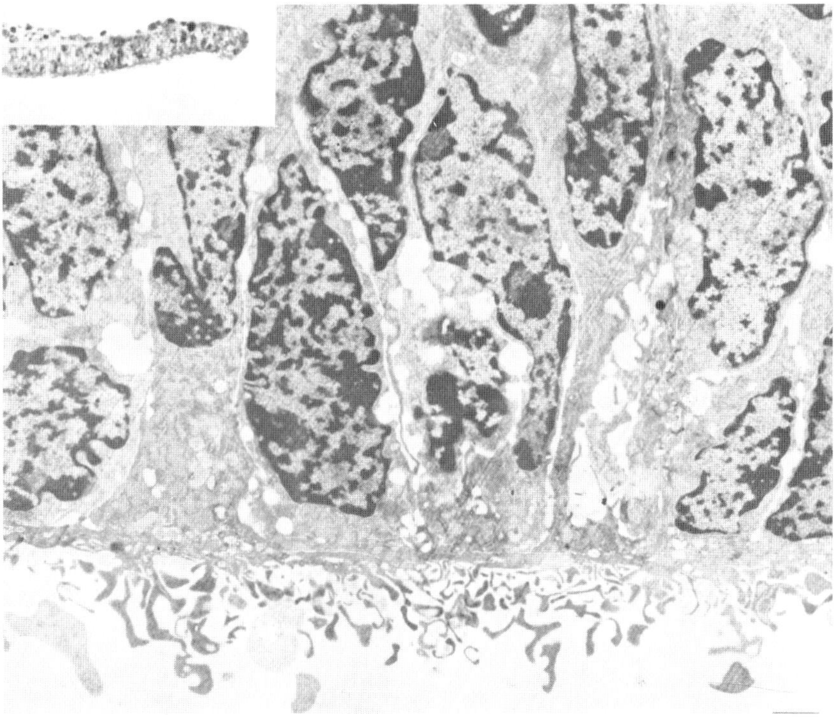

Fig. 7. Intact fetal tooth organs can readily be dissociated into epithelial and mesenchymal tissues following brief incubations with proteolytic enzymes. Following such treatment the basal lamina associated with the inner enamel epithelium is digested and significant "blebbing" of microvilli characterize the undersurface of this epithelium as visualized with electron microscopy (bar line = 1.0 μm). The insert is a light photomicrograph of the epithelial tissue following dissociation procedures.

organ morphogenesis [4, 5, 43]. A preponderance of data has been assembled which demonstrates the essential necessity for heterotypic tissue interactions leading to differentiation, histogenesis, and morphogenesis [4, 10, 11].

What is the nature of these interactions? What is the developmental lexicon from which these interactions are translated into various cellular responses? What are the "signals" generated by these interactions, and how are these signals translated from the external milieu of the tissue into intracytoplasmic biochemical information to which the cell responds? What levels of biological organization are significant in epithelial-mesenchymal interactions? As a direct consequence of *mesenchymal signals,* for example, do epithelial cells utilize pretranscriptional, transcriptional, translational, or posttranslational *responses* (see Fig. 9)?

Recently, our laboratory described a series of experiments showing that mesenchymal signals were impotent with respect to causing an epithelium to differentiate along a developmental sequence which would be complementary to that associated with the mesenchyme. Dr. Hata and myself (1978) have shown that fetal mouse molar tooth mesenchyme *did not cause* recombined avian limb epithelium to differentiate into secretory ameloblasts [44]. Instead of demonstrating "mesenchymal specificity," we have shown that the stage 22 avian limb epithelium caused de novo translation of type II collagen in the mouse tooth

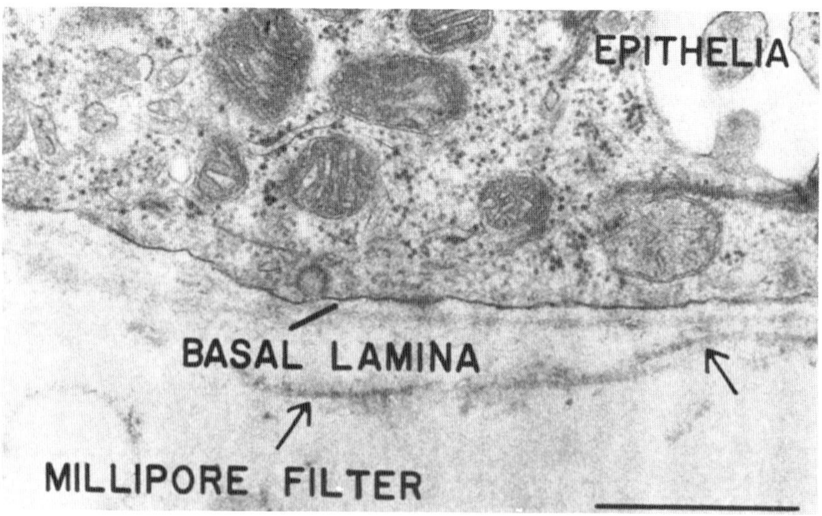

Fig. 8. Morphologic [39] and biochemical [29] studies indicate that enzymatically dissociated inner enamel epithelium, cultured for 48 hours on Millipore filter (0.45 μm pore size and 25 μm thickness), synthesize and secrete several different types of collagen; arrows indicate morphologic suggestions of type I collagen in addition to constituents within the basal lamina (bar line = 1.0 μm).

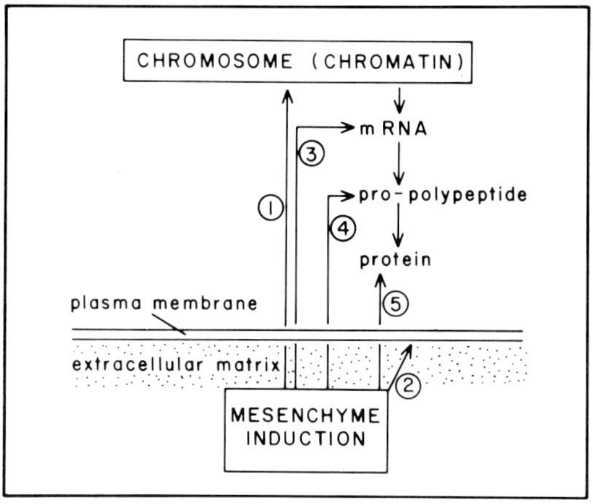

Fig. 9. Mesenchymal tissue, cells, subcellular fractions, or mesenchymal-derived factors [7] appear to be critically required for specific epithelial cytodifferentiation in vivo and in vitro. Mesenchyme instruction(s) or "induction" may 1) directly regulate differential gene expression within epithelial cells, 2) serve as a "signal" and engage epithelial cell surface receptors, 3) regulate transcription of unique mRNAs, 4) regulate translation, and/or 5) regulate posttranslational modifications of unique gene products (eg glycosylation, phosphorylation, etc).

mesenchyme. No type II collagen was detectable at the initiation of these experiments using immunologic and biochemical analyses in the tooth mesenchyme [44]. In vitro or as explants on the CAM, recombined heterologous epithelial-mesenchymal tissues formed masses of cartilage often in the form of a molar tooth organ (so-called "molariform"). These studies were the first to show that epithelial-mesenchymal interactions can affect de novo translation of gene products not present at the initiation of the experiment. Preexisting gene products were not merely amplified, but rather new gene products were detected within five days in culture.

Kollar and Baird showed that mouse tooth mesenchyme caused mouse foot pad epithelium to differentiate into a tissue analogous to secretory ameloblasts using conventional histologic criteria [36, 37]. It is not known, or as yet proven, that the foot pad epithelium synthesized and secreted new gene products not present at the initiation of the experiment. I sense we can safely assume, however, that it is likely that foot pad epithelium did not possess mRNAs for enamel proteins. These fascinating experiments, and others not mentioned, strongly suggest that epithelial-mesenchymal interactions may indeed mediate transcriptional and translational controls during development [44]. The advent of increasingly sensitive radioimmunoassays and the future employment of complementary DNA (cDNA) for enamel proteins, for example, should significantly stimulate advancement towards understanding the nature of these fascinating secondary embryonic tissue interactions.

Translational control describes the regulation of gene expression by controlling rates at which specific mRNA molecules are translated into gene products. It is now well established that numerous hormones, such as steroids, amplify preexisting mRNAs to translate increasingly elevated concentrations of gene product. Comparable controls seem to be associated with epithelial-mesenchymal interactions [7]. For example, total collagen synthesis was found to be amplified 20 times as a consequence of fetal epithelial-mesenchymal interactions during tooth morphogenesis in vitro relative to control isolated enamel organ epithelium or isolated dental papilla mesenchyme [29, 39, 44].

MESENCHYMAL-EPITHELIAL INTERACTIONS RESULTING IN EPITHELIAL DIFFERENTIATION: A DILEMMA

During embryogenesis all epithelium is essentially avascular; nutrients for epithelial cell metabolism are derived by diffusion from adjacent mesenchymal connective tissue stroma and more precisely mediated by the basal lamina located along the undersurface of all epithelia. Numerous investigations have repeatedly demonstrated that the mesenchymal connective tissue stroma is organ-specific; for example, fetal mouse tooth mesenchyme recombined with synergic foot pad epithelium will form a tooth organ expressing secretory ameloblasts, enamel matrix, and enamel mineralization and calcification [22]. The source of the mesenchyme *instructs* a dividing population of cells within an epithelial tissue to differentiate complementary to the specificity of the mesenchyme. This has even been demonstrated across vertebrate species; for example, in the classical studies which showed that embryonic avian skin dermis, isolated from the integument in which feather formation normally occurs, instructed mouse epithelium (isolated from a nonkeratinized portion of the fetal integument) to participate in the formation of feather morphogenesis [10, 11]. In the reciprocal experiments the fetal mouse dermis instructed the avian epithelium to participate in the formation of a nonkeratinized epidermis.

It is evident that our current "state of the art" methodology can provide permissive in vitro environments for the morphogenesis, histogenesis, and differentiation of numerous organ rudiments. These permissive in vitro environments can be chemically defined and may even support morphogenesis without the addition of serum and various growth promoting factors [9]. However, it is well appreciated that the intact fetal organ or a dissociated and reconstituted organ rudiment will advance developmentally in culture, whereas isolated tissues, epithelium, or mesenchyme removed from their respective complementary heterotypic tissue generally fail to differentiate and often no longer maintain the phenotypic characteristics attained at the initiation of the experiment [11–15, 21, 22].

Therefore, as might be predicted, in vitro organ cultures were found to be permissive for intact embryonic and fetal organ explants, whereas these same in vitro conditions were found not to be permissive for inner enamel epithelial differentiation into secretory ameloblasts; homotypic tissue explants known to be determined for a particular phenotype did not differentiate into terminally differentiated cells in vitro. Dissociated cell suspensions made from homotypic tissue isolates, either epithelium or mesenchyme, did not differentiate into ameloblast or odontoblast cells, respectively. If the pH, atmospheric conditions, relative humidity, ascorbic acid concentration, temperature, volume of medium, and medium constituents were found to be permissive for intact tooth organ explant morphogenesis, histogenesis, and cytodifferentiation in vitro, why were these "permissive conditions" found not to be permissive for either isolated homotypic tissue explants or primary cell cultures? Perhaps intact fetal tooth organs have very different nutrient requirements than do isolated fetal tooth tissues or primary cell cultures of homotypic tooth tissues.

SUMMARY AND PROSPECTS FOR FUTURE RESEARCH

Modern embryology has shown that metabolic processes also have very important morphologic characteristics since borders of metabolic fields within the developing embryo or fetus may be identified and delineated spatially and temporally. In a metabolic field, metabolic gradients, often of rather ubiquitous nutrients, occur in a spatial and temporal order and can be demonstrated by a comparison of sequential developmental stages. The positional, morphologic, and structural changes measurable in the metabolic fields of growing and proliferating cells and cell aggregations are always movements away from equilibrium. In a tissue, cells are interconnected by spatially ordered movements of matter of different orders of magnitude. Cells within a tissue constitute a unit of biologic organization which is definable both morphologically and kinetically (ie in time and space). Within and amongst tissues, especially when considering developing epidermal organ systems, *differences exist* which explain, for example, the numerous and different phenotypes expressed by regions of the integument (eg hair and tooth morphogenesis, keratinized and nonkeratinized epithelia, glandular epithelium in thymus, salivary, sebaceous, and mammary gland morphogenesis, etc). These issues confound attempts to formulate instructive and permissive in vitro conditions for various types of epidermal organs, tissues, and epithelial cells.

In considering congenital craniofacial malformations it becomes readily apparent that these relatively common occurrences are not inborn errors of metabolism and are not the result of unique structural gene deletions; rather these conditions – cleft lip and/or palate, for example – represent polygenic disorders resulting from as yet poorly understood interactions between the genome and the environment during the Embryonic Period of gestation [1]. It is not known whether these malformations express transcriptional, translational, posttranslational, or other levels of aberrant biologic regulation. Further, it is not known whether these malformations should best be studied using epithelial cell cultures in vitro.

Of the many important questions associated with human congenital craniofacial malformations, which question or questions might be directly answered using human studies, which using animal studies, which using mouse mutant studies, which using fetal organ cultures, tissue cultures and, finally, cell cultures? As these questions become better defined, complementary methodology will be employed in the research strategy. Recent advances in immunogenetics [45], the characterization of the dentition of inbred strains of mice [46], the identification of mouse mutants which possess unique dental aberrations [47], the recent advances in the biochemistry of tooth development in vivo and in vitro [48, 49], the availability of antisera cross-reactive with mouse fetal enamel proteins [50], and man's insatiable curiosity should provide answers and solutions to these significant health problems in the near future.

ACKNOWLEDGMENT

I would like to take this opportunity to thank Mrs. Peggy Meek for her untiring secretarial assistance in preparing this manuscript.

REFERENCES

1. Slavkin HC: "Developmental Craniofacial Biology." Philadelphia: Lea and Febiger, 1979.
2. Blechschmidt E: "The Beginnings of Human Life." New York: Springer-Verlag, 1977.
3. Rugh R: "The Mouse, Its Reproduction and Development." Minneapolis: Burgess Publishing Co, 1968, pp 227–236.
4. Grobstein C: Mechanisms of organogenetic tissue interaction. Natl Cancer Inst Monogr 26:279–299, 1967.
5. Grobstein C: Developmental role of intercellular matrix: Retrospective and prospective. In Slavkin HC, Greulich RC (eds): "Extracellular Matrix Influences on Gene Expression." New York: Academic Press, 1975, pp 9–16.
6. Roth S: A molecular model for cell interactions. Q Rev Biol 48:541–563, 1973.
7. Pictet RL, Rutter WJ: The molecular basis of the mesenchymal-epithelial interactions in pancreatic development. In Karkinen-Jääskeläinen M, Saxén L, Weiss L (eds): "Cell Interactions in Differentiation." New York: Academic Press, 1977, pp 339–350.
8. Hay ED: Cell-matrix interaction in embryonic induction. In Brinkley BR, Porter KR (eds): "International Cell Biology 1976–1977." New York: Rockefeller University Press, 1977, pp 50–57.
9. Slavkin HC: The nature and nurture of epithelial-mesenchymal interactions during tooth morphogenesis. J Biol Buccale 6:189–204, 1978.
10. Saxén L, Karkinen-Jääskeläinen M, Lehtonen E, Nordling S, Wartiovaara J: Inductive tissue interactions. In Poste G, Nicolson GL (eds): "The Cell Surface in Animal Embryogenesis and Development." Amsterdam: North-Holland Publishing Co, 1976, pp 331–407.
11. Slavkin HC: Embryonic tooth formation: A tool for developmental biology. Oral Sci Rev 4:1–136, 1974.
12. Ruch JV, Karcher-Djuricic V, Gerber R: Les déterminismes de la morphogenèse et des cytodifférenciations des ébauches dentaires de souris. J Biol Buccale 1:45–56, 1973.
13. Ruch JV, Karcher-Djuricic V: On odontogenic tissue interactions. Supra #5, pp 549–554.

14. Smith CE, Warshawsky H: Quantitative analysis of cell turnover in the enamel organ of the rat incisor. Anat Rec 187:63–98, 1977.
15. Thesleff I: Tissue interactions in tooth development in vitro. Supra #7, pp 191–207.
16. Thesleff I, Lehtonen E, Saxén L: Basement membrane formation in transfilter tooth culture and its relation to odontoblast differentiation. Differentiation 10:71–79, 1978.
17. Wolters JM, van Mullem PJ: Electron microscopy of epithelio-mesenchyme intercellular communication in trans-filter cultures of rat tooth germs. Arch Oral Biol 22:705–709, 1977.
18. Pannese E: Observations on the ultrastructure of the enamel organ. III. Internal and external enamel epithelia. J Ultrastruct Res 6:186–204, 1962.
19. Gaunt WA: An analysis of the growth of the cheek teeth of the mouse. Acta Anat (Basel) 54:220–259, 1963.
20. Kallenbach E: Electron microscopy of the differentiating rat incisor ameloblast. J Ultrastruct Res 35:508-531, 1971.
21. Koch WE: Tissue interaction during in vitro odontogenesis. In Slavkin HC, Bavetta LA (eds): "Developmental Aspects of Oral Biology." New York: Academic Press, 1972, pp 151–164.
22. Kollar EJ: Histogenetic aspects of dermal- epidermal interactions. Ibid, pp 125–149.
23. Miller WA: Inductive changes in early tooth development. I. A study of mouse tooth development on the chick chorioallantois. J Dent Res 48 Spec Suppl):719–725, 1969.
24. van der Linder FPGM, Duterloo HS: "Development of the Human Dentition." New York: Harper & Row, 1976.
25. Kraus BS, Jordan RE: "The Human Dentition Before Birth." Philadelphia: Lea & Febiger, 1965.
26. Nery EB, Kraus BS, Croup M: Timing and topography of early human tooth development. Arch Oral Biol 15:1315–1326, 1970.
27. Slavkin HC, Trump GN, Schonfeld S, Brownell A, Sorgente N, Lee-Own V: Epigenetic regulation of enamel protein synthesis during epithelial-mesenchymal interactions. Supra #7, pp 209–226,
28. Bailey AF: Biosynthesis of collagen cross-links: Relationship of heritable disorders. In Holton JB, Ireland JT (eds): "Inborn Errors of Skin, Hair, and Connective Tissue." Baltimore: University Park Press, 1975, pp 105–118.
29. Dorfman A: Genetic defects of the degradation of glycosaminoglycans: The mucopolysaccharidoses. Ibid, pp 163–177.
30. McKusick VA: "Heritable Disorders of Connective Tissue," 3rd Ed. St. Louis: CV Mosby, 1966.
31. Trelstad RL, Slavkin HC: Collagen synthesis by the epithelial enamel organ of the embryonic rabbit tooth. Biochem Biophys Res Commun 59:443–449, 1974.
32. Slavkin HC, Trump GN, Brownell A, Sorgente N: Epithelial-mesenchymal interactions: Mesenchymal specificity. In Lash JW, Burger MM (eds): "Cell and Tissue Interactions." New York: Raven Press, 1977, pp 29–46.
33. Kallenbach E: Fine structure of differentiating ameloblasts in the kitten. Am J Anat 145:283–318, 1976.
34. Slavkin HC, Bringas P Jr: Epithelial-mesenchyme interactions during odontogenesis. IV. Morphological evidence for direct heterotypic cell-cell contacts. Dev Biol 50:428–442, 1976.
35. Koch WE: In vitro differentiation of tooth rudiments of embryonic mice. I. Transfilter interaction of embryonic incisor tissues. J Exp Zool 165:155–170, 1967.
36. Kollar EJ, Baird GR: Tissue interactions in embryonic mouse tooth germs. I: Reorganization of the dental epithelium during tooth-germ reconstruction. J Embryol Exp Morphol 24:159–171, 1970a.

37. Kollar EJ, Baird GR: Tissue interactions in embryonic mouse tooth germs. II. The inductive role of the dental papilla. J Embryol Exp Morphol 24:173–186, 1970b.
38. Croissant R, Guenther H, Slavkin HC: How are embryonic preameloblasts instructed by odontoblasts to synthesize enamel? Supra #5, pp 515–521.
39. Slavkin HC, Matosian P, Wilson P, Bringas P, Mino W, Croissant RD, Guenther H: Epithelial-specific extracellular matrix influences on mesenchyme collagen biosynthesis in vitro. Supra #5, pp 515–521.
40. Hay ED, Revel JP: Fine structure of the developing avian cornea. Monogr Dev Biol 1:1–144, 1969.
41. Dodson JW, Hay ED: Secretion of collagen by corneal epithelium. II. Effect of the underlying substratum on secretion and polymerization of epithelial products. J Exp Zool 189:51–72, 1974.
42. Trelstad RL, Hayashi K, Toole BP: Epithelial collagens and glycosaminoglycans in the embryonic cornea. Macromolecular order and morphogenesis in the basement membrane. J Cell Biol 62:815–830, 1974.
43. Grobstein C: Reflections and summary. Supra #5, pp 809–814.
44. Hata R, Slavkin HC: De novo induction of a gene product during heterologous epithelial-mesenchymal interactions in vitro. Proc Natl Acad Sci USA 75:2790–2794, 1978.
45. Klein J: "Biology of the Mouse Histocompatibility-2 Complex." New York: Springer-Verlag, 1975, pp 521–536.
46. Wickramaratne GA de S: The "skeletal profile" and dentition of some inbred strains of mice. J Anat 117:565–573, 1974.
47. Sofaer JA: Aspects of the tabby-crinkled-downless syndrome. II. Observations on the reaction to changes of genetic background. J Embryol Exp Morphol 22:207–227, 1969.
48. Guenther HL, Croissant RD, Schonfeld SE, Slavkin HC: Identification of four extra-cellular-matrix enamel proteins during embryonic-rabbit tooth-organ development. Biochem J 163:591–603, 1977.
49. Slavkin HC, Weliky B, Stellar W, Slavkin MD, Zeichner-Gancz M, Bringas P Jr, Hyatt-Fischer H, Shimizu M, Fukae M: Ameloblast differentiation: Protein synthesis and secretion in fetal New Zealand white rabbit molar tooth organs and isolated epithelia in vitro. J Biol Buccale 6:309–326, 1978.
50. Hyatt-Fischer H, Chrispens J, O'Keefe D, Slavkin HC: An antisera for the fluorescent labeling of mouse amelogenins. In Termine J, Nylen M (eds): "Third International Symposium of Tooth Enamel." J Dent Res 58(9):1008–1009, 1979.

Human Newborn Urine as a Source of Epithelial Cells

Jeanette S. Felix, PhD, and John W. Littlefield, MD

Skin biopsy is the routine approach for obtaining a cell sample for in vitro growth. Using standard cell culture procedures, the fibroblast population present in most tissue biopsies rapidly overgrows the epithelial cell component. Pure cultures of dividing epithelial cells have been difficult to achieve until recently. As discussed elsewhere in this volume, there are now technical modifications which selectively suppress the proliferation of fibroblasts from certain tissues. As research evolves to include many different cell types for the study of inherited diseases and birth defects, there will be an increased need for routine biopsy techniques to obtain epithelial cells. One possibility is the culture of urinary tract lining epithelial cells which can be recovered from the urine [1, 2, 3].

Several epithelial cell types, as well as red and white blood cells, are found in the urinary sediment. These epithelial cells include renal tubular epithelial cells; transitional cells from the renal pelvis, the ureters, and the bladder; and squamous epithelial cells from the anterior urethra. Since only epithelial cells line the urinary tract, the sediment is unlikely to contain fibroblasts. There is constant, slow renewal of this cell population, resulting in continuous exfoliation from the urinary tract surface lining into the urine. Desquamation of this epithelial lining seems to be increased as a result of inflammation, neoplastic changes, and renal disease, and following vigorous exercise. Normally, the mean daily rate of excretion of cells measured in normal adult males and in children 4–12 years of age is 6×10^5 to 1×10^6 cells per day [4]. However, urine from a newborn baby contains a significantly higher number of cells, possibly the result of continued rapid growth and development of the urinary tract until several months after birth.

We will review our findings on cell cultures derived from human newborn urine [3, 5]. The urine specimens were obtained from 1-day-old to 3-month-old infants in the full-term and intensive care nurseries by the nursing staff. Although sterile preparatory techniques were used in collecting the urine, approximately 25% of these specimens showed gross bacterial or fungal contamination after 1–2 days in culture, even when maintained with penicillin and streptomycin in the medium.

Birth Defects: Original Article Series, Volume XVI, Number 2, pages 231–237

Cultures were initiated by centrifuging the specimen and resuspending the entire sediment in culture medium (Eagle's Minimal Essential Medium plus 15% fetal calf serum). The cell suspension was plated into standard plastic culture vessels and incubated at 37°C in 5% CO_2.

Less than 1% of the cells attached to the dish surface and only a small number of the attached cells divided to form colonies. Among the specimens which yielded cell cultures, there was an average of 3 macroscopic colonies formed per ml of specimen during the first 2 weeks of culture. Cell growth occurred in 51% of the uncontaminated specimens from infants younger than 1 week compared to 25% from infants older than 1 week. When primary colonies were subcultured, the dispersed cell population usually doubled every 24 hours until the culture began to grow slowly and then ceased to divide. Some cultures could be passed up to 6 times using trypsin to suspend the cells. Final populations of 10^8 cells could be achieved from 10-ml specimens. As many as 25 cell population doublings were achieved in the more vigorous cultures. This estimate of population doublings was calculated assuming one starting cell per initial colony and knowing the final cell number obtained. When the cells ceased dividing, they remained attached and flat. If not subjected to further trypsinization, the cells appeared healthy for several more weeks and only slowly acquired the appearance of degenerating or dead cells. Near-confluent monolayers of nondividing urinary cells have been maintained for up to 4 months with regular medium changes. At early passages, the colony-forming efficiency of cells was as high as 15%. Cultures could be frozen in medium containing 10% dimethyl sulfoxide and successfully recovered after thawing.

The morphology of the majority of cultured urinary cells from newborns is shown in Figure 1 and was designated Type I. These cells grew as monolayers, adhering firmly to the culture surface. The primary colonies formed contiguous groups of bipolar cells which were much less spindle-shaped than are fibroblasts. Cells at the edge of a colony also remained in close contact with the central area of the colony, instead of moving to unoccupied areas. Neither the dense center of the colony nor confluent mass culture formed parallel arrays of cells as do fibroblasts; instead the cells were randomly arranged.

Type II cells (Fig. 2) were a minor component of the cellular growth derived from urine. These colonies were seen in 10% of the urine cultures and when present represented only 2–4% of the total colonies in that culture. These colonies formed very compact monolayers of small cells which typically grew as a uniform sheet and often formed dense swirls of cells throughout the colony. Urine collected from newborns who were being treated with the diuretic furosemide formed large numbers of Type II colonies. These cultures yielded 30–60 colonies per ml instead of the usual 3 per ml, and 50–95% of these were Type II. This increase in viable urinary cells may reflect excessive cell loss due to the presumed action of furosemide at the Henle's loop.

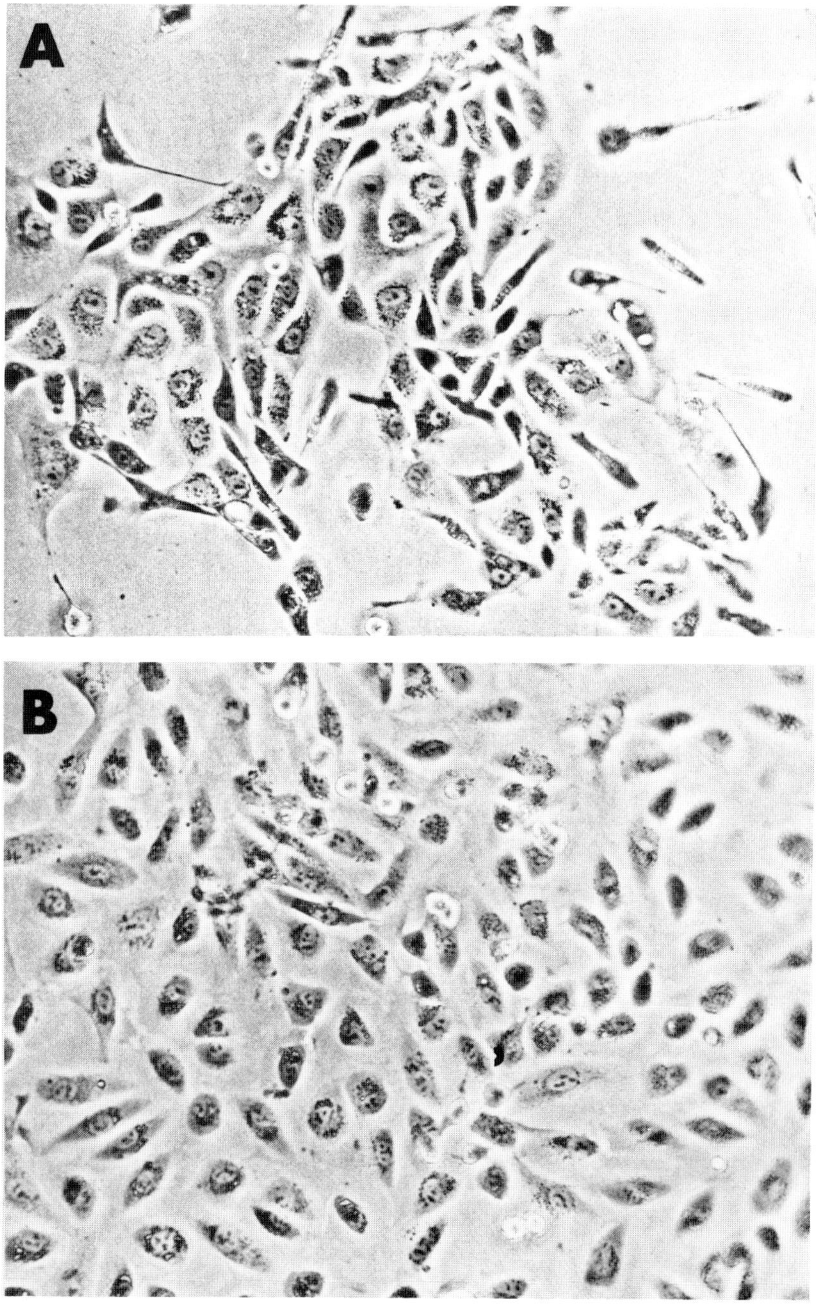

Fig. 1. A) A colony of Type I urinary cells. The majority of cells cultured from urine form primary colonies with this morphology. The cells are bipolar but much less elongated than typical human diploid fibroblasts. Peripheral cells remain in close contact with each other around a confluent central area. Phase contrast view of living cells. B) A confluent area of Type I urinary cells.

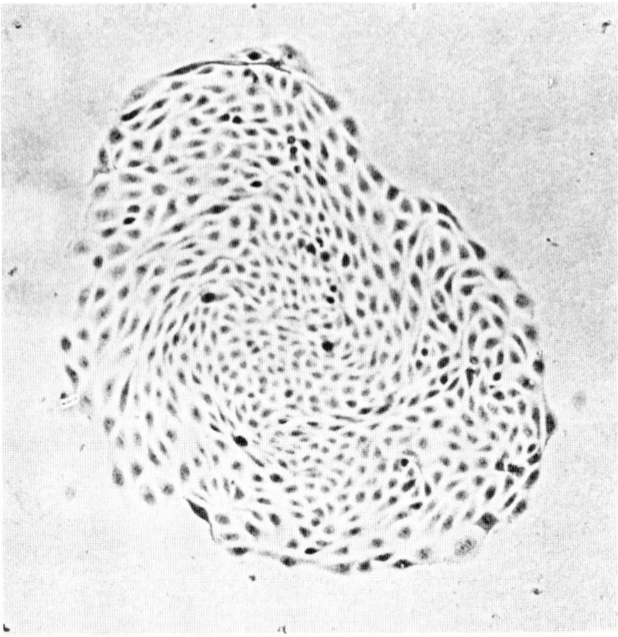

Fig. 2. A colony of Type II urinary cells. Less than 5% of colonies derived from normal newborn urine are of this morphology. The colony grows as a sheet of cells with a smooth edge. Phase contrast view of living cells.

We have tried to optimize culture procedures for maximum growth of urine cells and for maximum recovery of viable cells from the urine [5]. Our goal is to derive large urinary tract cell populations from any single individual. The following variables were evaluated by determining their effect on several growth parameters: 1) number of colonies initiated per specimen, 2) growth rate, 3) colony-forming efficiency of early passage cells, and 4) culture life-span. Various media, sera, supplements of amino acids, polyamines, hormones, and growth factors were tested, as well as feeder layers, conditioned media, and specially treated culture surfaces. There was no improvement in culture success with any of these modifications, but further examination of culture conditions or specimen collection might be useful. Thus, at present, newborn urinary cell cultures can be derived following culture procedures which are standard for establishing cell cultures from amniotic fluid. Neither feeder cell layers nor fibroblast inhibitors have been necessary, and mitogens active on some epithelial cells have not been effective.

Two epithelial properties have been demonstrated in these urinary cell cultures: keratin production and plaque formation by BK virus. Keratin production by cultured cells can be demonstrated with immunofluorescent techniques using antibody prepared against a group of keratins purified from human stratum corneum [6]. This antibody has identified keratin filaments in skin keratinocytes and various other stratified epithelia, but not in connective tissue or cultured mesenchymal cells. Also the ability to produce keratin is retained during serial cultivation of human epidermal cells [7]. In studies done with Dr. T.-T. Sun, we found that many newborn urinary cells stained positively for keratin, as shown in Figure 3, even though these cells do not form stratified cultures [5]. Since there were some negative cells in the cultures, it was necessary to determine if these cells had lost the ability to produce keratin, or if there was a mixed population of keratin-producing and nonproducing cells which could be separated by looking at colonies. Primary colonies from 2 cultures were examined. Six colonies were examined from 1 culture, 4 of which had only positively staining cells while 2 had only negatively staining cells. In 3 colonies examined from a second culture, only keratin-positive cells were seen. Therefore, cells in the urine apparently are either keratin-positive or keratin-negative and this phenotype is stably maintained in culture, resulting in pure positive colonies and pure negative colonies. When positive and negative colonies from these 2 cultures were pooled, and then grown through 4 passages, both keratin-producing and keratin-negative cells were observed. Thus, a specific differentiated function has been retained over many cell divisions in culture. Since it appears that all cells which line the urinary tract, including renal tubular cells, produce keratin, as seen in stained tissue sections [8], the identity of the negative urinary cells is unclear. These cultures contained cells only of Type I morphology, suggesting that further classification of cultured urinary cells is necessary. Indeed, among those cells producing keratin, some have keratin filaments in radial arrays around the nucleus and others have arrays of longitudinal filaments in the cells.

Another epithelial cell characteristic demonstrated in urinary cell cultures is the susceptibility to lytic infection by BK virus [9]. BK virus is a human papovavirus which was isolated from the urine of a kidney transplant patient [10]. BK virus specific antibodies are commonly found in human serum, and the virus is rarely connected with disease. BK can be grown but will not form plaques in Vero cells (African Green Monkey kidney cells). Primary cultures of human embryonic kidney cells allow BK plaque formation while neither human fibroblasts nor established nonkidney cells support growth of this virus. Our results show that confluent monolayers of human newborn urinary cells develop plaques as the result of focal lytic infection by BK virus. After exposing the cell monolayer to a suspension of virus, the cultures are overlaid with agar and incubated for an additional 2 weeks, then neutral red dye is added to the medium. This vital dye is transported into living cells, while colorless areas indicate groups of nonviable cells. Virus-infected cultures have clear plaques quantitatively proportional to the dilution of the virus suspension. With time, the plaques increase in size. BK virus was twice plaque-purified by picking virus from a single plaque, regrowing

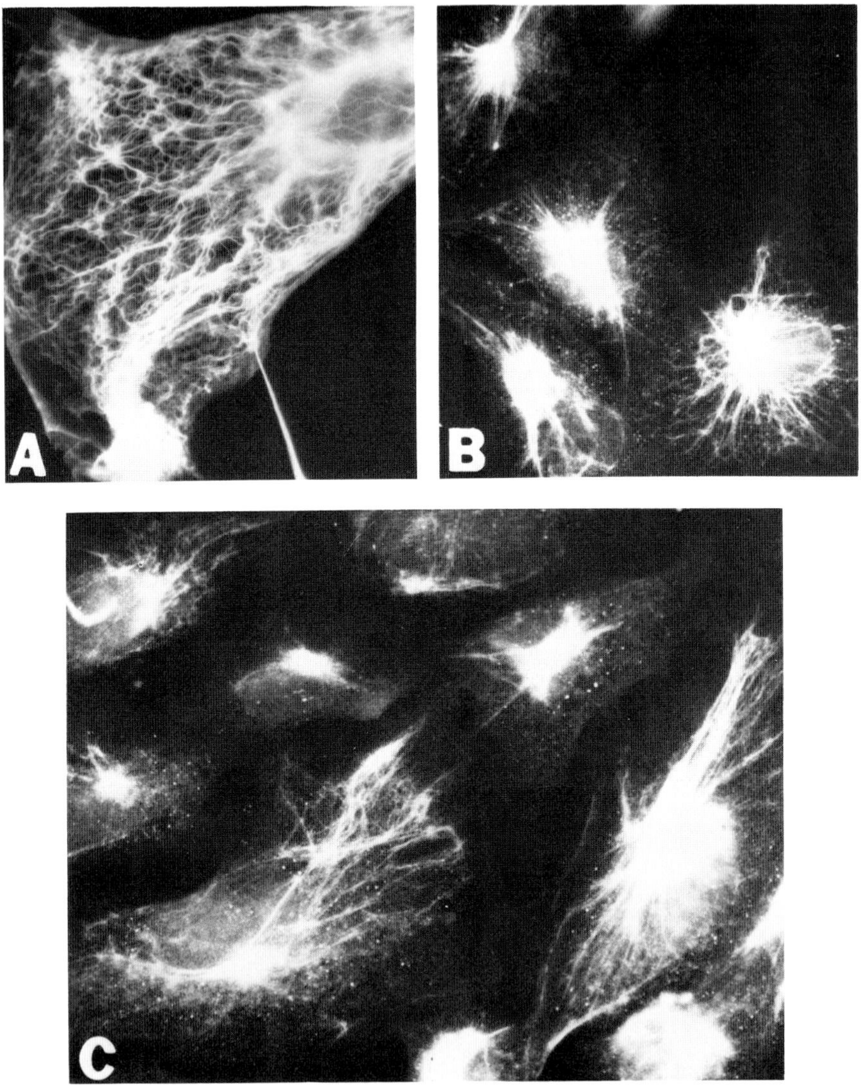

Fig. 3. Immunofluorescent staining of cultured urinary cells by antikeratin antibody. A culture of cells derived from human newborn urine was fixed and stained with antikeratin antiserum. A) Brightly stained filaments of keratin are clearly evident in the cytoplasm of this single urinary cell. B and C) Urinary cells from secondary cultures produced keratin during 4 serial passages over a 4-week period.

the virus in Vero cells, again infecting urinary cell monolayers to produce plaques, and then repeating this process. Ten independent newborn urine cultures have yielded BK plaques. From the distribution and shape of plaques all cells in the monolayer seem equally susceptible to BK virus infection.

In summary, urinary cell cultures can be viewed as a mixture of at least 2 types of epithelial cells. These cells can be grown without the use of feeder layers or fibroblast inhibitors. No fibroblasts have been identified yet in any culture. These cultures could be useful in several ways. First, they can reflect the status of the urinary tract cells in vivo, as shown by cell number and cell type present in the urine. A urinary tract-specific metabolic function, perhaps of the kidney or of the bladder, might be expressed in these cultured cells. Second, genetic metabolic diseases might be defined whose defects are generally evident in all surface epithelia, but not in fibroblasts. Urine cells would provide an easy means for screening individuals, especially if uncultured cells could be tested. Third, problems of cellular differentiation and neoplasia would be appropriately studied in urinary cell cultures.

An important aspect of urine cell culture is that it is accomplished through a totally atraumatic, noninvasive means for cell sampling. The ability to grow cells from adult urine also suggests that this approach could be used to sample persons of any age, although cultures from adults are more difficult to establish at this time. In both newborns and adults, several specimens might be needed to ensure that a viable culture is obtained.

REFERENCES

1. Sutherland GR, Bain AD: Culture of cells from the urine of newborn children. Nature 239:231, 1972.
2. Linder D: Culture of cells from the urine and bladder washings of adults. Somatic Cell Genet 2:281–283, 1976.
3. Felix JS, Littlefield JW: Urinary tract epithelial cells cultured from human urine. Int Rev Cytol (In press).
4. Strauss MB, Welt LG: "Diseases of the Kidney," 2nd Ed. Little, Brown & Co., 1971.
5. Felix JS, Littlefield JW: Evaluation of growth requirements for keratinocytes and other epithelial cells cultured from human urine. (In preparation.)
6. Sun T-T, Green H: Immunofluorescent staining of keratin fibers in cultured cells. Cell 14:469–476, 1978.
7. Sun T-T, Green H: Keratin filaments of cultured human epidermal cells: Formation of intermolecular disulfide bonds during terminal differentiation. J Biol Chem 253:2053–2060, 1978.
8. Sun T-T, Shih C, Green H: Keratin cytoskeleton in epithelial cells of internal organs. Proc Natl Acad Sci USA (In press).
9. Sack GH Jr, Felix JS: Studies on BK virus cloned in human urinary epithelial cells. (In preparation.)
10. Gardner SD, Field AM, Coleman DV, Hulme B: New human papovavirus (B.K.) isolated from urine after renal transplantation. Lancet 1:1253–1257, 1971.

Selection of Epithelial Cells in Culture by D-Valine Medium*

Barbara R. Migeon, MD

We have reported a nutrient medium specifically enabling the growth, in vitro, of normal epithelial cells of human and rodent origin [1, 2]. The basis of the selection is the ability of some epithelial cells to utilize D-amino acids. When D-valine (D-VAL) is substituted for L-valine (L-VAL) in the medium, only those cells having D-amino acid oxidase can convert the D-amino acid into its essential L-enantiomer (Fig. 1). Using medium containing D-VAL instead of L-VAL and serum dialyzed to remove L-VAL, we have been able to propagate epithelial cell populations having the pertinent enzyme and to inhibit the growth of fibroblasts and other cells which do not. The ability of D-VAL medium to inhibit fibroblasts in cultures derived from kidneys has enabled selection of renal epithelial cells in the absence of fibroblast overgrowth. The cells selected in D-VAL transmit to progeny not only their epithelial morphology but also their ability to synthesize

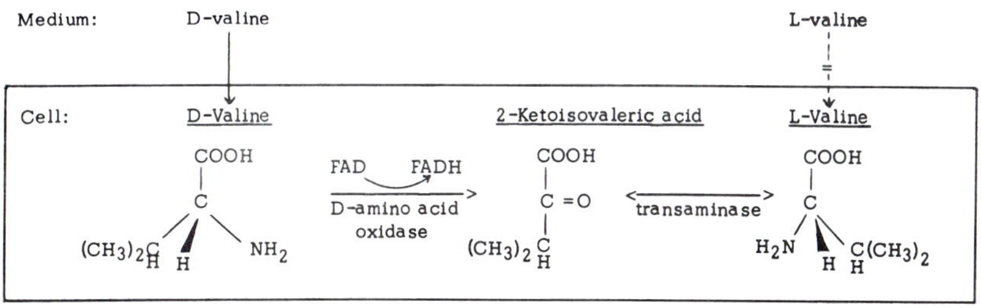

Fig. 1. Basis of chemical selection for cells with D-amino acid oxidase. Essential L-VAL, omitted from the nutrient medium is replaced by D-VAL. Epithelial cells with D-amino acid oxidase convert D-VAL to L-VAL and therefore can proliferate while fibroblasts, lacking this enzyme, cannot. (Figs. 1 and 4 from Gibert SF, Migeon BR: D-valine as a selective agent for normal human and rodent epithelial cells in culture. Cell 5:11-17, © 1975 by The MIT Press, with permission.)

*Supported by NIH grant HD 05465.

Birth Defects: Original Article Series, Volume XVI, Number 2, pages 239–247

TABLE 1. Summary of Activity of Renal Enzymes in Human and Mouse Cells in Culture

Renal Enzyme	Assays	Cells Assayed										
		Human					Mouse					
		Kidney			Skin	Lung	Kidney		Lung		3T3	RAG
		Fetal D-VAL	Adult D-VAL	Fetal L-VAL	Adult L-VAL	Fetal L-VAL	Fetal D-VAL	Adult D-VAL	Adult D-VAL	Adult L-VAL		
D-Amino Acid Oxidase	Growth in D-VAL	+	+		−		−	+	+		−	−
	Growth in 2-KIVA	+			+							
	Histochemical	+			−			+				
Carbonic Anhydrase		+		−				+	+	−	−	−
Alkaline Phosphatase	Histochemical				−			+				
	Spectrophotometric				−			+				
Lactate Dehydrogenase	Electrophoretic*	+		−	−	−						

*Kidney specific.

From Gilbert SF, Migeon BR: Renal enzymes in kidney cells selected by D-valine medium. J Cell Physiol 92:161–168, 1977, with permission.

"differentiated cell" enzymes in vitro. The selected cells have D-amino acid oxidase, carbonic anhydrase, high levels of alkaline phosphatase, and the renal specific pattern for lactate dehydrogenase [2] (Table 1). The presence of these renal enzymes suggests that the selected epithelial cells are of renal tubular origin and indicates that these differentiated functions are retained in cultured cells.

D-AMINO ACID OXIDASE ACTIVITY OF SELECTED CELLS

There is considerable evidence the D-amino acid oxidase is present in the D-VAL selected cells. Cells which proliferate in D-VAL cannot divide in valine-*free* medium. On the other hand, those cells unable to proliferate in D-VAL can do so if provided the product of the D-amino acid oxidase reaction, 2-ketoisovaleric acid (Fig. 2). Cells from fetal mouse kidney, known to lack D-amino acid oxidase are unable to proliferate in D-VAL. Lastly, D-amino acid oxidase activity has been detected histochemically (based on the reduction of tetrazolium to an insoluble product) in D-VAL selected cells from adult mouse and fetal human kidneys, but not in human skin fibroblasts incubated in the same reaction mix [1].

Studies of carbonic anhydrase activity in the D-VAL selected kidney cells indicate that the specific activity of the enzyme in the cultured cells is less than that in fresh kidney cells prior to culture [2] (Fig. 3). Furthermore, although the enzyme

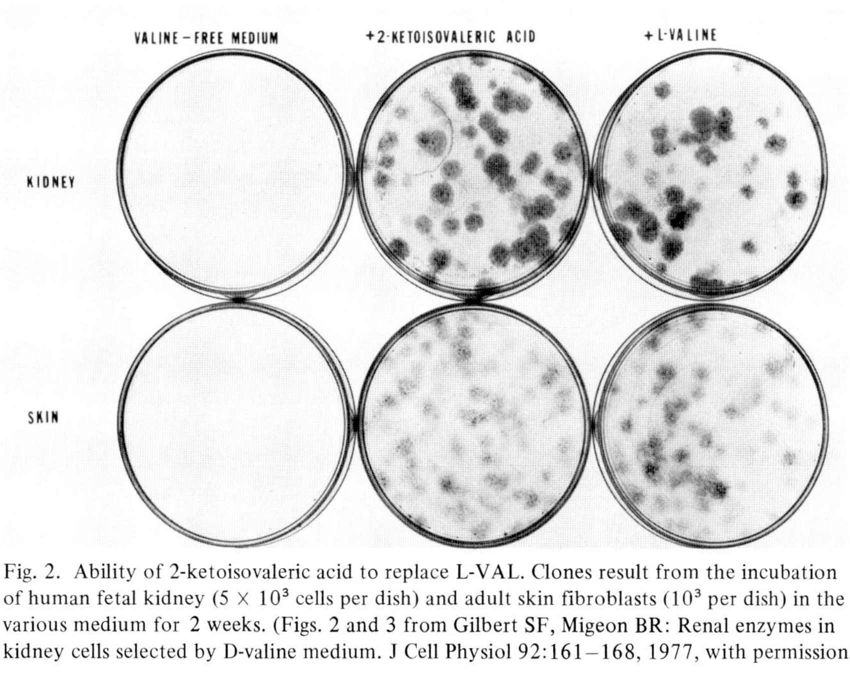

Fig. 2. Ability of 2-ketoisovaleric acid to replace L-VAL. Clones result from the incubation of human fetal kidney (5×10^3 cells per dish) and adult skin fibroblasts (10^3 per dish) in the various medium for 2 weeks. (Figs. 2 and 3 from Gilbert SF, Migeon BR: Renal enzymes in kidney cells selected by D-valine medium. J Cell Physiol 92:161–168, 1977, with permission.)

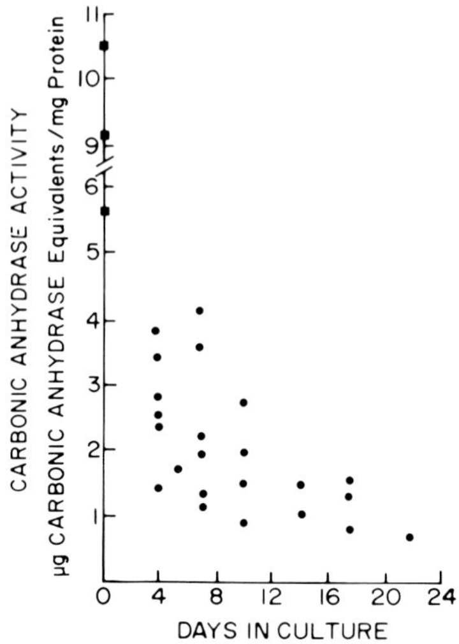

Fig. 3. Carbonic anhydrase activity of D-VAL selected mouse renal cells as a function of time in culture. Activity was estimated from a standard curve, using mouse carbonic anhydrase II. Circles represent individual dishes of D-VAL selected cells. Squares at day 0 indicate activities of the initial suspensions (free of red blood cells) from which cells were plated.

is readily detectable in the cells throughout the period of observation, the activity decreases with time in culture. This decrease in activity occurs even when the growth of less specialized cells has been inhibited, so that it cannot be attributed merely to the dilution of specialized enzymes by proteins from other cell types. It is possible that cells in vitro have a limited capacity to synthesize these specialized enzymes. Alternatively, the medium or substrate may not be adequate to maintain renal functions in vitro for long periods of time.

POTENTIAL FOR GROWTH

We have observed that these epithelial cells, although able to give rise to clones, do not survive many cell transfers subsequently. The ability to proliferate in D-VAL requires the continuous expression of a differentiated function, so that the loss of proliferative ability may result from dedifferentiation rather than from cell senescence. On the other hand, the nutrient medium used for the isolation of these differentiated cells is far from optimal as serum must be dialyzed to eliminate an important source of L-VAL. Dialysis removes other small molecules which may be essential for growth of these cells. Nonetheless, it is conceivable that these D-VAL selected cells are undergoing a programmed senescence. Epithelial cell populations derived by non-selective means from urine [3] and semen [4] also exhibit a limited potential for growth. It may be that most euploid cells carrying on differentiated functions have a restricted capacity for proliferation.

EPITHELIAL CELLS SELECTABLE IN D-VAL

The selective medium was designed as a means of obtaining pure populations of renal epithelial cells, because these cells were known to have D-amino acid oxidase. Our initial studies indicated as expected, that cells from human adult and fetal kidneys and from rodent adult kidneys could proliferate in D-VAL, while those from rodent fetal kidneys, known to lack D-amino acid oxidase, could not (Table 1). Subsequent studies have indicated, however, that some cells from tissues not known to have the pertinent enzyme, can proliferate in the selective medium. It seems that cell growth is a more sensitive indicator of the presence of the enzyme than biochemical assays. D-amino acid oxidase was long thought to occur only in kidney and liver where racemation of D-amino acids has been observed, but has more recently been detected in human cerebellum and neutrophils. Our bioassay has enabled us to infer the presence of D-amino acid oxidase in cells of human fetal lung (Fig. 4), umbilical cord, and cerebellum. Others have been able to select proliferating epithelial cell populations from the mouse mammary gland [5] and rat adrenal cortex [6].

Unfortunately, there does not seem to be any D-amino acid oxidase in epithelial cells from dermal biopsies. The growth of epithelial cells as well as fibroblasts from these skin explants is completely inhibited in D-VAL. Other cells which lack the ability to proliferate in D-VAL include fetal cells derived from intestine and cartilage (Migeon, unpublished observations) and EB-transformed lymphoid cell lines [7].

In our hands D-VAL selection must be maintained to inhibit fibroblasts in mixed populations of fibroblast and epithelial cells or in dishes containing explants. Although many of the fibroblasts in D-VAL detach from the dish, the few which remain, even after weeks of L-VAL deprivation, are capable of proliferation when L-VAL is supplied. We have also encountered problems with the transfer of epithelial colonies; many of the cells do not survive the transfer.

Despite the difficulties in propagation, the fact that D-VAL selected cells retain certain differentiated functions for weeks in culture has encouraged us to look at the possibility of selecting cells from the amniotic fluid which might express urea cycle enzymes.

SELECTION OF AMNIOCYTES

The prenatal diagnosis of inborn errors has generally been limited to those diseases where the defect is demonstrable in fibroblasts. Unfortunately, many enzyme deficiencies responsible for metabolic errors are not demonstrable in fibroblasts. Included among these are the inborn errors classified as hyperammonemias involving

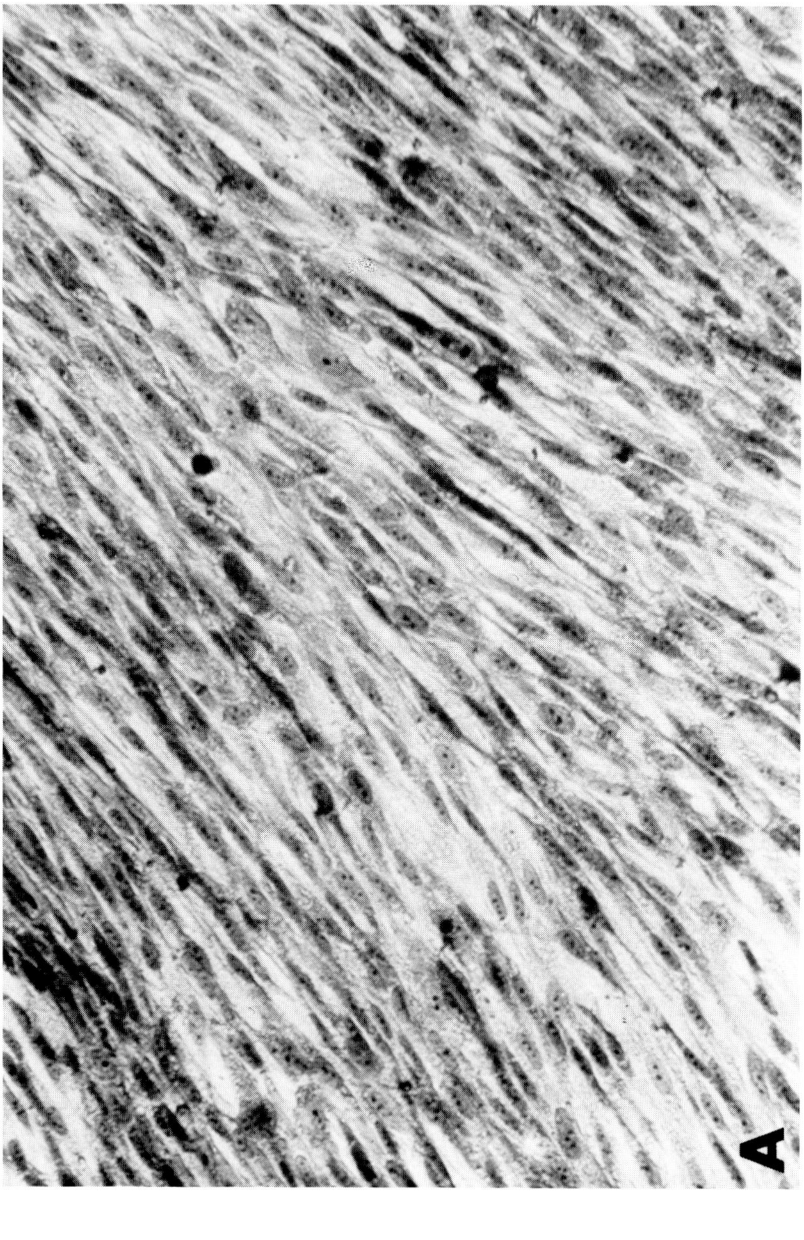
A

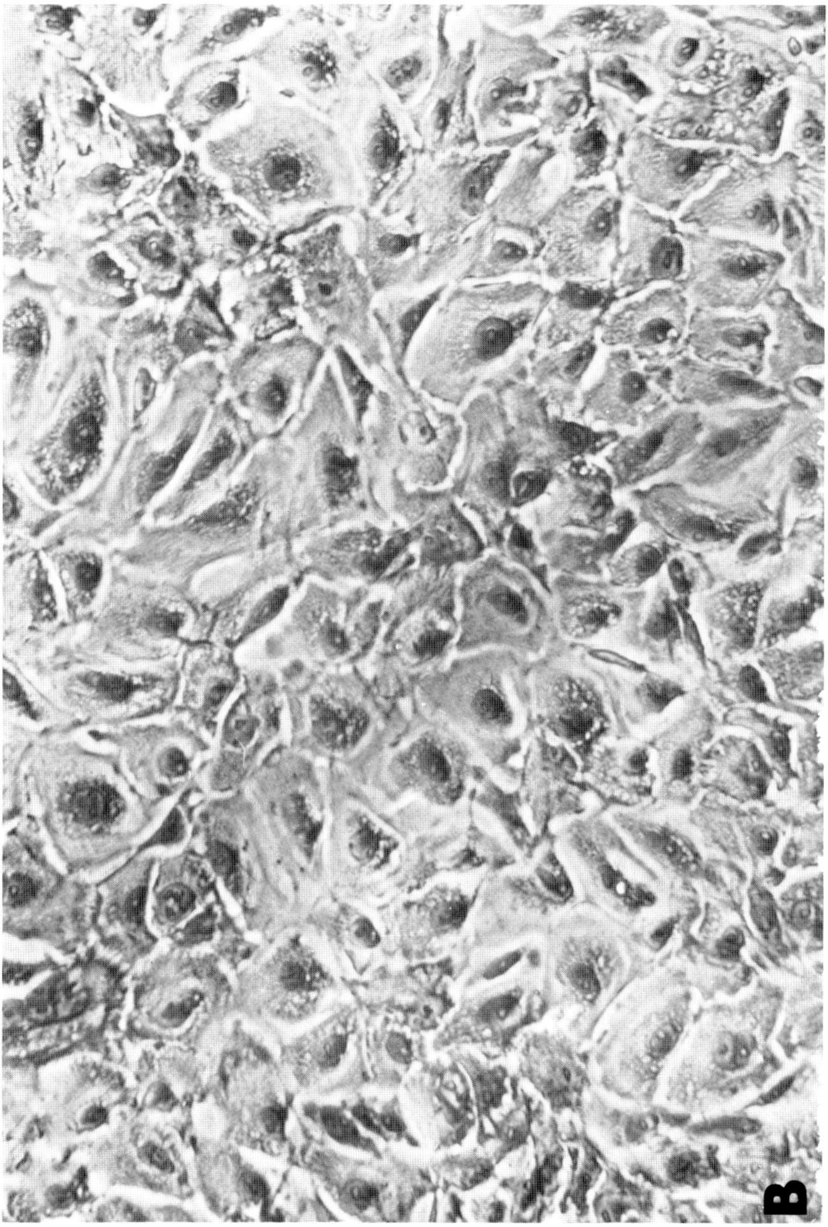

Fig. 4. Outgrowths from explants of human fetal lung after 2 weeks in L-VAL or D-VAL. Note proliferation of A) fibroblasts in L-VAL and B) epithelial cells in D-VAL.

deficiencies of enzymes in the urea cycle. Although some of these enzymes may be found in skin fibroblasts, the complete cycle occurs only in liver and kidney cells. Ornithine transcarbamoylase and carbamoyl phosphate synthetase are found only in differentiated cells.

Although the majority of amniotic fluid cells may be derived from fetal membranes as evidenced by production of human chorionic gonadotropin [8, 9], it is likely that cells from the fetus also contribute to the composition of the heterogenous cell population. We expect that cells from the gastrointestinal and urinary tracts might be found among the amniocytes. Although clones of epithelial cells are often obtained from cultures of amniotic fluid, these are usually overgrown by fibroblasts which proliferate at a faster rate. Therefore, if there are cells which have an intact urea cycle, they would be obscured by those that do not.

We have been attempting to enrich for such differentiated amniocytes by discouraging the proliferation of fibroblasts using D-VAL selection [10]. We obtained amniotic fluid from women undergoing elective termination of pregnancy in the Fertility Control Clinic of The Johns Hopkins Hospital. Cells were pelleted by centrifugation and the pellet was resuspended and distributed into plastic tissue culture dishes containing either MEM enriched with nonessential amino acids and 20% fetal calf serum or MEM D-VAL (GIBCO) containing 20% dialyzed fetal calf serum. Cultures were maintained in 5% CO_2 at 37° with medium changes twice weekly. After 2–3 weeks, there were abundant colonies (ie 10–12) proliferating in each control dish. These colonies were of mixed morphology – some fibroblastic, others with epithelial morphology. In the dishes maintained in D-VAL, there were 1–4 colonies per dish. All of the colonies were of epithelial morphology and were considerably less dense than those in control dishes, presumably in part attributable to the dialyzed serum. These colonies were subcultured in situ in the dish to disperse the cells from the clones into monolayers. The D-VAL selected cells, along with those maintained in nonselective medium, were assayed for the presence of ornithine transcarbamoylase, using spectrophotometric assays. We did not detect any activity of this enzyme in either the D-VAL selected cells from the mouse in control amniocytes maintained under nonselective conditions.

The fact that we were not able to obtain ornithine transcarbamoylase activity in these D-VAL selected amniocytes does not preclude their renal origin, as activity of this enzyme was not detectable in D-VAL selected cells from the mouse kidney. This may be attributable to the fact that the specific activity of the enzyme in kidney cells is only 1–3% of that in liver cells. Therefore, more sensitive assays may be necessary to detect urea cycle enzymes in anmiocytes of renal origin. Although the derivation of these D-VAL selected cells has not been established, it is clear that one can select for amniocytes able to utilize D-amino acids. When the identity of these cells is established, it may be possible to utilize them for prenatal diagnosis of inborn errors not demonstrable in fibroblasts.

ACKNOWLEDGMENTS

The author wishes to acknowledge contributions to the work described in this paper by Dr. Scott F. Gilbert, Dr. Saul W. Brusilow, Mr. Tai T. Do, and Ms. Joyce A. Sprenkle.

REFERENCES

1. Gilbert SF, Migeon BR: D-valine as a selective agent for normal human and rodent epithelial cells in culture. Cell 5:11–17, 1975.
2. Gilbert SF, Migeon BR: Renal enzymes in kidney cells selected by D-valine medium. J Cell Physiol 92:161–168, 1977.
3. Felix JS, Littlefield JW: Human newborn urine as a source of epithelial cells. This volume.
4. Phillips SG, Phillips DM, Kabat EA, Miller OJ: Human semen as source of epithelial cells for culture. In Vitro 14:639–650, 1978.
5. White MT, Hu ASL, Hamamoto ST, Nandi S: In vitro analysis of proliferating epithelial cell populations from the mouse mammary gland: Fibroblast-free growth and serial passage. In Vitro 14:271–281, 1978.
6. Liles S, Ramachandran J: Regulation of delta 5–3 beta-hydroxysteroid dehydrogenase-isomerase activity in adrenocortical cell cultures by adreno-corticotropin. Biochem Biophys Res Commun 79:226–233, 1977.
7. Benke PJ, Dittmar D: Human lymphocyte response to D-valine media, Biochim Biophys Acta 451:635–637, 1976.
8. Priest JH, Priest RE, Sgoutas DS: Production of hormone by cells cultured from human amniotic fluid (Abstract) Am J Hum Genet 29:88A, 1977.
9. Priest RE, Marimuthu KM, Priest JH: Origin of cells in human amniotic fluid cultures: Ultrastructural features. Lab Invest 39:106–109, 1978.
10. Migeon BR, Sprenkle JA, Do TT, Brusilow SW: Selective propagation of epithelial cells from amniotic fluid, based on retention of differentiated function. (In preparation).

Cultured Pulmonary Epithelial Cells: Clonal Isolation of Human Fetal Alveolar Type II Cells*

A. Keith Tanswell, MB, MRCP (UK), FRCP (C) and Barry T. Smith, MD, FRCP (C)

In recent years, cell culture techniques previously utilized primarily by cell biologists and cytogeneticists have increasingly been developed to provide information regarding physiologic and pathophysiologic behavior of differentiated cell types in vivo. In heterogeneous organs such as lung this is a particularly important approach since, theoretically, it should be possible to isolate, maintain in vitro, and determine the function of a variety of different cell types in an unequivocal fashion. Nevertheless, a number of problems remain. This paper will attempt to identify one of these: in vivo, various adjacent cell types function in an organized, harmonious fashion; in vitro, such relationships are increasingly lost with increasing "refinement" of the culture system.

NEONATAL RESPIRATORY DISTRESS SYNDROME AS A BIRTH DEFECT

Neonatal respiratory distress syndrome (RDS) is the single largest cause of mortality and morbidity in the neonatal period and a major contributor to subsequent neurologic handicap. It represents delivery of the fetus prior to functional maturation of the lung adequate to allow normal postnatal gas exchange [1]. Central to the disorder is inadequate development of the pulmonary surfactant, a complex lipoprotein required to stabilize the lung during gaseous (postnatal) respiration [2]. Under normal circumstances, regulatory control provides for appearance of the pulmonary surfactant prior to the onset of labor, so that the central defect might be regarded as dysfunction in the regulation of these 2

*Supported by a grant (MA 5757) from the Medical Research Council of Canada.

Birth Defects: Original Article Series, Volume XVI, Number 2, pages 249–259

events expressed either as premature labor or delayed lung maturation. Evidence for familial [3] and racial [4] difference in the timing of lung maturation point to genetic determination of this process, a factor which has received inadequate attention.

The pulmonary surfactant is produced and secreted by the pulmonary alveolar epithelial Type II cell. Spurred on by the clinical relevance of Type II cell function to RDS and aided by the fact that a relatively large proportion (ca 15%) of lung cells are represented by the Type II cell population, a number of in vitro Type II cell models have been developed [5–10].

CLONAL ISOLATION OF HUMAN FETAL ALVEOLAR TYPE II CELLS: EVIDENCE FOR CELL INTERACTIONS AND GROWTH

Lung tissue was obtained at autopsy, within 2 hours of death, from a 32-week-gestation anencephalic female infant who died just prior to delivery. The tissue was dispersed into an isolated cell population by trypsinization as previously described [11]. This population was implanted in culture [11] and the supernatant medium removed after 2 hours, at which time only fibroblasts had attached to the substrate [12]. The supernatant, now relatively enriched in nonfibroblastic elements, was then placed in a fresh flask and maintained in mixed monolayer culture for 1 week. At this time the population was mixed [11], consisting of fibroblasts, endothelial and epithelial cells. This population was trypsinized, counted, and diluted to a concentration of 2 cells/ml. Some of this suspension (0.5 ml), theoretically containing 1 cell, was placed in each of 192 Microtest growth wells. After 2 hours, at which time implanted cells had settled to the growth surface, but before mitosis could occur, each well was scanned by phase contrast microscopy to determine the actual number of cells implanted. A total of 188 cells were identified (mean 0.98/well) with a range of 0–5 cells/well. Since single cells cannot be reliably identified as to type by phase microscopy, this was inferred by the pattern of subsequent growth.

After a 14-day growth period, without media change, the wells were re-examined. Of the 45 wells successfully implanted with a single cell, 25 (56%) showed fibroblastic growth while 20 showed no growth. Thus, our aim to clone alveolar Type II cells was not realized. We reasoned that of the cells present in the initial cell population, only fibroblasts clone under these conditions. If all implanted fibroblasts grew (subsequent experiments with these fibroblast clones show plating efficiencies greater than 90%), it can be assumed that 56% of the cells in the original population were fibroblastic in nature.

Examination of wells implanted with more than one cell was of particular interest, for here a third growth pattern was seen. In addition to fibroblastic growth or no growth, some wells showed a mixed growth pattern consisting of fibroblasts and another cell type. We then reasoned that coincubation of the non-fibroblast cell types with a fibroblast might have accounted for the growth of the other cell types. Assuming the initial population had 56% fibroblasts as above, it was possible to compare observed frequencies of the 3 outcomes with predicted frequencies as calculated using Bayes' theorem [13]. As shown in Table 1, the observed and predicted frequencies of the 2-cell well correlate well, supporting the concept of fibroblast support of nonfibroblast growth under these conditions. Nevertheless, this relationship could be due to chance alone. However, if 3-cell wells are similarly analyzed (Table 1), the predicted frequencies are quite different but, again, observed and predicted frequencies show a very close relationship. Although the number of 4-cell (6) and 5-cell (3) wells was too small to allow reliable probability analysis the outcome in each case was mixed growth. With 4 or more cells, this outcome would be predicted to occur in greater than 80% of cases.

Despite our failure to isolate alveolar Type II cells by cloning single cells, each of the 15 "clones" giving mixed growth from wells initially implanted with 2 cells was subcultured and studied, since it was reasoned that each subpopulation arose from a single cell and therefore represented a true clone. One of these cultures (9LAE11) showed the morphology depicted in Figure 1, a population of rounded-up, birefringent cells overlying a typical fibroblast monolayer. By electron microscopy, this population contained osmiophilic lamellar bodies characteristic of the alveolar Type II cell. Since the rounded-up epithelial elements were less firmly attached to the substratum than the fibroblasts, they could be selectively removed by vigorously agitating the flasks and transferring the supernatants to fresh growth flasks. After this procedure was repeated 4 times at weekly intervals, the epithelial element (fetal lung epithelial cells [FLE]) was isolated free of fibroblastic contamination (Fig. 2).

This population has been maintained in minimum essential medium containing 10% fetal calf serum. It has both morphologic (Fig. 3) and biochemical (Table 2) characteristics of the alveolar Type II cell. After the 10th–15th population doubling level, the cells assume a more pavement-like configuration (Fig. 4), but

TABLE 1. Probability Analysis of 2- and 3-Cell Wells

	Possible initial cell types	Growth pattern	Predicted frequency (%)	Observed frequency (%)
2-Cell wells	2 fibroblasts	fibroblastic	31	34
	1 fibroblast, 1 other	mixed	49	43
	2 nonfibroblasts	none	19	23
3-Cell wells	3 fibroblasts	fibroblastic	18	23
	at least 1 fibroblast, 1 other	mixed	74	69
	3 nonfibroblasts	none	8	8

their biochemical characteristics are essentially unchanged (Table 2). A similar morphologic change, but over a shorter time span, has been noted with cultured adult rabbit alveolar Type II cells [7]. The FLE cells have retained a normal diploid female karyotype for up to 30 population doublings to date.

These results suggest that pulmonary fibroblasts exert a positive influence upon the growth of other lung cells from low cell density. This interaction is not obligatory, however, since the clonal alveolar Type II cell population (FLE) can be maintained in pure cell culture, providing a minium cell density (ca 5×10^3 cells/cm^2) is maintained.

CELL-CELL INTERACTIONS MODULATING DEVELOPMENTAL EFFECTS OF HORMONES

The above results suggest that cell-cell interactions may regulate pulmonary cell growth and, since alveolar Type II cells can be cloned by the cylinder method where all cells share a common medium [8], infer that soluble mediators may be involved.

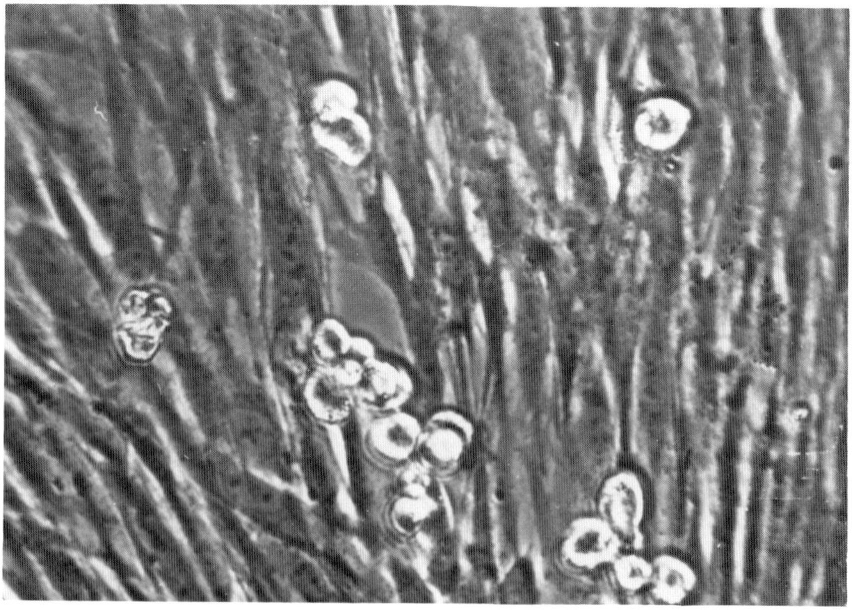

Fig. 1. Culture (9LAE11) isolated from cloning well initially seeded with 2 human fetal lung cells. Consists of a population of rounded-up, granular cells overlying a typical fibroblast monolayer (original magnification, × 200).

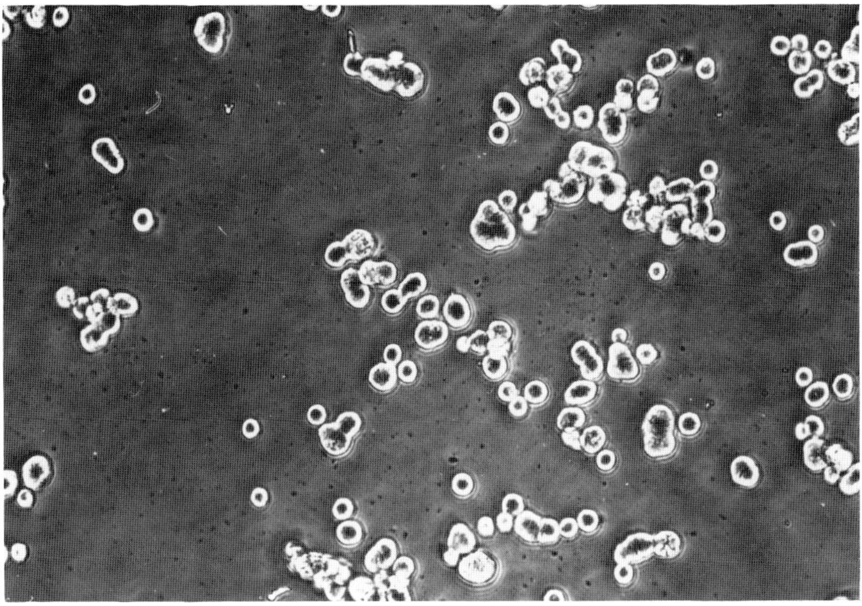

Fig. 2. Purified Type II alveolar cell (FLE) population isolated from the culture shown in Fig. 1. The cells (population doubling 8) remain rounded up (original magnification × 100).

Direct observations suggest that soluble factors may also regulate pulmonary cellular differentiation. Glucocorticoids are known to be involved in the regulation of fetal lung maturation [16] and, in mixed cell cultures, enhance the production of surfactant by the alveolar Type II cell [11, 17]. However, no such effect of glucocorticoids could be observed with the clonal alveolar Type II cells (FLE), unless the cells were reconstituted with the fibroblast cell population [18]. This is due to production, by the fetal lung fibroblast in response to glucocorticoid, of a soluble, low molecular weight polypeptide, fibroblast-pneumonocyte factor [18]. Indeed, a partially purified preparation of fibroblast-pneumonocyte factor has been shown to accelerate fetal lung maturation in vivo [19].

CULTURED EPITHELIAL CELLS: AN INTERMEDIATE GOAL

In view of the above observations, it rational to attempt to isolate and culture pure epithelial cell populations? We believe it is, for it allows further study of the type of interaction noted above. Furthermore, phenotypic expression observed in such cultures can be unequivocally assigned to the cell type in question. Here,

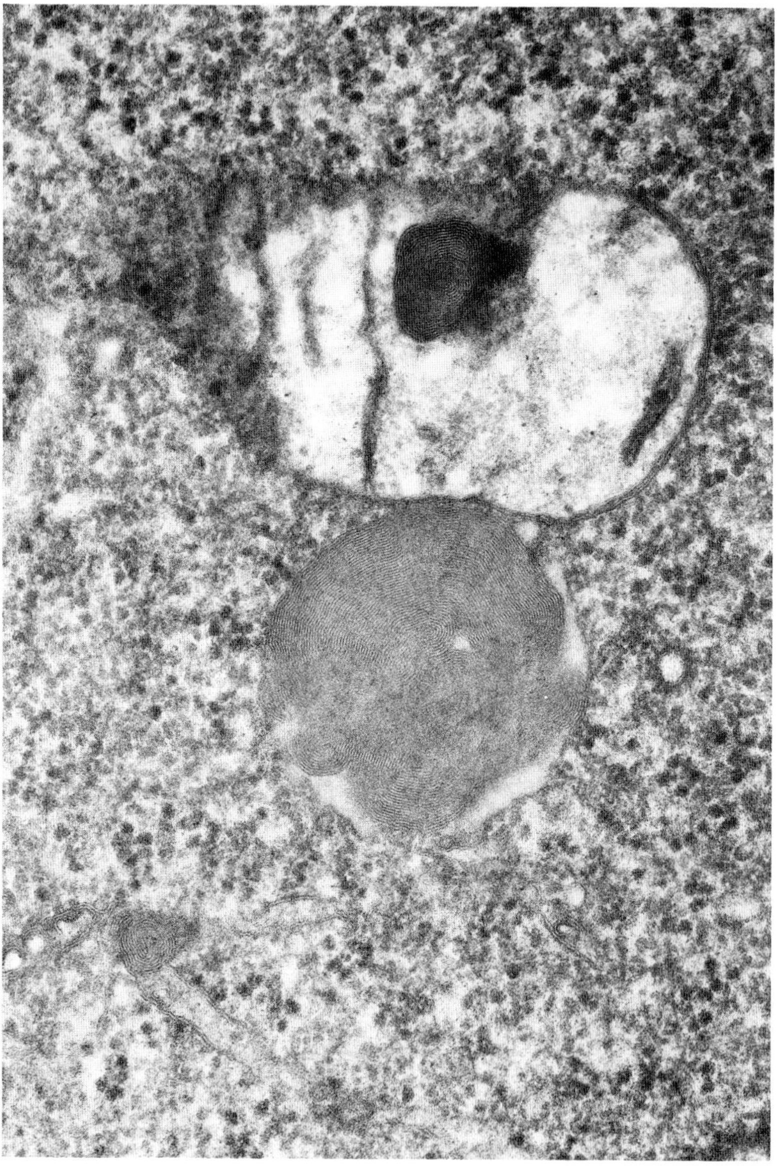

A

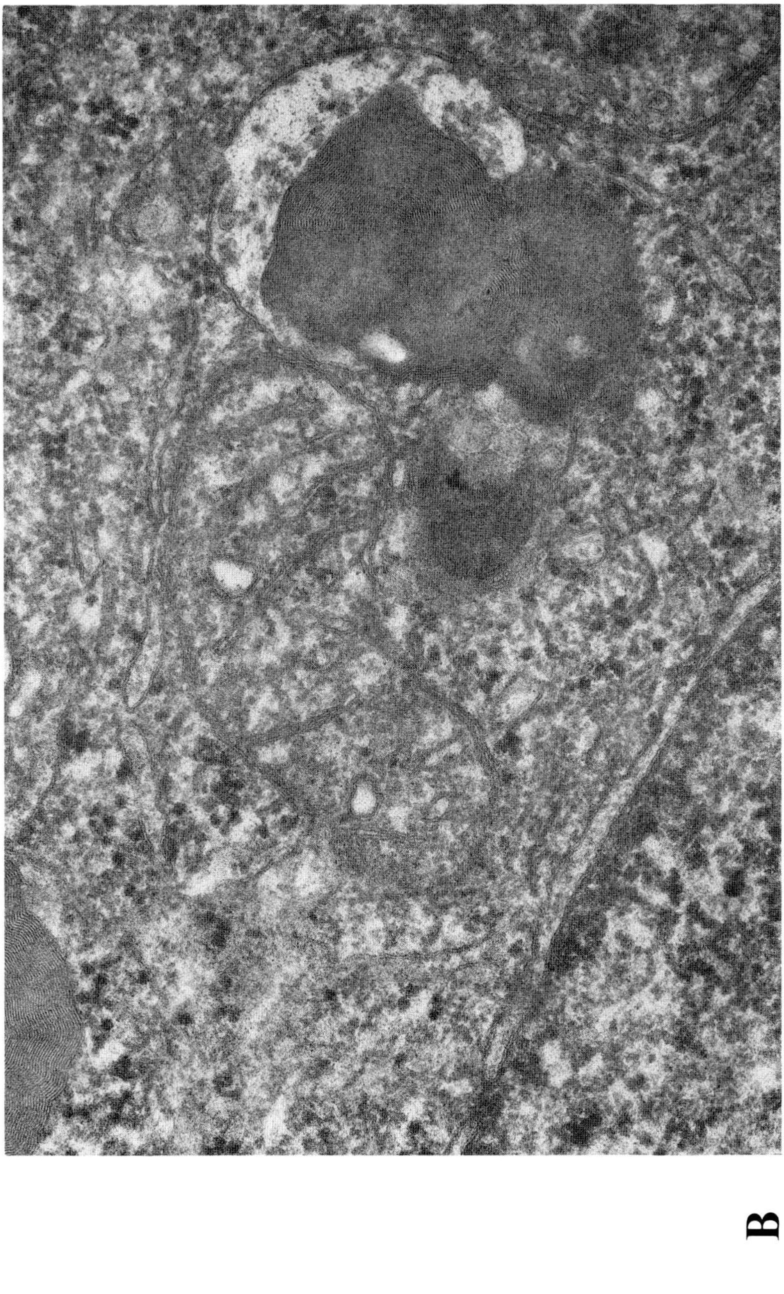

B

Fig. 3. Electron photomicrographs of FLE cells (population doubling 9) shown in Fig. 2. Morphology has been enhanced by the tannic acid technique [14]. A) A mature lamellar body is seen adjacent to a mitochondrion containing a developing lamellar inclusion [15]. Also note the lamellar structure in the cisternae of rough endoplasmic reticulum (original magnification, × 64,000). B) Fusion of a multivesicular body to a large lamellar body [15] is shown. Note the small lamellar inclusion in the mitochondrion at the lower right (original magnification, × 64,000).

TABLE 2. % Total Lipid Phosphorus in FLE Cells (means of 4 determinations)

Phospholipid species	Passage 10 (rounded-up)	Passage 20 (pavement-like)
phosphatidylcholine		
total	76.8	75.4
desaturated	26.9	26.1
phosphatidylethanolamine	12.6	10.4
phosphatidylglycerol	4.8	3.5
sphingomyelin	2.4	2.1
lysophosphatidylcholine	0.8	1.2
other	2.5	6.5

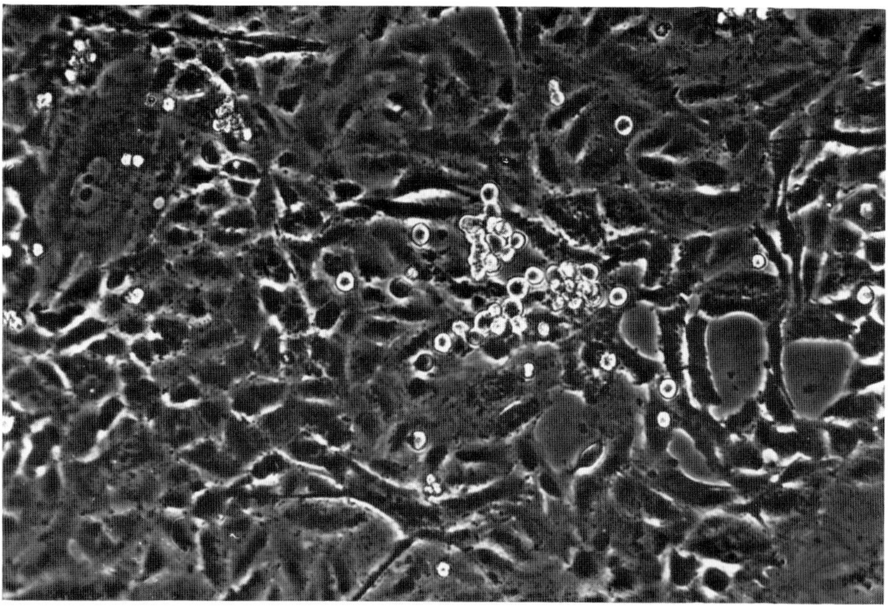

Fig. 4. FLE cells at population doubling level 15. The cells have now assumed a more typical pavement-like configuration (original magnification, × 100).

though, a further proviso must be recognized: *negative results (in isolation) are relatively meaningless,* since they may simply represent loss of phenotypic expression due to the unphysiologic nature of the preparation. In contrast, however, those phenotypic characteristics which are expressed almost certainly represent potential characteristics in vivo, for it is exceedingly rare for in vitro systems to gain new phenotypic characteristics.

Thus, the study of cultured epithelia can provide useful information, but it is best to test hypotheses so generated in more complex (hence more physiologic) systems. It represents but part of the classic biologic approach of parsing complex systems into their component parts followed by controlled reassembly.

EPITHELIAL CELL CULTURE AND PULMONARY BIRTH DEFECTS

The complexity of lung morphology and the diversity of its epithelia make it likely that a number of pulmonary birth defects can be studied in that they do or may represent dysfunction of one or more epithelial cell types. As noted above, culture of alveolar epithelium has provided information of relevance in the understanding of neonatal RDS.

The airway epithelium may be amenable to similar study. Indeed, airway epithelium is well maintained in organ culture systems [20–22]. It has been possible to enzymatically separate and maintain in culture airway epithelial sheets for many decades, and such an approach has given clear evidence of epithelial-mesenchymal interactions regulating airway embryogenesis [23, 24]. Nevertheless, the airway epithelium differentiates into a variety of specialized epithelial cell types. Thus, isolation and study of mucous-secreting cells [25] may have relevance in our understanding of disorders such as cystic fibrosis, while study of ciliated cells may provide information relating to defects of ciliary assembly and function such as are seen in Kartagener syndrome [26].

A more demanding task, in view of their small numbers, will be the isolation and study of pulmonary APUD (amine precursor uptake and decarboxylation) cells, known as Kulchitsky cells [27]. These very specialized cells have been shown to be hypoxia-sensitive [28] and possibly mediate intrapulmonary adjustments to balance local perfusion and ventilation. Thus, their proposed role in protecting against disordered ventilation/perfusion may provide information to aid our understanding of developmental defects such as apnea of prematurity and sudden infant death syndrome.

Finally, epithelial cell cultures alone, and as elements for recombination with other pulmonary cell types, may be useful tools in understanding the complex problems of lung growth [29] related to such defects as Potter syndrome [30] (renal agenesis) and diaphragmatic hernia [31].

CONCLUSION

The complex cellularity of the lung renders isolation and culture of many pulmonary epithelial cells a prodigious task. Nevertheless, it can be expected that such study will yield commensurate rewards.

ACKNOWLEDGMENTS

We thank Miss Susan Walker and Dr. John Shelbourn, Department of Pathology, Duke University Medical Center, for preparing the electron photomicrographs.

REFERENCES

1. Farrell PM, Avery ME: Hyaline membrane disease. Am Rev Resp Dis 111:657–688, 1975.
2. Avery ME, Mead J: Surface properties in relation ot atelectasis and hyaline membrane disease. Am J Dis Child 97:517–523, 1959.
3. Graven SN, Misenheimer HR: Respiratory distress syndrome and the high risk mother. Am J Dis Child 109:489–494, 1965.
4. Olowe SA, Akinkugbe A: Amniotic fluid lecithin/sphingomyelin ratio: Comparison between an African and North American community. Pediatrics 62:38–41, 1978.
5. Mason RJ, Williams MC, Greenleaf RD, Clements JA: Isolation and properties of type II alveolar cells from rat lung. Am Rev Resp Dis 115:1015–1026, 1977.
6. Frosolono MF, Kress Y, Wittner M, Rosenbaum RM: Culture characteristics of cells derived from type II pneumocyte enriched fractions from rabbit and rat. In Vitro 12: 708–717, 1976.
7. Diglio CA, Kikkawa Y: The type II epithelial cells of the lung. IV. Adaptation and behavior of isolated type II cells in culture. Lab Invest 37:622–631, 1977.
8. Douglas WHJ, Kaighn ME: Clonal isolation of differentiated rat lung cells. In Vitro 10:230–237, 1974.
9. Douglas WHJ, Teel RW: An organotypic in vitro model system for studying pulmonary surfactant production by type II alveolar pneumonocytes. Am Rev Resp Dis 113:17–23, 1976.
10. Smith BT: Cell line A 549: A model system for the study of alveolar type II cell function. Am Rev Resp Dis 115:285–293, 1977.
11. Smith BT, Torday JS, Giroud CJP: Evidence for different gestation-dependent effects of cortisol on cultured fetal lung cells. J Clin Invest 53:1518–1526, 1974.
12. Smith BT, Giroud CJP: Effects of cortisol on serially propagated fibroblast cell cultures derived from the rabbit fetal lung and skin. Can J Physiol Pharmacol 53:1037–1041, 1975.
13. Colton T: "Statistics in Medicine." Boston:Little Brown & Co, 1974, p 71.
14. Kalina M, Pease DC: The preservation of ultrastructure in saturated phosphatidyl cholines by tannic acid in model systems and type II pneumocytes. J Cell Biol 74:726–741, 1977.
15. Callas G, deGroot WJ: Fine structural observations on the origin and development of lamellar bodies in alveolar Type II pneumocytes. In Sanders CL, Schneider RP, Dagle GE, Ragan HA (eds): "Pulmonary Macrophage and Epithelial Cells." Springfield:National Technical Information Service, 1977, pp 192–204.
16. Smith BT: Prevention of hyaline membrane disease: An attempt to mimic a physiologic process. In Moss AJ (ed): "Pediatrics Update." New York:Elsevier North-Holland, 1979, pp 151–167.
17. Torday JS, Smith BT, Giroud CJP: The rabbit fetal lung as glucocorticoid target tissue. Endocrinology 96:1462–1467, 1975.
18. Smith BT: Fibroblast-pneumocyte factor: Intercellular mediator of glucocorticoid effect on fetal lung. In Stern L, Oh W, Friis-Hansen B (eds): "Intensive Care in the Newborn, II." New York:Masson Publishing USA, 1978, pp 25–32.

19. Smith BT: Lung maturation in the fetal rat: Acceleration by injection of fibroblast-pneumocyte factor. Science (In press).
20. Guerrero RR, Rounds DE, Booher J: An improved organ culture method for adult mammalian lung. In Vitro 13:517–524, 1977.
21. Adamson IYR, Bowden DH: Reaction of cultured adult and fetal lung to prednisolone and thyroxine. Arch Pathol 99:80–85, 1975.
22. Rose GG, Yajima T: Fetal mouse lung in circumfusion system cultures. In Vitro 13: 749–768, 1977.
23. Grobstein C: Tissue interaction in the morphogenesis of mouse embryonic rudiments in vitro. In Rudnick R (ed): "Aspects of Synthesis and Order in Growth." Princeton: Princeton University Press, 1954, pp 233–256.
24. Alescio T, Dani AM: Hydrocortisone-increased glycogen deposition and its dependence on tissue interactions in mouse embryonic lung developing in vitro. J Embryol Exp Morphol 27:155–162, 1972.
25. Boat TF, Cheng PW: Mucous glycoproteins. In Mangos JA, Talamo RC (eds): "Cystic Fibrosis: Projections into the Future." New York: Stratton Intercontinental Medical Book Corp, 1976, pp 165–177.
26. Kartagener M, Stucki P: Bronchiectasis with situs inversus. Arch Pediatr 79:193–207, 1962.
27. Cutz E, Chan W, Wong V, Conen PE: Endocrine cells in rat fetal lungs. Ultrastructural and histochemical study. Lab Invest 30:458–464, 1974.
28. Lauweryns JM, Cokelaere M, Deleersnyder M, Liebens M: Intrapulmonary neuro-epithelial bodies in newborn rabbits. Cell Tissue Res 182:425–440, 1977.
29. Thurlbeck WM: Postnatal growth and development of the lung. Am Rev Resp Dis 111: 803–844, 1975.
30. Potter EL, Bohlender G: Intrauterine respiration in relation to development of the fetal lung. Am J Obstet Gynecol 42:14–22, 1941.
31. Areechon W, Reid L: Hypoplasia of lung with congenital diaphragmatic hernia. Br Med J 1:230–232, 1963.

intestinal goblet cells, it could be assumed that mucous cells elsewhere in the CF patient, under the same genetic influence, would be similarly affected. Clarification of the defect in intestinal cells might lead to rational therapeutic approaches to respiratory or reproductive dysfunction. The use of rectal mucosa in the search for a goblet cell defect has several advantages: goblet cells are most abundant in the rectal epithelium, accounting for about 1 out of every 4 epithelial cells [14] (Figs. 1–3); the rectal mucosa is safely and painlessly biopsied with a minimum of inconvenience to the patient; and rectal mucosal biopsies may be maintained in vitro for 24–48 hours, due to the development of intestinal organ culture techniques.

DEVELOPMENT OF ORGAN CULTURE METHODS FOR INTESTINAL BIOPSIES

Early attempts at maintaining intestinal mucosa in vitro utilized small fragments of tissue immersed in tissue culture medium, usually with continual shaking and oxygenation [15–17]. Under these conditions, survival times, as judged by ^{3}H-thymidine incorporation and preservation of histologic structure, varied from 2.5 to a maximum of 19 hours. The survival of human mucosal tissue in vitro was significantly extended, however, when the organ culture method originated by Trowell [18] was adapted by Trier and his colleagues [19, 20] for mucosal biopsies, first from small intestine [19] and later from rectum [20]. This method provides excellent preservation of epithelial cell morphology and function for 24–48 hours, and it remains the technique of choice at this writing.

Very briefly, mucosal biopsies are not immersed but are mounted, epithelium up and cut side down, on screens which are floated on the surface of culture medium in a humid, well-oxygenated atmosphere. The tissue is never agitated; medium diffuses through the underlying connective tissue to the epithelium. As in all culture systems, the choice of medium is crucial and Trowell's T8 medium, which contains insulin (50 mg/liter) and large amounts of glucose (4 gm/liter), was empirically found to be optimal for human mucosa.

Shortly after this method was introduced, it was reported that rectal mucosal biopsies were well-preserved histologically for up to 90 hours in a similar organ culture system from which insulin was deleted and to which hydrocortisone (5–10 μg/ml) was added [21]. Unfortunately, no illustrations of the tissue were provided, no subsequent publications using this modified method have appeared, and the results were not confirmed by pilot studies in Trier's laboratory [20].

CURRENT ORGAN CULTURE METHOD FOR HUMAN RECTAL BIOPSIES

Biopsies are obtained using a single port multipurpose suction biopsy tube (Quinton Instruments, Seattle, WA) positioned in the rectum 7–10 cm from the

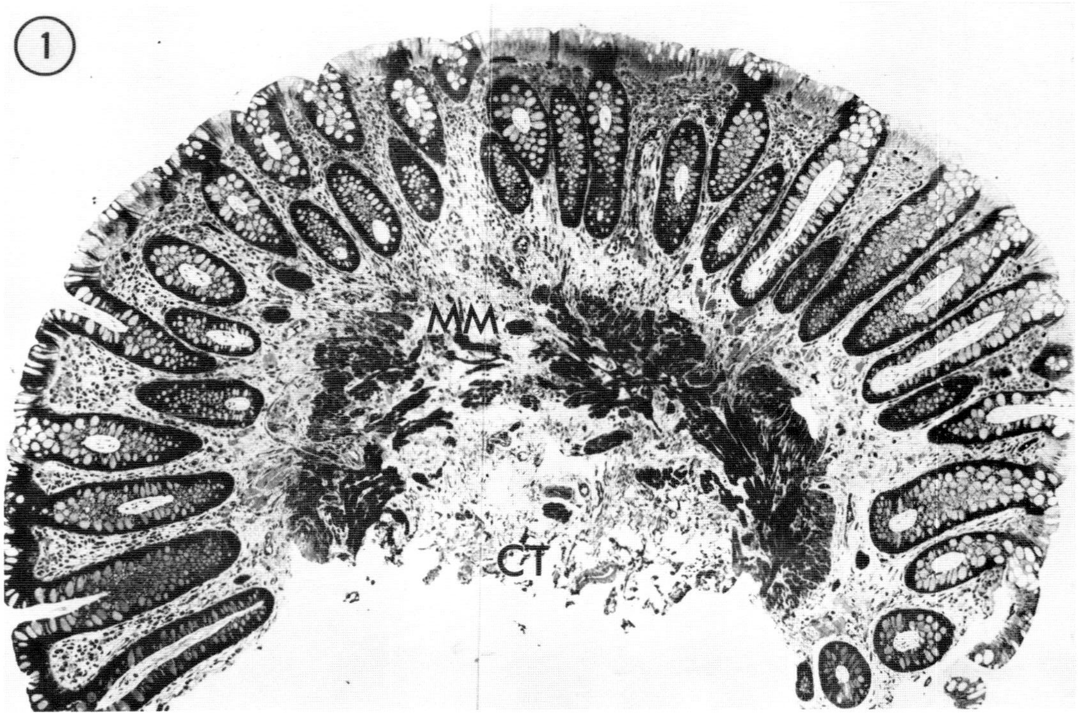

Fig. 1. Biopsy of rectal mucosa from a normal adult volunteer, as seen in a one micron plastic section stained with periodic acid-Schiff and iron-hematoxylin. When the biopsy is placed in organ culture, the contracted muscularis mucosae (MM) and a thin layer of submucosal connective tissue (CT) will directly contact the nutrient medium. The mucosal glands and surface epithelium, exposed to a humid, oxygenated atomosphere in the culture system, will sustain many of their metabolic processes for at least 24 hours (X 91).

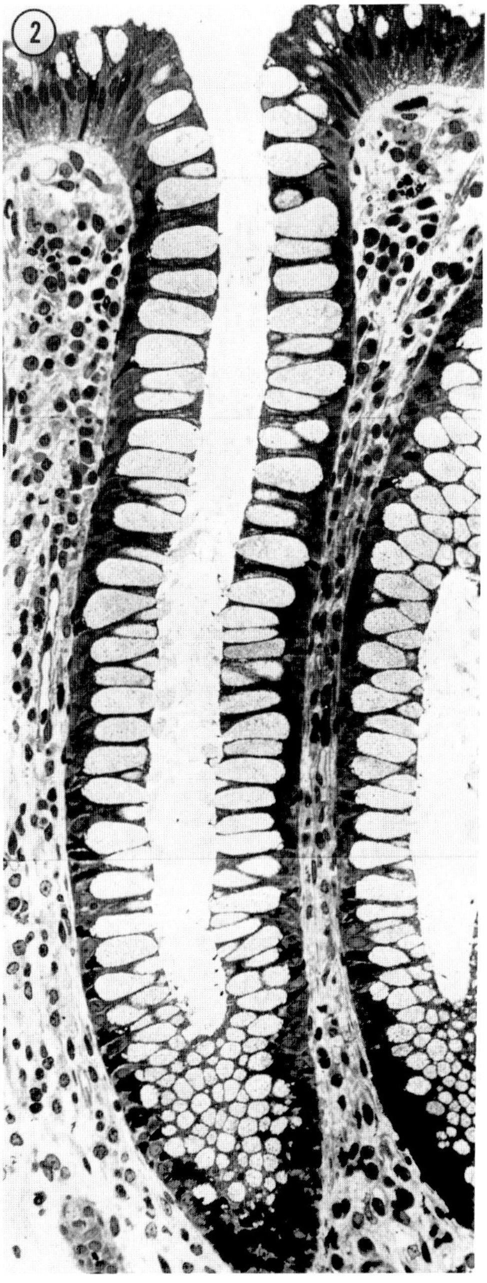

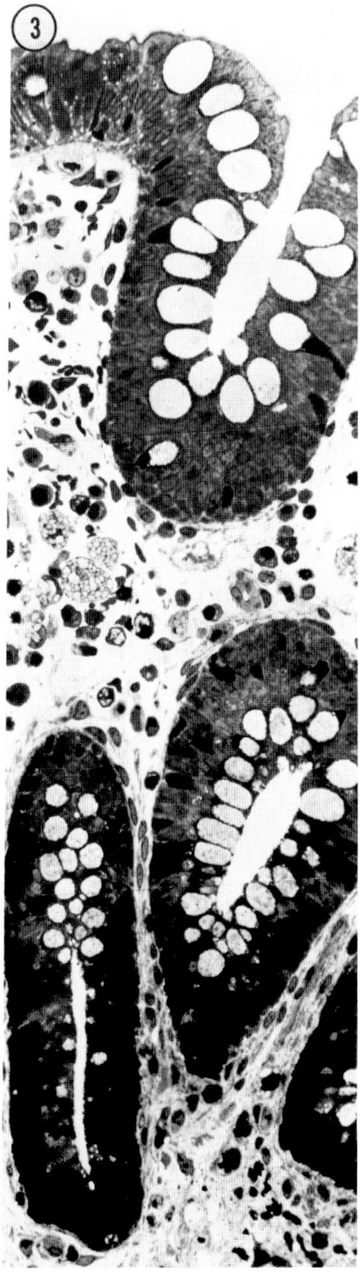

Fig. 2. A rectal mucosal gland from a CF patient prior to organ culture. The epithelium is rich in goblet cells, all of which are active in the synthesis and secretion of mucus. The biopsy procedure itself does not induce massive mucous secretion, and the epithelial cells are viable and intact (× 367).

Fig. 3. A rectal mucosal gland from a normal sib volunteer, maintained in organ culture for 24 hours. The glands, sectioned tangentially, are well-maintained, but intracellular mucus stores in goblet cells are diminished, especially in the lower crypt regions (× 400).

anus. Biopsies measure 2–4 mm in diameter and include the full thickness of the mucosa with little or no submucosal connective tissue (Fig. 1). They are recovered within 5–10 seconds and are immediately mounted, cut surface down, on stainless steel screens over the center well of an organ culture dish (Falcon Plastics, Los Angeles, CA). The central well is then filled with sterile, oxygenated culture medium until the screen begins to float and the dish is covered. Humidity is maintained by a saturated felt ring which encircles the central well. The medium consists of 90% Trowell's T8 medium and 10% fetal calf serum (both from Grand Island Biological Co., Grand Island, NY). In studies using small and large intestinal biopsies from normal individuals and from patients with celiac disease or ulcerative colitis, bacterial growth was adequately controlled by the addition of penicillin (10,000 units/ml) and streptomycin sulfate (10 mg/ml). In later studies using rectal biopsies from CF patients, microorganisms were more effectively controlled by adding gentamicin (100 μg/ml) and mycostatin (60 units/ml).

Radioactive compounds may be conveniently and economically added to the culture medium to provide a precisely controlled pulse of radioactive precursor. The chase is accomplished without disturbing the tissue by drawing off the labeled medium and replacing it with a medium containing an excess of unlabeled precursor.

Culture dishes are then placed in a McIntosh jar (Torsion Balance Co., Clifton, NJ), gassed with a mixture of 95% O_2 and 5% CO_2, and placed in an incubator at 37°C. The jar is again gassed at 6- or 12-hour intervals. At the end of the culture period, biopsies are either fixed, embedded, and sectioned for histologic, ultrastructural, and autoradiographic studies or are homogenized and fractionated for biochemical analysis. Labeled macromolecules released into the culture medium may also be separated and biochemically characterized.

RESULTS

Normal Mucosa

Initial studies using cultured biopsies of human gastric fundus and antrum, duodenum-jejunum, colon, and rectum were designed to test the ability of the epithelium to sustain metabolic activities in vitro. These and subsequent studies up to the year 1976 were summarized by Trier [22]. The survival of human mucosal biopsies from various regions of the GI tract, as well as of biopsies taken from the comparable regions of different species, was found to vary unpredictably. Whereas human gastric fundus degenerates rapidly, human antrum, small intestine, colon, and rectum are well maintained. Rabbit mucosa from all GI areas cultures well, whereas, rat, mouse, and hamster small intestine mucosae do not.

Successful maintenance of epithelial cells in cultured biopsies was determined primarily by careful light and electron microscopic study. In addition, biochemical analyses of ^{3}H-leucine-labeled biopsies showed that synthesis of protein in human small and large intestinal biopsies continued at steady state rates during the first 24 hours of culture [23]. DNA synthesis, detected autoradiographically as incorporation of ^{3}H-thymidine into the nuclei of proliferating cells, also continued for 24 hours. Since comparable protein and DNA synthetic activity were measured in human and in rabbit mucosal biopsies, rabbit mucosa provides a convenient model for pilot studies. Such studies have shown that protein [24] and glycoprotein synthesis and secretion [25] and secretory IgA synthesis and transport [26, 27] continue in culture for at least 24 hours. Normal human rectal biopsies studied autoradiographically after ^{3}H-glucosamine incorporation showed synthesis, transport, and secretion of both brush border glycoproteins in columnar cells and mucous glycoproteins in goblet cells during the same time period [28]. In separate studies, the incorporation of ^{3}H-glucosamine into brush border glycoproteins by human small intestinal biopsies was investigated with biochemical methods using peroral biopsies and operative material [29]. The rate of overall ^{3}H-glucosamine incorporation remained constant during a 48-hour culture period, and the glycoproteins produced and inserted into the brush borders included disaccharidases, enterokinase, and alkaline phosphatase.

Having established the viability of biopsies in short-term organ culture, the system is now being used to clarify the factors which control normal epithelial function. Uptake of ^{3}H-glucosamine into secretory glycoproteins of rabbit colonic biopsies was enhanced by cyclic AMP and by agents which elevate intracellular cyclic AMP levels [30]. In other studies, cyclic AMP elevation was associated with inhibition of DNA synthesis [31]. Organ culture studies of gastric mucosa confirmed the ability of this tissue to synthesize G-17 gastrin in vitro [32], and showed that gastrin and other secretagogues directly stimulate gastric protein secretion. The trophic effect of gastrin on the mucosa, an important phenomenon which had previously been demonstrated in vivo [33], was thus confirmed in organ culture.

Intestinal Mucosa in Disease States

When intestinal dysfunction occurs in a hereditary disease such as cystic fibrosis, it is difficult to determine whether this is due to a defect in the intestinal cells themselves or is secondary to an abnormal humoral or luminal environment. In such cases, organ culture may allow us to differentiate intrinsic from extrinsic influences. Published studies of 2 nonhereditary diseases, celiac sprue and ulcerative colitis, serve to illustrate this point. Intestinal mucosa in celiac sprue patients consistently shows damaged surface epithelial cells with a compensatory enhancement of crypt mitotic index, but in organ culture without luminal contents, the epithelium reverts to normal within 24 hours [34]. This improvement in surface cell morphology and function is prevented by the addition of gluten peptides to the culture medium [35]. In the case of ulcerative colitis, however, the accelerated rates of cell proliferation and glycoprotein synthesis which accompany the disease in vivo are not reversed in organ culture [36]. In this case, intestinal epithelial malfunction, at least on a short-term basis, does not depend on extramucosal factors.

Both intrinsic and extrinsic factors have been invoked in attempts to explain the "mucous secretion defect" of cystic fibrosis. On the intrinsic side, it was postulated that CF goblet cells hypersecrete mucous glycoproteins and that this may be due to defects in the intracellular regulation of secretion or to high levels of glycosyltransferase activity. It was impossible to determine in vivo whether individual CF mucous cells were actually hypersecreting, however, since an increase in cell numbers could account for increases in both synthetic enzymes and secretory products. To determine whether CF intestinal goblet cells have an "intrinsically" rapid rate of secretion, we compared the cells of CF, sib control, and adult control rectal biopsies in organ culture [28]. Nascent secretory glycoproteins were pulse-labeled with ^{3}H-glucosamine and maintained on chase medium for various time intervals up to 24 hours before fixation, histologic processing, and autoradiographic analysis (Fig. 4). We found that, although the movement of labeled mucous granules varied widely among individual goblet cells within any one tissue sample

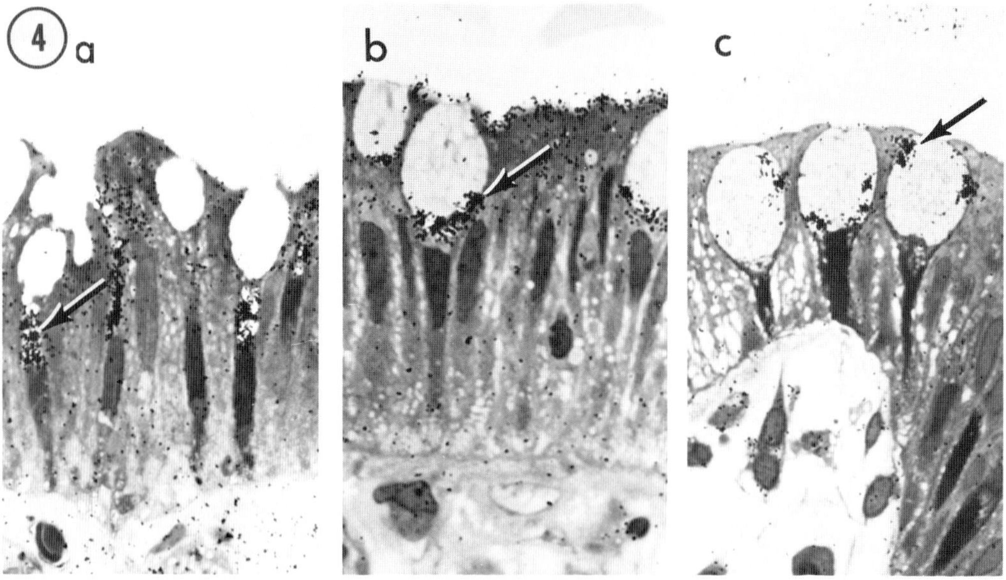

Fig. 4. Human goblet cells continue to synthesize and secrete mucous glycoprotein for at least 24 hours in organ culture. During this time, intracellular migration of a cohort of ^{3}H-glycosamine-labeled mucous granules (arrows) may be followed by autoradiography. a) At 2 hours after a 20-minute radioactive pulse, labeled mucus is located above the nucleus (× 840). b) At 4 hours the label has moved apically (× 840). c) At 20 hours, separate groups of labeled granules have migrated variable distances toward the epithelial surface (× 630).

(Fig. 4c), average transport rates were remarkably uniform among all biopsies studied. In particular, rates in CF and sib control biopsies did not differ significantly from those of adult controls. Furthermore, the patterns of incorporation of 4 different glycoprotein precursors (^{3}H-glucosamine, ^{3}H-fucose, ^{35}S-sulfate, and ^{3}H-N-acetylmannosamine) into various mucosal cell types were identical in all biopsies. We concluded that 1) the intrinsic, baseline rate of mucous secretion is not elevated in CF goblet cells, 2) no gross abnormalities in the carbohydrate composition of CF secretions are detectable by autoradiography, and 3) baseline secretory rates in organ culture are uniform. Thus, the response of goblet cells to secretagogues can be validly tested in this system.

The possibility remains that hypersecretion does occur in CF mucosa in situ, perhaps due to elevated hormone or transmitter levels or to luminal factors such as immune complexes or bacterial products. We are currently testing the effects of potential secretagogues on colonic mucosal cells in organ culture using autoradiographic methods and ultrastructural analysis. Secretion of glycoproteins can also be assessed biochemically, but autoradiography allows us to precisely visualize the movement of labeled material within individual cells and differing cell types even before it is released into the culture medium, and allows us to study changes in intracellular membrane systems in very small samples of the same tissues. Furthermore, newly secreted mucous glycoproteins tend to form a gel-like layer on the mucosal surface and in the crypts. Material secreted into this gel may not be detected by biochemical analysis of the culture medium but it is readily detected by autoradiography (Fig. 5). On the other hand, autoradiography does not allow us to quantitatively relate glycoprotein production to mucosal unit weight since the penetration of labeled precursor through the tissue is variable, and counting the densely clustered silver grains that appear over labeled mucous cells is unreliable.

Recent experiments in our laboratory (with Dr. R. Specian) have shown that the earliest response of goblet cells to secretagogues (at 2–5 minutes) is detectable only by electron microscopy (EM). A more extensive secretory response is detected both by EM and by autoradiography by 5–20 minutes, and a dramatic response is evident at 30 minutes to 1 hour. Only at much later time intervals (such as 3, 5, and 24 hours) have secreted glycoproteins in the culture medium been measured biochemically using this culture system [25, 29, 30].

LIMITATIONS OF INTESTINAL ORGAN CULTURE METHODS

Although organ culture methods have been improved and are widely used, intestinal mucosal survival is still limited to 24–48 hours. Studies concerning cell migration and turnover are thus complicated by a relatively early and poorly defined onset of degeneration. The earliest signs of epithelial cell death, often noted prior to 24 hours, appeared in immature crypt cells in the central region of the biopsy, presumably because they were poorly perfused by the unagitated

5

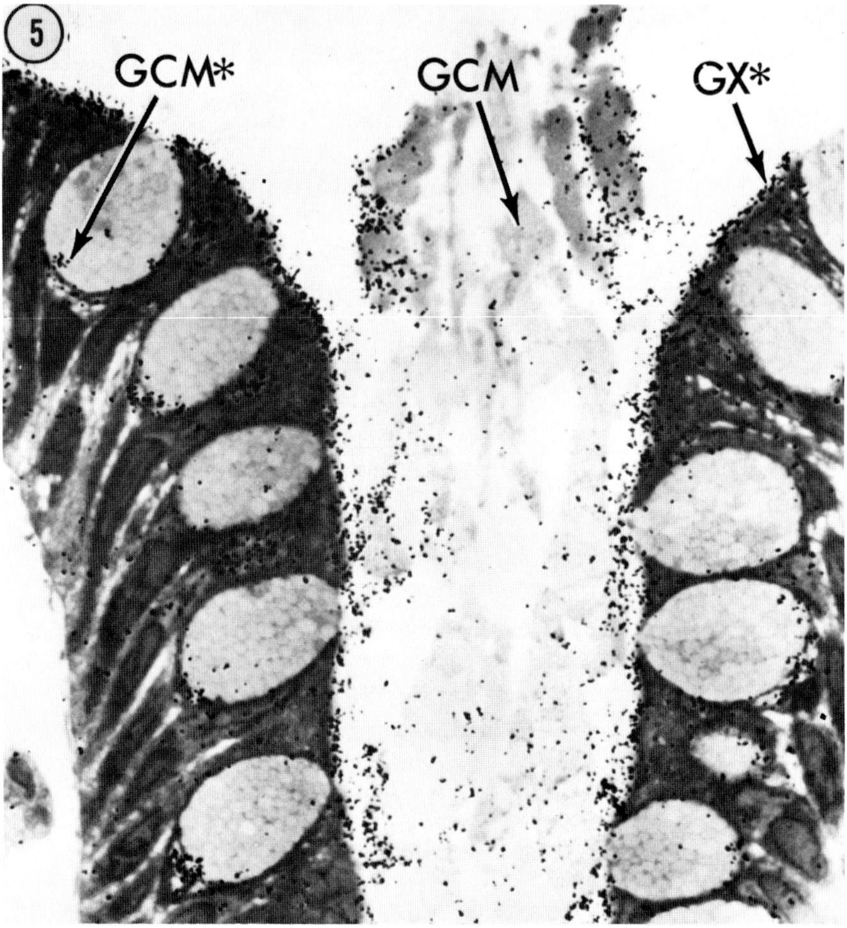

Fig. 5. Autoradiograph of the mouth of a rectal crypt from a normal sib volunteer, 6 hours after a pulse of ^{3}H-glucosamine. Unlabeled, secreted goblet cell mucus (GCM) fills the crypt lumen and protrudes onto the surface, while the mucus which was labeled by the pulse (GCM*) has not yet been secreted. Radioactive columnar cell glycoproteins, presumably released from the radiolabeled glycocalyx (GX*) precipitate in association with secreted mucus and both cell products tend to adhere to the mucosal surface (× 1116).

medium. In cultured human rectal biopsies, goblet cells deep in the crypts throughout the biopsy appeared to synthesize and secrete mucus normally during the first 12 hours, but at later times, their intracellular mucus stores were rapidly depleted and the cells became unrecognizable [20, 28] (Fig. 3). Upper crypt and surface goblet cells maintained normal morphology and synthetic and secretory activity for 24 hours (Fig. 4). Fortunately, this and many other metabolic processes are rapid enough to be validly studied within a few hours. Strictly speaking, the current method should be termed "organ maintenance." The epithelium undergoes limited proliferation [20] but does not give rise to a stable, differentiated epithelial cell line. This limitation may be inherent in intestinal tissue since these epithelial cells even in vivo have a life-span of only 4–6 days.

A second limitation is inherent in the complexity of mucosal tissue. Intercellular junctions among epithelial cells, epithelial-mesenchymal interactions, and the presence of residual nerve terminals and immunologically competent cells in the adherent lamina propria may serve to maintain a functional epithelium, but they also may complicate the interpretation of experimental data. For example, it is difficult to determine whether goblet cells respond directly to secretagogues or whether their response is mediated, perhaps via gap junctions, by the columnar cells which surround them and which are known to carry cell surface receptors [37]. Isolated cell populations may be necessary to resolve such questions.

CURRENT AND FUTURE STUDIES ON CYSTIC FIBROSIS

Despite its limitations, the organ culture method has opened up a new phase in our ability to investigate normal and abnormal intestinal epithelial function. To date, cystic fibrosis is the only inherited disease to which the method has been applied. Recently, the surface cells of biopsies from CF patients were found to accumulate lipid and glycogen in organ culture, while their counterparts from normal individuals did not. While this may be an artifact produced by the in vitro environment, it also may reflect an underlying alteration in CF nonmucous cells [14]. Organ culture methods will allow us to compare the responsiveness of CF mucous and nonmucous cells to secretagogues and inhibitors with that of their counterparts from normal individuals. At the same time, the intracellular membrane events involved in the goblet cell's secretory process may be systematically studied in cultured normal human mucosa [38] and then in CF mucosa to determine whether CF mucous cells carry out exocytosis in a normal fashion.

REFERENCES

1. Staehelin LA: Structure and function of intercellular junctions. Int Rev Cytol 39: 191–283, 1974.
2. Kaye GI, Lane N, Pascal RR: Colonic pericryptal fibroblast sheath: Replication, migration, and cytodifferentiation of a mesenchymal cell system in adult tissue. Gastroenterology 54:852–865, 1968.
3. Marsh MN, Trier JS: Morphology and cell proliferation of subepithelial fibroblasts in adult mouse jejunum. Gastroenterology 67:622–635, 636–645, 1974.

4. Mathan M, Hermos JA, Trier JS: Structural features of the epithelio-mesenchymal interface of rat duodenal mucosa during development. J Cell Biol 52:577–588, 1972.
5. di Sant' Agnese PA, Davis PB: Research in cystic fibrosis. N Engl J Med 295:481–485, 534–541, 597–602, 1976.
6. Wood RE, Boat TF, Doershuk CF: Cystic fibrosis. Am Rev Respir Dis 113:833–878, 1976.
7. Mangos JA, Bargman GJ, Martinez JR Jr, Rennert OM: Physiology and pharmacology of secretion and cystic fibrosis. In Mangos JA, Talamo RC (eds): "Cystic Fibrosis, Projections Into the Future." New York: Stratton Intercontinental Medical Book Corp, 1976, pp 311–336.
8. Sturgess J, Reid L: An organ culture study of the effect of drugs on the secretory activity of the human bronchial submucosal gland. Clin Sci 43:533–543, 1972.
9. Sturgess J, Reid L: Secretory activity of the human bronchial mucous gland in vitro. Exp Mol Pathol 16:362–381, 1972.
10. Boat TF, Kleinerman JI: Human respiratory tract secretions. 2. Effect of cholinergic and adrenergic agents on in vitro release of protein and mucous glycoprotein. Chest 67: 32S–34S, 1975.
11. Coles SJ, Reid L: Glycoprotein secretion in vitro by human airway: Normal and chronic bronchitis. Exp Mol Pathol 29:326–341, 1978.
12. Boat TF, Cheng PW: Mucous glycoproteins. Supra #7, pp 165–177 .
13. Butcher FR: Relevance of cyclic nucleotides and calcium to cystic fibrosis. Supra #7, pp 243–258.
14. Neutra MR, Trier JS: Rectal mucosa in cystic fibrosis. Morphological features before and after short term organ culture. Gastroenterology 75:701–710, 1978.
15. Deschner E, Lewis CM, Lipkin M: In vitro study of human rectal epithelial cells. I. Atypical zone of H^3-thymidine incorporation in mucosa of multiple polyposis. J Clin Invest 42: 1922–1928, 1963.
16. Shorter RG, Spencer RJ, Hallenbeck GA: Kinetic studies of the epithelial cells of the rectal mucosa in normal subjects and patients with ulcerative colitis. Gut 7:593–596, 1966.
17. Galand P, Mainguet P, Arguello M, Chretien J, Douxfils N: In vitro autoradiographic studies of cell proliferation in the gastrointestinal tract of man. J Nucl Med 9:37–39, 1968.
18. Trowell OA: The culture of mature organs in a synthetic medium. Exp Cell Res 16: 118–147, 1959.
19. Browning TH, Trier JS: Organ culture of mucosal biopsies of human small intestine. J Clin Invest 48:1423–1432, 1969.
20. Eastwood GL, Trier JS: Organ culture of human rectal mucosa. Gastroenterology 64: 375–382, 1973.
21. Johansen PG: An in vitro system for studying mucus secretion and other physiological activities in human intestinal mucosa. Experientia 26:130–131, 1970.
22. Trier JS: Organ-culture methods in the study of gastrointestinal-mucosal function and development. N Engl J Med 295:150–155, 1976.
23. Trier JS: Organ culture of intestinal mucosa. In Hekkens WTJM, Peña AS (eds): "Coeliac Disease." Proceedings of the Second International Coeliac Symposium, Noordwijkerhout, The Netherlands, 1974. Leiden: HE Stenfert Kroese BV, 1974, pp 81–90.
24. Sutton DR, Donaldson RM Jr: Synthesis and secretion of protein and pepsinogen by rabbit gastric mucosa in organ culture. Gastroenterology 69:166–174, 1975.
25. MacDermott RP, Donaldson RM Jr, Trier JS: Glycoprotein synthesis and secretion by mucosal biopsies of rabbit colon and human rectum. J Clin Invest 54:545–554, 1974.
26. Kagnoff MF, Donaldson RM Jr, Trier JS: Organ culture of rabbit small intestine: Prolonged in vitro steady state protein synthesis and secretion and secretory IgA secretion. Gastroenterology 63:541–551, 1972.

27. Kagnoff MF, Serfilippi D, Donaldson RM Jr: In vitro kinetics of intestinal secretory IgA secretion. J Immunol 110:297–300, 1973.
28. Neutra MR, Grand RJ, Trier JS: Glycoprotein synthesis, transport, and secretion by epithelial cells of human rectal mucosa: Normal and cystic fibrosis. Lab Invest 36:535–546, 1977.
29. Hauri HP, Kedinger M, Haffen K, Freiburghaus A, Grenier JF, Hadorn B: Biosynthesis of brush border glycoproteins by human small intestinal mucosa in organ culture. Biochim Biophys Acta 467:327–339, 1977.
30. LaMont JT, Ventola A: Stimulation of colonic glycoprotein synthesis by dibutyryl cyclic AMP and theophylline. Gastroenterology 72:82–86, 1977.
31. Alpers DH, Philpott GW: Control of deoxyribonucleic acid synthesis in normal rabbit colonic mucosa. Gastroenterology 69:951–959, 1975.
32. Harty RF, Van der Vijver JC, McGuigan JE: Direct demonstration of gastrin synthesis by antral mucosal explants in organ culture. (Abstract) Clin Res 24:285A, 1976.
33. Johnson LR: The trophic action of gastrointestinal hormones. Gastroenterology 70:278–288, 1976.
34. Trier JS, Browning TH: Epithelial-cell renewal in cultured duodenal biopsies in celiac sprue. N Engl J Med 283:1245–1250, 1970.
35. Falchuk ZM, Gebhard RL, Sessoms C, Strober W: An in vitro model of gluten-sensitive enteropathy: Effect of gliadin on intestinal epithelial cells of patients with gluten-sensitive enteropathy in organ culture. J Clin Invest 53:487–500, 1974.
36. Eastwood GL, Trier JS: Epithelial cell renewal in cultured rectal biopsies in ulcerative colitis. Gastroenterology 64:383–390, 1973.
37. Walker WA, Field M, Isselbacher KJ: Specific binding of cholera toxin to isolated intestinal microvillous membranes. Proc Natl Acad Sci USA 71:320–324, 1974.
38. Neutra MR, Schaeffer SF: Membrane interactions between adjacent mucous secretion granules. J Cell Biol 74:983–991, 1977.

Establishment of Human Colonic Mucosal Culture Strains From Colonoscopy Specimens

B. Shannon Danes, MD, PhD

In vitro studies of human colonic pathology have been limited by the unavailability of culture lines or stains of human colonic epithelial cells. This paper reports the establishment of such epithelial strains established from biopsies of colonic mucosa taken at colonoscopy from either normals or patients with adenomatosis of the colon and rectum (ACR). The basic methods used were in vitro enrichment [1, 2] to select for epithelial cells with subculturing by the nonenzymatic passing method [3].

MATERIALS AND METHODS

Through the colonoscope, specimens (2 X 3 mm) of colonic mucosa or ACR polyp were obtained. Each specimen was immediately placed in a tube containing 50 ml reinforced Eagle's medium (pH 7.4) with 10% (vol) fetal bovine serum and 50 μg/ml of gentamicin and Fungizone. The tube was shaken vigorously to wash the mucosal surface and then placed at 4°C for 24 hr.

The biopsy specimen was then cut into small fragments (approximately 4). Two fragments were placed in each Petri dish (28 cm^2) containing just enough Eagle's minimum essential medium with 20% (vol) fetal bovine serum to cover the explant (approximately 1 ml) and grown in a humidified atmosphere of 5% CO_2 in air [4]. It was found that if the fragment was allowed to rest on the culture floor with the meniscus of the medium just covering its upper surface, a sheet of epithelium invariably appeared within the first culture week. Thereafter, the volume of medium used was 5 ml and was changed completely every 7 days.

After 4–6 culture weeks this primary culture was trypsinized [4] and the cells which lost their surface attachment were discarded. This was repeated once a week for the next 3–4 weeks.

*This study was supported by a grant from the National Large Bowel Cancer Project of the National Cancer Institute Division of Cancer Research (R26 CA 15973), and supported in part by the Danes Medical Research Fund, Cornell University Medical College, and the Zemurray Foundation.

Birth Defects: Original Article Series, Volume XVI, Number 2, pages 275–281

At the end of 3 culture months the cell population in the primary culture appeared to be predominantly epithelium. To subculture, the nonezymatic passing method [3] was used to dissociate the epithelial cells. All subsequent subcultures were established using this methodology.

OBSERVATIONS

After 5 months of such in vitro enrichment program (see Materials and Methods), culture strains were obtained which contained predominantly cells with the features of epithelial cells: 1) The cells grew in clusters of small "sheets" (Figs. 1 and 2); a pattern distinct from the whorls formed by the parallel arranged fibroblasts. 2) Individual cells had a polygonal shape with many cytoplasmic connections (Fig. 3) rather than the spindle-shape of the fibroblast. 3) Subculture by trypsinization was not possible as they did not lose their adherence from the plastic surface, whereas fibroblasts did in the presence of trypsin. 4) Subculture by nonenzymatic passing method [3] was routinely effective as the epithelial cells rather than the fibroblasts rounded up first and lost their surface attachment. 5) Surface topographies by scanning electron microscopy [5] of the epithelial cells and the fibroblasts were distinctly different (Fig. 3).

After 5–6 culture months the few fibroblasts present appeared to undergo senescence (mitoses were rarely observed; the relative number in an individual subline decreased). There was no such evidence for senescence for the epithelial cell population.

The establishment of strains and growth characteristics of the strains established from colonic mucosa from normals and colonic polyps from ACR patients were indistinguishable. There did appear to be one striking morphologic feature between these strains. The epithelial cells from normals had small distinct nucleoli, whereas those from ACR polyps had very prominent, large nucleoli (Figs. 1 and 2). The difference was noted in both the living (Figs. 1 and 2) and stained preparations.

DISCUSSION

Tissue specimens of colonic mucosa obtained during colonoscopy have proven to be a source of viable mucosa which in vitro reproducibly yielded culture strains of epithelial cells.

During this research it became apparent that the following 8 technical aspects, which influenced the number of epithelial cells present in the primary explant cultures, had to be followed:

1) Immediate washing of the biopsy in chilled culture media containing antibiotics (gentamicin and Fungizone) to reduce cell trauma and/or multiplication of microbial contaminants.

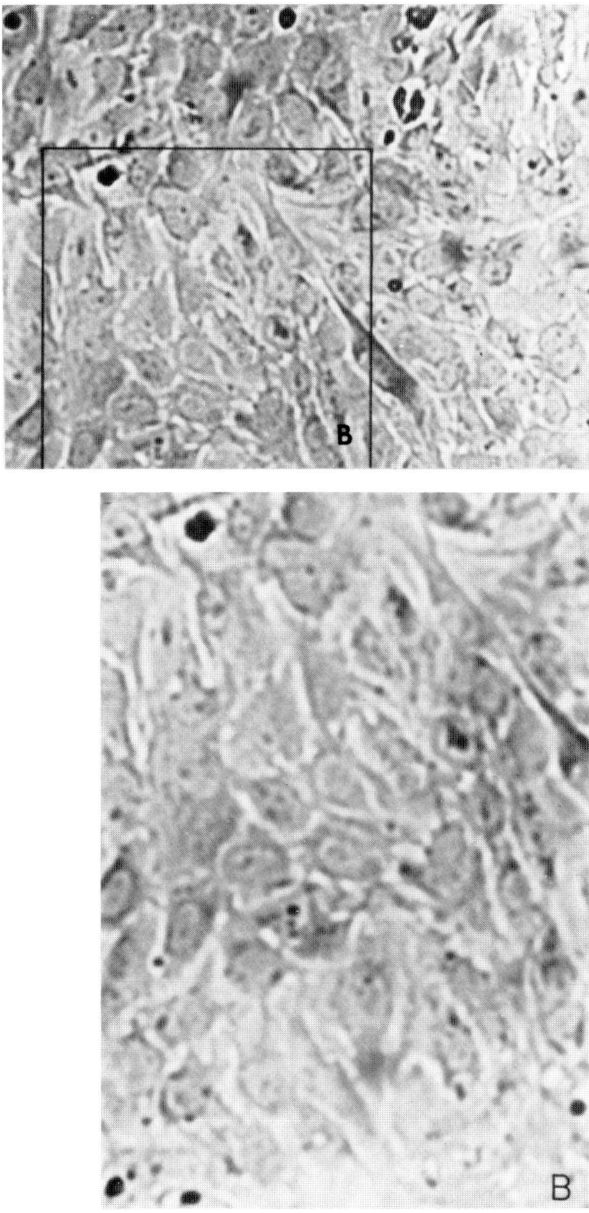

Fig. 1. Monolayer of epithelial cells growing in a flask culture. Culture established from a colonic mucosa biopsy taken during colonoscopy of a normal individual. Cell population selected by in vitro enrichment [1, 2] with subculturing by nonenzymatic passing method [3] over a 5-month period. Living culture photographed under light microscopy [A) × 250; B) × 500].

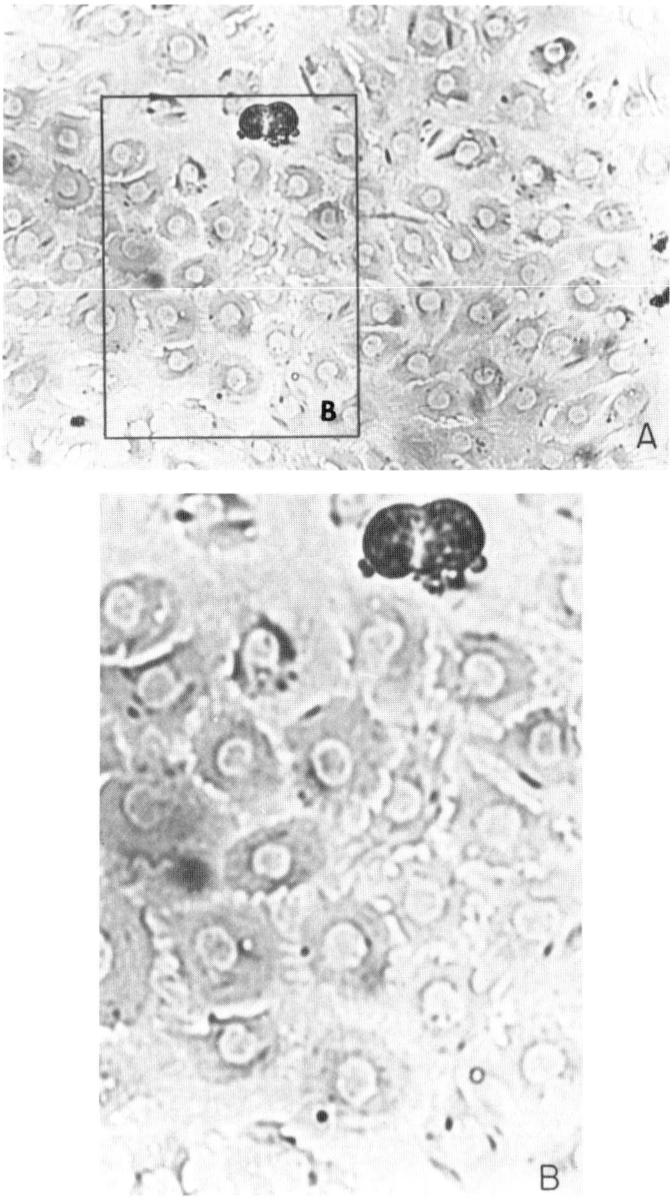

Fig. 2. Monolayer of epithelial cells growing in a flask culture. Culture established from a colonic polyp taken during colonoscopy of a patient with adenomatosis of the colon and rectum. Culture and photographic procedures used were the same as described in Figure 1 [A) × 250; B) × 500].

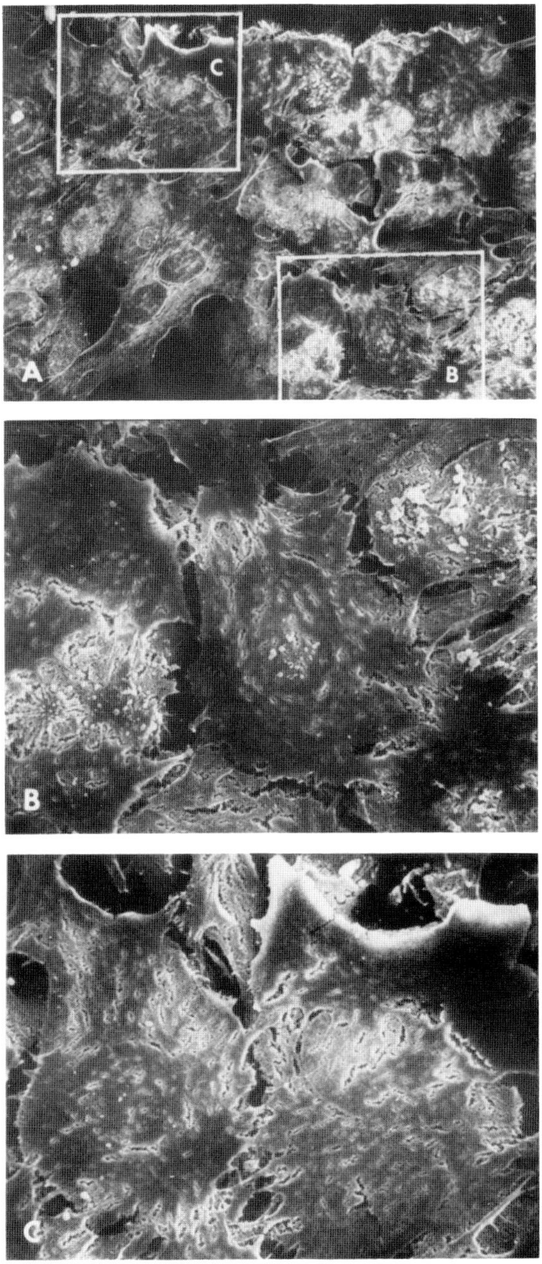

Fig. 3. A scanning electron micrograph of a monolayer of epithelial cells established from normal colonic mucosa as described in Figure 1 [A) × 350]. Higher magnifications (× 1,000) of areas (B) and (C) showing the cell surface topography to be smooth with a few stubby microvilli and numerous cytoplasmic connections.

2) Continued storage at 4°C for 24 hours prior to culture to abolish microbial contaminants.

3) Inclusion of antibiotics in medium for the initial 14 culture days.

4) Biopsy cut into small fragments and each fragment allowed to rest on culture floor. (Scoring of a tissue fragment to the plastic floor reduced the uniform migration of epithelium from the explant.)

5) A minimum amount (1 ml/28 cm^2) of medium during the initial 7–14 culture days. (Meniscus of medium acted as a position force in relation to culture surface and perhaps produced conditions, ie oxygen tension, amenable for mucosal migration [6, 7]; however, this has not yet been substantiated by experimental data.)

6) Gradual reduction of the fibroblast population through weekly trypsinization prior to any attempts at subculturing epithelium, irrespective of the ratio of the 2 cell types within a single culture. (The mutual interdependence of the stroma and epithelia in any tissue has been assumed since the work of Grobstein [8] on the importance of stroma in embryonic growth and development. This interrelationship appeared to be a factor in the initial culture period of the colonic tissue.)

7) Selection of epithelial cells by use of a nonenzymatic passing method [3]. (In a mixed cell population the epithelial cell loses its attachment more readily in this system than the fibroblast. This gives a second cell selection system yielding an increasing uniform cell population in subcultures.)

8) Subculture only when the cell population covered the culture surface (28 cm^2). Subculturing prior to an adequate cell sample delayed growth in subcultures or ran the risk of culture loss.

The cell population established from colonic biopsies by enrichment methods have been designated cell strains rather than lines as defined by the Tissue Culture Association (definitions: "A cell strain is derived either from a primary culture or a cell line by the selection . . . of cells having specific properties . . ."; "A cell line arises from a primary culture at the time of the first subculture" and "consists of numerous lineages of cells originally present in the primary culture" [9]). As the cells subcultured were selected for by an enrichment method (see Materials and Methods) [1, 2], these cultures are by the above definitions human colonic strains.

Strains of colonic mucosal cells have been established from normals and colonic polyps from ACR patients. So far, the morphologic characteristics of the cultured mucosal cells have been similar with one exception. The nucleoli in the strains derived from ACR polyps were very large and prominent as compared to the discrete nucleoli in the cells derived from the normal colonic mucosa (Figs. 1 and 2). Studies on these 2 strains should demonstrate whether this difference has relevance to the changes that have been reported to occur [10] during the formation of a colonic polyp in vivo.

By following the methodology described above, it has been possible to reproducibly establish epithelial strains from colonic mucosal biopsies taken at colonoscopy. The cell population composing each cell strain retained their epithelial phenotype in culture (Figs. 1–3). The cell origin of the epithelial population comprising each strain established has not as yet been determined. As the morphologic appearance of the culture population derived from each biopsy of normal colonic mucosa appeared to be the same, it has been assumed that mucosal cells with the ability to proliferate under the in vitro culture conditions established have been selected for. Further studies should reveal if such epithelial cells represent the "stem cell line" of colonic columnar epithelium.

ACKNOWLEDGMENTS

The author wishes to acknowledge the invaluable assistance of Erika Sutanto and Irene Tsalapatanis.

REFERENCES

1. Williams GM, Weisburger EK, Weisburger JH: Isolation and long-term cell culture of epithelial-like cells from rat liver. Exp Cell Res 69:106–112, 1971.
2. Kasten FH: Rat myocardial cells in vitro: Mitosis and differentiated properties. In Vitro 8:128–150, 1972.
3. Lechner JF, Narayan KS, Ohnuki Y, Babcock MS, Jones LW, Kaighn ME: Replicative epithelial cell cultures from normal human prostate gland: Brief communication. J Natl Cancer Inst 60:797–801, 1978.
4. Danes BS, Bearn AG: Cystic fibrosis of the pancreas. A study in cell culture. J Exp Med 129:775–793, 1969.
5. Anderson TF: Techniques for the preservation of three-dimensional structure in preparing specimens for the electron microscope. Trans NY Acad Sci 13:130–134, 1951.
6. Ham RG: Cloning of mammalian cells. In Prescott DM (ed). "Methods in Cell Physiology," vol V. New York: Academic Press, 1972, pp 37–74.
7. Taylor WG, Richter A, Evans VJ, Sanford KK: Influence of oxygen and pH on plating efficiency and colony development of WI-38 and Vero cells. Exp Cell Res 86:152–156, 1974.
8. Grobstein C: Cytodifferentiation and its control. Science 143:643–650, 1964.
9. Schaeffer WI: Proposed usage of animal tissue culture terms. (Revised 1978.) Tissue Culture Association (TCA) Manual 4:779–792, 1978.
10. Lane N, Fenoglio CM, Kaye GI, Pascal RR: Defining the precursor tissue of ordinary large bowel carcinoma: Implication for cancer prevention. In Lipkin ML, Good RA (eds): "Gastrointestinal Tract Cancer." New York: Plenum, 1978, pp 295–324.

Liver Cell Culture: Current Status and Prospects for the Study of Inherited Diseases

D. Montgomery Bissell, MD and Alexander G. Bearn, MD

The inherited diseases of the liver range in severity from clinically trivial to devastating. At a clinical level, the more serious of these disorders represent difficult problems in management, and investigation is directed at early diagnosis and (if feasible) treatment. At a more general level, all of the inherited defects of parenchymal liver function provide a unique opportunity to probe a discrete aspect of hepatic physiology, potentially with ramifications well beyond the clinical problem per se. In some of these (Table 1) the genetic defect is known, but the pathogenesis of the liver disease is unclear, eg hereditary fructose intolerance. In others, the hereditary abnormality – in molecular terms – is obscure, although its consequences are known and therapy is available, eg hemochromatosis. For all of these diseases, studies at the cellular level are of great interest if not indeed essential for their elucidation.

What might liver cell culture offer in this area of investigation? With regard to the identification of persons carrying specific gene defects, cultured skin fibroblasts or formed blood elements have served well and are much more accessible than hepatic cells. Thus, hepatocyte culture may be of limited value at the clinical level. Rather, it may be viewed as a potentially important tool in dissecting the pathophysiology of those diseases in which the genetic defect is expressed solely or predominantly as altered liver function. No other approach permits direct analysis at the cellular level with a homogeneous population of hepatic parenchymal cells, providing precise control over experimental variables and accurate kinetic data. Culture also permits – at least theoretically – relatively long-term preservation of human cells with unique defects.

Widespread acceptance of liver cell culture at the present time is tempered by the view that hepatocytes are difficult to maintain in culture and that, when cultured, they soon cease to exhibit many of the characteristic features of intact liver. The former concept is inaccurate; numerous studies have documented straight-

Birth Defects: Original Article Series, Volume XVI, Number 2, pages 283–291

TABLE 1. Some Inherited Diseases Involving the Liver

Disease or syndrome	Biochemical defect	Clinical features of liver disease
Glycogen storage diseases		
Type I (von Gierke)	Glucose-6-phosphatase deficiency	Hepatomegaly
Type II (Pompe)	α-1,4-glucosidase deficiency	Hepatomegaly
Type III(Cori)	Amylo-1,6-glucosidase deficiency	Hepatomegaly
Type IV	α-1,4-glucan: α-1,4-glucan-6 glucosyl transferase deficiency	Hepatomegaly, cirrhosis
Hereditary fructose intolerance	Fructose-1-phosphate aldolase deficiency	Jaundice, cirrhosis
Galactosemia	Galactose-1-phosphate-uridyl transferase deficiency	Hepatomegaly, jaundice, ascites
Wilson disease	Unknown	Cirrhosis, hepatic failure
Hemochromatosis	Unknown	Cirrhosis, hepatoma
Hereditary tyrosinemia	Unknown	Cirrhosis, hepatoma
α_1-antitrypsin deficiency	Unknown	Cirrhosis
Wolman disease	Acid cholesterol-ester hydrolase deficiency	Hepatomegaly, cirrhosis
Cystic fibrosis	Unknown	Cirrhosis
Porphyrias		
Acute intermittent	Uroporphyrinogen-I-synthetase deficiency	None
Coproporphyria	Coproporphyrinogen oxidase deficiency	None
Variegata	Unknown	None
Protoporphyria	Ferrochelatase deficiency	Jaundice, cirrhosis (rare)
Cutanea tarda	Uroporphyrinogen decarboxylase deficiency	Cirrhosis, iron excess
Hyperbilirubinemias		
Unconjugated (Gilbert)	Unknown (probably multiple)	Mild jaundice
Conjugated (Dubin-Johnson, Rotor)	Unknown	Mild-to-moderate jaundice
Acatalasemia	Catalase deficiency	None

forward methods (including serum-free conditions) for hepatocyte culture [1–7]. On the other hand, functional change in cultured liver cells is an important phenomenon, affecting short-term primary culture as well as serially propagated liver-derived cell lines; this problem will be reviewed in some detail. Finally, the possibilities and priorities for further studies with hepatocyte culture will be discussed.

Phenotypic change in cultured liver cells.

Numerous permanent cell lines derived from normal liver or from hepatomas have been characterized, with documentation of selected specific liver functions [1]. However, in general, liver-derived cells (normal or neoplastic) in serial culture fail to exhibit the complete spectrum of characteristics of hepatic parenchymal cells in vivo. Even in those cell lines with demonstrable hepatic properties (eg albumin synthesis), the level of function (quantitatively) may be far different from that of the parent organ [1].

It was unclear previously whether altered function represented phenotypic change in the cultured cells or was due solely to genetic factors; chromosomal abnormalities in serially propagated liver cells are common [8]. The question has been answered, in part, by recent studies of adult rat hepatocytes in nonproliferating primary monolayer culture. Details of this method are available in recent publications [2–7]. Briefly, hepatic parenchymal cells are obtained by collagenase perfusion of rat liver and purified by sedimentation. These are used for the preparation of mass cultures, in which cells attach to the substratum within 4 hours of plating and form a confluent monolayer after 12–20 hours. In general, cultures are utilized within one week after plating.

With primary culture of adult rat hepatocytes, the magnitude of early phenotypic change varies with the process under study but may be striking. An example of alteration with significant secondary effects is a decrease in the level of the microsomal cytochrome(s) known as P-450. During the first 24 hours after plating, the concentration of cytochrome P-450 in culture declines to 10–20% of that in the parent liver [9, 10]. The regulation of this process is under study in several laboratories [10–13]. The initial event in culture appears to be increased dissociation of the heme and protein moieties of cytochrome P-450. A heme-replete state in the cell ensues, and this has a number of secondary effects, as shown diagrammatically in Figure 1. The basal activity or δ-aminolevulinic synthetase – which is known to be subject to regulation by cellular heme – is reduced, as is its response to inducing agents such as barbiturates [10]. In addition, heme degradation is increased, and heme oxygenase – the enzyme system mediating the conversion of heme to bile pigment – is stimulated [8, 10]. Saturation of apo-tryptophane pyrrolase by heme (Fig. 1) has not been examined as yet in culture but would be predicted from studies in vivo [14]. These spontaneous changes in culture closely mimic the response of the liver in vivo to a heme load, either exogenous or endogenous [15, 16]. Thus, what appears to be initially a perturbation confined to a single microsomal system impinges secondarily on several hepatic functions.

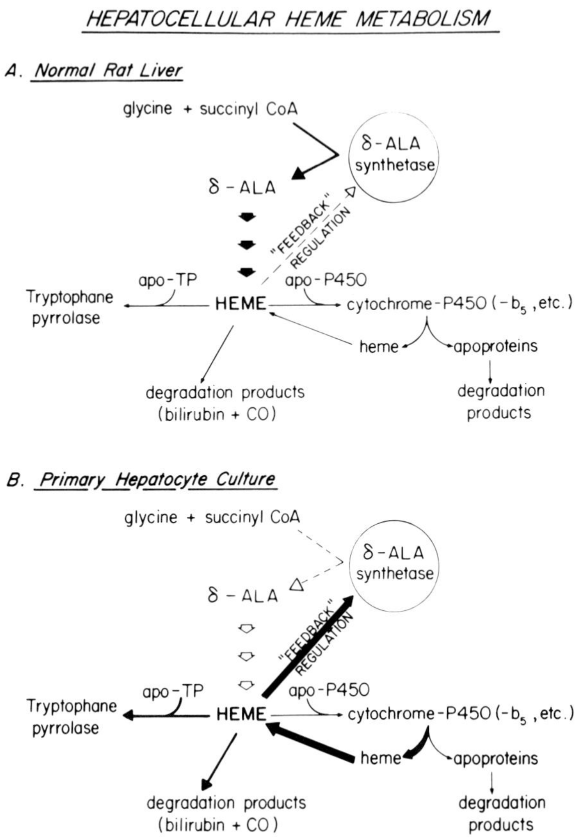

Fig. 1. Postulated pathways of heme metabolism in A) normal intact rat liver and B) rat hepatocytes in primary monolayer culture.

RELEVANCE OF PHENOTYPIC CHANGE TO THE STUDY OF HUMAN GENETIC DISEASES

The above example was selected to illustrate that phenotypic change occurs, may be relatively rapid, and is metabolically significant. The studies cited above were carried out with rat liver and, to date, it is unknown whether human liver cells in primary culture exhibit a similar change in cytochrome P-450. If so, their usefulness would be compromised for examination of certain of the hereditary diseases, specifically the hepatic porphyrias. The heme-synthetic pathway in human liver is known to be senstive to heme [17]. Thus, a heme-replete state (secondary to accelerated degradation of cytochrome P-450) would be associated with altered regulation of the pathway, as shown in Figure 1. In light of this problem, it seems reasonable that, for the present, studies of this area of metabolism in cultured hepatocytes should focus on the basis for the change in cytochrome P - 450 rather than on mechanisms of porphyrinogenesis.

On the other hand, the secondary effects of heme repletion, while multiple, will be limited and may not impinge on the study of other inherited diseases. For example, controversy exists as to the presence of an abnormality in the uptake or transport of iron in the liver of persons with hemochromatosis [18]. The available information indicates that transport processes, in general, are well preserved in primary hepatocyte culture [19], and this encourages study of iron transport. Wilson disease and Menke syndrome, 2 diseases of copper metabolism, also would benefit from analysis at both the organ and cellular level [20]. The fate of copper (free or bound) in liver cells or fibroblasts is unknown. Although the half-life of Cu^{67} is short (57 hours), it allows tracking of the radioactive label, and such an experiment would prove informative. Menkes syndrome [20, 21], an X-linked inherited disease associated with defective absorption of copper but not affecting the liver, could be illuminated by studies in both fibroblast and organ culture. Preliminary data [22] indicate the absorption of copper is normal but transport through the cell and delivery to tissues is defective. Studies in human fibroblasts [23] also indicate a disturbance in transport. Overall, it seems likely that hepatocyte culture will prove to be an elegant and definitive approach in the investigation of many of the diseases listed in Table 1.

PRESERVATION OF GENETICALLY DEFECTIVE HUMAN LIVER CELLS

Cell culture is widely perceived as a technique for propagating and thereby indefinitely preserving cells of a specific type. This is particularly desirable for genetic diseases which themselves are rare or in which the initial supply of tissue may be limited to a few milligrams provided by needle biopsy. At the present time, neither cell lines from normal liver nor primary hepatocyte culture meets this need satisfactorily. Propagation per se of cells from liver tissue is achieved reliably [1]; however, as noted above, cultures obtained in this manner on the whole fail to retain the phenotype of the liver in vivo. While only a few serial cultures have been prepared from adult human liver [1], the experience suggests that large-scale attempts to propagate cell lines with specific metabolic attributes will be unproductive. Primary cultures, while attractive in many respects, present the difficulty that relatively large amounts of cellular material are required. Moreover, primary cultures either are short-lived or evolve as a cell line, losing liver-specific functions in the process. Preservation of fresh cellular material in frozen storage for later primary culture is a possibility that should be explored. Human fetal liver cells may be frozen in an isotonic solution containing 10% dimethyl sulfoxide and fetal calf serum for a period of several weeks and, after thawing and washing, will form cultures comparable to those of the parent liver [23]; whether hepatocytes survive this form of storage for longer periods of time remains to be investigated.

AREAS FOR FURTHER INVESTIGATION

Phenotype change in primary hepatocyte culture occurs in a highly ordered, reproducible manner. Because the cells are freshly derived from the organism, it is likely that the regulatory mechanisms called into play and mediating phenotypic change are those of the intact liver. In the area of heme metabolism, this postulate is supported by recent studies in which rat hepatocytes in primary culture were compared with the liver in vivo [8]. Thus, study of phenotypic change may be expected to yield important insight into the regulation of those metabolic processes exhibiting culture-adaptive changes, as well as measures for reversing or preventing the appearance of the phenomenon.

For primary culture of human liver, sources of tissue and methods of dissociation need to be examined. Needle biopsy provides too little cell material for analyses in primary culture, and surgical liver biopsies may not be available. As success in hepatic transplantation improves, large amounts of genetically altered liver may become available. It is generally assumed that postmortem liver is unsuitable for culture because the organ undergoes autolysis, although that assumption has not been widely tested. The possibility of studying fetal tissues should be considered if the ethical issues surrounding its use can be resolved. With prenatal diagnosis becoming relatively common, providing the option for early abortion, fetal liver may be increasingly available as a source of tissue with specific gene defects. The behavior of human fetal liver in primary culture has been investigated relatively little [1]; in animal systems, the findings suggest that differentiation of fetal liver towards the adult phenotype continues – possibly at an accelerated pace – in culture [24, 25].

Another interesting approach to the expression of human hepatic genes in cultured cells is that employing cell hybridization. Mouse hepatoma cells fused to diploid human cells of various origins form proliferating hybrid cells that are capable of producing several human serum proteins [26, 27]. The elicitation of hepatic specific traits from the human genome in the hybrid provides a source of material for the analysis of gene expression. Hybrid cells also permit the establishment of cells from patients with genetic defects of the liver as "immortal" cell lines.

Most of the diseases listed in Table 1 are believed to involve the parenchymal cell population of the liver, reflecting the fact that relatively little study has been devoted to the nonparenchymal cells (the several types of sinusoidal lining, particularly Kupffer cells, and biliary epithelial cells). Not only may these cells be the focus of genetic disease (as in the lipid-storage diseases), but they may interact metabolically with the parenchymal cell population. The nonparenchymal cells of the liver constitute part of the unique pericellular environment of the hepatocyte and may be important determinants of hepatocellular function [28]. With methods now available for preparing and culturing nonparenchymal cells – including techniques for obtaining relatively pure subfractions of nonparenchymal cells [29] – mixed cell cultures may be constructed in a controlled fashion and the interaction of the various cell types in the liver studied. The pericellular environment of the hepatocyte includes also bile, contiguous with one face of the cell and possessing unique lipid-solubilizing properties. Preliminary studies with cultured rat hepatocytes have suggested that bile (or bile acid micelles) is required for the export of conjugated bilirubin from hepatocytes to extracellular fluid [30]. These data raise the possiblity that bile also is an important determinant of hepatocyte function. It is as yet unclear if genetic defects of the pericellular environment exist or if disruption of this environment in the preparation of isolated hepatocytes is responsible in part for phenotypic change in culture. Further investigation of these questions is needed.

CONCLUSION

Thus far, in studies of human genetic diseases, serially propagated cells from liver have provided little insight. Although the construction of fibroblast-hepatoma hybrids is a novel approach that needs to be explored, there are several reasons for emphasizing the use of primary hepatocyte culture in the study of inherited diseases at the cellular level. Primary cultures are temporally and metabolically close to the intact liver and, therefore, are more likely than are cell lines to yield physiologic information. For those areas of investigation in which phenotypic change poses a problem, studies of phenotypic change per se should have a high priority, lending insight not only into the regulation of metabolic processes in culture but also in the intact liver. Finally, the need for a *broad* examination of liver functions in culture should be stressed. There is a tendency for investigators to select a few "key" functions and judge the stability and viability of a culture accordingly. This approach may be misleading, in as much as phenotypic change will involve only some – not all – cell functions. Of the diseases listed in Table 1, a number may be amenable to study. Examination in culture of the several areas of metabolism relevant to those conditons should prove fruitful.

REFERENCES

1. Bissell DM: Study of hepatocyte function in cell culture. Prog Liver Dis 5:69–82, 1976.
2. Bissell DM, Hammaker L, Meyer UA: Parenchymal cells from adult rat liver in non-proliferating monolayer culture. I. Functional studies. J Cell Biol 59:722–734, 1973.
3. Bonney RJ: Adult liver parenchymal cells in primary culture: Characteristics and cell recognition standards. In Vitro 10: 130–142, 1974.

4. Michalopoulos G, Pitot HC: Primary culture of parenchymal liver cells on collagen membranes. Morphological and biochemical observations. Exp Cell Res 94:70–78, 1975.
5. Seglen PO: Preparation of isolated rat liver cells. Methods Cell Biol 13:29–83, 1976.
6. Leffert HL, Moran T, Boorstein R, Koch KS: Procarcinogen activation and hormonal control of cell proliferation in differentiated primary adult rat liver cell cultures. Nature 267: 58–61, 1977.
7. Savage CR Jr, Bonney RJ: Extended expression of differentiated function in primary cultures of adult liver parenchymal cells maintained on nitrocellulose filters. I. Induction of phosphoenolpyruvate carboxykinase and tyrosine aminotransferase. Exp Cell Res 114: 307–315, 1978.
8. Schaeffer WI, Polifka MD: A diploid rat liver cell culture. III. Characterization of the heteroploid morphological variants which develop with time in culture. Exp Cell Res 95:167–175, 1975.
9. Guzelian PS, Bissell DM, Meyer UA: Drug metabolism in adult rat hepatocytes in primary monolayer culture. Gastroenterology 72:1232–1239, 1977.
10. Bissell DM, Guzelian PS: Ascorbic acid deficiency and cytochrome P-450 in adult rat hepatocytes in primary monolayer culture. Arch Biochem Biophys 192:569–576, 1979.
11. Guzelian PS, Bissell DM: Effect of cobalt on synthesis of heme and cytochrome P-450 in the liver: Studies of adult rat hepatocytes in primary monolayer culture and in vivo. J Biol Chem 251:4421–4427, 1976.
12. Decad GM, Hsieh DPH, Byard JL: Maintenance of cytochrome P-450 and metabolism of aflatoxin B_1 in primary hepatocyte cultures. Biochem Biophys Res Commun 78:279–287, 1977.
13. Paine AJ, Legg RF: Apparent lack of correlation between the loss of cytochrome P-450 in hepatic parenchymal cell culture and the stimulation of haem oxygenase activity. Biochem Biophys Res Commun 81:672–679, 1978.
14. Bissell DM, Hammaker LE: Effect of endotoxin on tryptophan pyrrolase and Δ-aminolaevulinate synthase: Evidence for an endogenous regulatory haem fraction in rat liver. Biochem J 166:301–304, 1977.
15. Bissell DM, Hammaker LE: Cytochrome P-450 heme and the regulation of hepatic heme oxygenase activity. Arch Biochem Biophys 176:91–102, 1976.
16. Bissell DM, Hammaker LE: Cytochrome P-450 heme and the regulation of δ-aminolevulinic acid synthetase in the liver. Arch Biochem Biophys 176:103–112, 1976.
17. Watson CJ: Hematin and porphyria. N Engl J Med 293:605–608, 1975.
18. Valberg LS: Tissue iron distribution in idiopathic hemochromatosis. Gastroenterology 75:915–916, 1978.
19. Kletzien RF, Pariza MW, Becker JE, Potter VR, Butcher FR: Induction of amino acid transport in primary cultures of adult rat liver parenchymal cells by insulin. J Biol Chem 251: 3014–3020, 1976.
20. Sass-Kortsak A, Bearn AG: Hereditary disorders of copper metabolism. In Stanbury JB, Wyngaarden JB, Fredrickson DS (eds): "The Metabolic Basis of Inherited Disease." New York: McGraw-Hill, 1978, pp 1098-1126.
21. Menkes JH, Alter M, Steigleder GK, Weakley DR, Sung JH: A sex-linked recessive disorder with retardation of growth, peculiar hair, and focal cerebral and cerebellar degeneration. Pediatrics 29:764–779, 1962.
22. Danks DM, Cartwright E, Stevens BJ, Townley RRW: Menkes' kinky hair diseases: Further definition of the defect in copper transport. Science 179:1140–1142, 1973.
23. Chan W-Y, Garnica AD, Rennert OM: Cell culture studies of Menkes kinky hair disease. Clin Chim Acta 88:495–507, 1978.

24. Bissell DM, Tilles JG: Morphology and function of cells of human embryonic liver in monolayer culture. J Cell Biol 50:222, 1971.
25. Burchell B, Dutton GJ, Nemeth AM: Development of phenobarbital-sensitive control mechanisms for uridine diphosphate glucuronyltransferase activity in chick embryo liver. J Cell Biol 55: 448–456, 1972.
26. Darlington GJ, Bernhard HP, Ruddle FH: Human serum albumin phenotype activation in mouse hepatoma-human leukocyte cell hybrids. Science 185:859–862, 1974.
27. Rankin JK, Darlington GJ: Expression of human hepatic genes in mouse hepatoma-human amniocyte hybrids. Somatic Cell Genet 1:1–10, 1979.
28. Wanson JC, Drochmans P, Mosselmans R, Knook DL: Symbiotic culture of adult hepatocytes and sinus-lining cells. In Wisse E, Knook DL (eds): "Kupffer Cells and Other Sinusoidal Cells." Amsterdam: Elsevier North-Holland, 1977, pp 141–150.
29. Knook DL, Blansjaar N, Sleyster E Ch: Isolation and characterization of Kupffer and endothelial cells from rat liver. Exp Cell Res 109:317–329, 1977.
30. Bissell DM, Deal DR, Hammaker LE: Determinants of bilirubin transport into bile. Gastroenterology 69:809, 1975.

Cell Culture Systems for Studies of Normal and Abnormal Endocrine Function

Harold M. Nitowksy, MD

GENETIC BASIS OF ENDOCRINE DISEASE

As with disease affecting other body systems, genetic factors play a significant role in the pathogenesis of many endocrine diseases. Although in many of these disorders genetic effects are clearly identifiable, the precise role of hereditary factors is not easily discerned, and the mechanisms involved remain obscure. In these instances, studies of epithelial cell cultures from endocrine glands and various target tissues may aid in elucidating pathogenetic mechanisms.

In a growing number of genetically determined diseases, it has been possible to demonstrate directly an abnormality or absence of a specific protein or enzyme [1]. In many or even most genetic disorders, only the distal physiologic effects of the gene mutation are recognizable, and the underlying or primary defect is unknown. Nevertheless, it is reasonable to assume that a single primary defect exists whenever a disease is transmitted by a single gene mechanism, and the various manifestations of the disease can be related to the mutational event by a more or less complicated "pedigree of causes." Studies on epithelial cultures from patients with endocrine disorders may help identify the primary defect and provide explanations for the biochemical and clinical aberrations associated with these diseases.

The cell culture system as a model for study of endocrine diseases may be useful in other ways. Recent studies of genetic disorders have generally shown that an entity that appears clinically uniform often reflects the end result of different gene mutations [2]. These may involve different mutant alleles at a single locus or the action of mutant genes at different gene loci. Considering the complex enzymatic control of metabolism, it is not surprising that interference with

Birth Defects: Original Article Series, Volume XVI, Number 2, pages 293–304

different metabolic steps necessary for a given function may lead to similar end results. Thus, the demonstration of molecular or biochemical differences at the cellular level may be useful for the demonstration and documentation of genetic heterogeneity in endocrine disorders.

The identification of a gene affecting a specific endocrine function usually can be inferred from genetic analysis of family pedigrees. Since at least 50 phenotypically distinct and simply inherited disorders of the endocrine glands are currently recognized [3], there must be at least a corresponding number of genes which affect endocrine function in a major way. Mutations of these genes cause endocrine dysfunction, which is manifested at different functional levels, including glandular differentiation and neoplasia; hormone synthesis, secretion, and transport; and hormone action at the target cell level.

In most endocrine disorders, elucidation of the molecular or biochemical abnormalities resulting from these gene mutations has not been achieved.

Several generalizations can be made regarding the relationship between molecular pathophysiology and the mechanism of inheritance in endocrine disorders. The endocrine neoplasia syndromes, such as multiple endocrine adenomatosis, familia hyperparathyroidism without other gland involvement, and the medullary thyroid carcinoma-pheochromocytoma syndromes, are each inherited as autosomal dominant traits, as is frequently the case for other heritable tumors [4]. As for most enzyme deficiency states in man, the disorders affecting hormone biosynthesis show an autosomal recessive pattern of inheritance [1]. Finally, it is noteworthy that the best documented examples of hormone resistance in man – eg vitamin D-resistant rickets, nephrogenic diabetes insipidus, and the testicular feminization syndrome – result from mutations involving different genes on the X chromosome [1].

Table 1 lists various endocrine disorders in which genetic factors have been demonstrated to play a significant role. An attempt has been made to classify these on the basis of available information or certain presumptions, into those disorders where the primary gene defect appears to be intrinsic to the endocrine gland and those where the target tissues or organs are refractory to hormone action.

CELL CULTURES IN ENDOCRINE RESEARCH

In recent years there has been increasing interest in the use of cell culture in endocrinology, both as a means of exploring endocrine phenomena in health and disease, as well as for the study of basic aspects of gene action and regulation [5]. This interest reflects in part the advances in cell culture techniques that permit the expression of differentiated function of endocrine cells in vitro. In addition, the development of sensitive analytic methods, such as radioimmunoassay, has made it possible to accurately and reproducibly measure levels of hormones synthesized by cells in culture. In its ultimate form, the ability of the cell culture system to sustain all tissue-specific functions and responses in vitro for an indefinite period of time under completely defined conditions would allow it to supercede a variety of other methods.

Unfortunately, few of the cell culture models of endocrine function currently in use provide a reliable facsimile of endocrine cells and tissues in vivo. In some instances, it has proved possible, by judicious selection of techniques to reproduce certain essential features of endocrine behavior for extended periods of time in vitro. Even when changes in functional activity occur as a result of culture, they may aid in elucidating the factors that regulate hormone synthesis, secretion, and action in vivo [6].

The general failure to demonstrate specialized functions of cells cultured in vitro led to the widely held view that such cells "dedifferentiate" in culture and that such a system was implicitly unsuited to studies of endocrine function and regulation [7]. However, recent observations may aid in dispelling this view, since many of the unsuccessful early attempts to maintain special function were shown to result from the overgrowth of cultures by adventitious cell types present in the original tissues, such as fibroblast-like cells, vascular endothelial cells, or pericytes [8].

Interest in cell culture in endocrine research has revived from the almost universal skepticism of a decade ago to the extent that numerous attempts are being made to derive significant information from almost all conceivable hormone-producing cells and tissues in vitro [5]. Thus, recent examples have included secretion of thyrotropin-releasing factor (TRF) [9] and vasopressin [10] by organ cultures of adult guinea pig hypothalamus. This system bears some resemblance to the established cell line from embryonic rat hypothalamus secreting both vasopressin and neurophysin [11] from which a series of subclones of neurosecretory and primitive nerve cell lines has been derived [12]. There are several reports of the secretion of anterior pituitary peptide and protein hormones, by established tumor cell lines and primary monolayer cultures of normal adult adenohypophyseal cells [13]. The latter have been used in the study of gonadotropin [14], growth hormone [15], prolactin [16], ACTH [17] and TSH [18] secretion. Similarly, studies have been reported on the secretion of insulin and glucagon by primary monolayer cultures of neonatal rat pancreas [19] and a hamster islet cell tumor line [20]. Gastrin secretion has been demonstrated in primary cultures of both rat [21] and human pancreas [22]. Studies have been reported on the secretion of proparathormone by cultures of human parathyroid adenomas [23], and a parathyroid-hormone-producing cell line has been derived following SV-40 viral transformation of a cultured parathyroid adenoma [24].

Studies of thyroid follicular cells in culture and their morphologic and functional responses have been particularly successful, probably because the gland lends itself well to the production by enzymatic dissociation of a high yield

TABLE 1. Endocrine Disorders Influenced by Genetic Factors

Endocrine Gland	Disorder	Genetic defect: Intrinsic	Genetic defect: Target
Pituitary	Diabetes insipidus		
	a) vasopressin sensitive	+	
	b) nephrogenic		+
	Dwarfism		
	a) familial panhypopituitarism	+	
	b) growth hormone deficiency	+	
	c) Laron dwarfism	+	
	d) Pygmy		+
	Hypogonadism		
	a) Kallmann syndrome	+	
	b) familial gonadotropin deficiency	+	
Parathyroid	Hypoparathyroidism		
	a) familial neonatal	+	
	b) familial with Addison disease and moniliasis	+	
	c) familial	+	
	d) Albright hereditary osteodystrophy		+
	Hyperparathyroidism		
	a) familial neonatal	+	
	b) familial with multiple endocrine adenomatosis	+	
	c) familial	+	
	d) vitamin D-resistant rickets		+
Thyroid	Hypothyroidism		
	a) iodine transport defect	+	
	b) failure to form organic iodine	+	
	c) failure to couple iodotyrosines	+	
	d) deficient iodotyrosine deiodase	+	
	e) abnormal thyroglobulin synthesis	+	
	f) abnormal serum iodinated polypeptides	+	
	g) Pendred syndrome	+	
	h) familial goiter	+	
	i) athyreosis	+	
	j) autoimmune thyroiditis	?	
	k) familial thyroid unresponsiveness		+
	l) familial thyrotropin deficiency	–	–
	Hyperthyroidism		
	a) familial	?	
	Serum thyroxine binding globulin		
	a) increase	–	–
	b) decrease	–	–
Adrenal	Adrenal hyperplasia		
	a) 21-hydroxylase deficiency	+	
	b) 11-hydroxylase deficiency	+	

TABLE 1 (cont'd)

Endocrine Gland	Disorder	Genetic defect	
		Intrinsic	Target
	c) 3β-hydroxysteroid dehydrogenase deficiency	+	
	d) 17-hydroxylase deficiency	+	
	e) 20, 22-desmolase deficiency	+	
	f) 17, 20-desmolase deficiency	+	
	Adrenal insufficiency		
	a) congenital adrenal hypoplasia	+	
	b) familial Addison disease	+	
	c) Wolman disease	+	
	d) familial ACTH unresponsiveness		+
	e) Schmidt syndrome	?	
	f) familial aldosterone deficiency	+	
	Other		
	a) Bartter syndrome	–	–
	b) familial variations in corticosteroid-binding globulin	–	–
Pancreatic islets	Diabetes mellitus		
	a) juvenile diabetes	?	?
	b) maturity onset diabetes	?	?
	c) others		
	Hypoglycemia (primary)		
	a) leucine sensitivity	?	
	b) glucagon deficiency	+	
	c) multiple endocrine adenomatosis	+	
Gonad	Gonadal differentiation		
	a) familial XX gonadal dysgenesis	+	
	b) familial XY gonadal dysgenesis	+	
	c) familial hermaphroditism	+	
	d) familial male hypogonadism	+	
	e) Sertoli-cell only syndrome	+	
	f) Stein-Leventhal syndrome	+	
	Sexual development		
	a) complete testicular feminization		+
	b) familial incomplete male pseudohermaphroditism, Type 1		+
	c) familial incomplete male pseudohermaphroditism, Type 2		+
	d) incomplete testicular feminization		+
	e) familial sexual precocity	–	–
Multiple glands	Endocrine tumors		
	a) multiple endocrine adenomatosis	–	–
	b) familial medullary thyroid carcinoma-pheochromocytoma syndromes	–	–

of epithelial cells which can be readily identified by a characteristic morphologic response to thyrotropin in the formation of follicle-like structures [25]. Recent reports have dealt with the regulation of thyrotropic receptors in primary monolayer cultures of dog, bovine, and human follicular cells [26], as well as thyrotropic stimulation of cyclic adenosine 3′,5′-monophosphate (cAMP) in primary cultures of human cells [27] and proliferated secondary cultures of dog follicular cells [28]. Verrier et al [29] prepared cultures of porcine follicular thyroid cells in sufficient quantities to permit preparation of purified membranes and the study of hormonally activable adenylate cyclase, thereby placing cell cultures in a similar category with other in vitro systems for the biochemical analysis of mechanisms of hormone action. Primary monolayer cultures of adult human thyroid have been utilized for measurements of secretion of thyroxine and triiodothyronine [30].

Recent studies of primary monolayer cultures of adult [31] and fetal human adrenocortical cells have been carried out to measure steroid production [32]. Similarly, studies have been made of primary monolayer cultures of adult rat [33] and human [34] testicular interstitial cells. Among other findings, these have shown an effect of follicle stimulating hormone (FSH) in the secretion of estrogen [35], as well as androgen binding protein [36] by primary cultures of Sertoli cells. Ovarian steroidogenic cells have been successfully cultured, and recent studies have dealt with progesterone [37], androgen [38], estrogen [39], and HCG receptor activity [40] as functional parameters using both theca and granulosa cell types.

This brief and incomplete list of recent reports amply demonstrates the application of cell culture systems to studies of basic aspects of endocrine function and regulation. In general, the culture system, methodology, media, and experimental procedures have varied according to the aims and objectives of the experimental approach. Similarly, the period of culture has varied from a few days to many weeks or months. It is undoubtedly premature to specify the precise conditions under which an indefinite retention of functional activity by normal endocrine cells may be achieved for most endocrine tissues in culture, if indeed, this will ever be possible.

SPECIFIC APPLICATIONS OF CELL CULTURE METHODS

The significance and relevance of many of these studies to endocrine function in vivo or to the pathogenesis of endocrine disease remains obscure. Indeed, the disparity between the effects of certain pituitary tropic hormones in vitro and their presumed action in vivo has raised fundamental questions regarding certain generally accepted hormonal interrelationships. For example, studies of the effect of ACTH on growth of cultured adrenal cells have yielded unexpected results.

A major problem in cell biology is the nature of the mechanisms regulating cell proliferation. A vast body of information has accumulated in recent years on factors that influence the growth of cells in monolayer culture. For the most part, however, established cell lines and/or their transformed counterparts have been used in these studies, and the validity of these models in relation to the growth of normal cells in vivo remains a subject for speculation. Nonetheless, it appears that a wide variety of factors, including cell contact, density, nutrient supply, serum, hormones and proteins, cyclic nucleotides, etc, all directly or indirectly influence the rate at which cultured cells divide. However, in studying the specific regulation of growth by cultured endocrine cells, there is concern not so much with these general effects but with the tissue-specific proliferative responses that occur in endocrine cells and tissues in vivo and whether they can be reproduced in vitro. The establishment of a valid in vitro model of in vivo endocrine growth would in turn greatly facilitate the study of the possible aberrations in growth control in various hyperplastic and neoplastic conditions.

As yet, no in vitro system has effectively reproduced in the long-term the proliferative behavior of endocrine cells in vivo. The relationship between ACTH and the growth of adrenocortical cells affords a good example of the paradoxes that have been observed.

The first observation to be made on the growth of adrenocortical cells in culture was the inhibitory effect of ACTH on the proliferation of the Y-1 adrenal tumor cell line [41]. Since it was known that ACTH inhibits the growth of adrenocortical tumors in vivo [42], this response of the cultured cells occasioned little surprise and was attributed to their neoplastic origin. However, when methods for the culture of normal adult rat adrenal cells were developed, it was clear that ACTH also inhibited the proliferation of nonneoplastic cells [43]. In view of the known effect of ACTH in raising intracellular adrenal cyclic AMP levels and the large body of literature documenting the predominantly inhibitory effects of cyclic AMP on the proliferation of all types of cultured cells, it appeared that the inhibition was due to the cyclic nucleotide. Indeed, similar inhibitory effects on growth in culture have been noted with other endocrine cell types in which a tropic hormonal stimulus acts to raise cyclic AMP levels [44]. Here then is the essential paradox: administration of ACTH in vivo results in adrenal hyperplasia, yet in vitro its effects are inhibitory.

One possibility is that the recently discovered higher molecular weight forms of ACTH [13] are responsible for the growth response. No evidence for or against this possibility has yet been documented, and it is a valid solution only if the hormone(s) acts in some way not directly involving cyclic AMP. Related to this suggestion is a possible role for a variety of polypeptides that have been isolated from both the pituitary and the brain. Thus, fibroblast growth factor (FGF) stimulates the growth of adrenal Y-1 tumor cells [45]. FGF, however, lacks the necessary specificity for a tropic adrenal growth-promoting hormone. A related polypeptide, ovarian growth factor, has also been isolated from the pituitary and shown to possess some degree of specificity in stimulating proliferation in an ovarian cell line [46]. Indeed, a number of growth-promoting factors not identical with known pituitary hormones appear to occur in the pituitary and often occur as impurities in classical hormone preparations. It has, therefore, been suggested that these may be the true growth-stimulating hormones of the pituitary [47]. However, their distribution in vivo (brain as well as pituitary), as well as their general lack of specificity, argues against this hypothesis, and their true physiologic role may be similar to that of the somatomedins and insulin rather than the highly specific, classical pituitary hormones.

The inhibitory response obtained with cyclic AMP in vitro, could be an artifact of culture due to the abnormal environment of the cells. Although cyclic AMP will ameliorate adrenal weight loss in hypophysectomized animals [48], there is no evidence that it will stimulate growth in vivo. Indeed the similar behavior of the epidermis in vitro and in vivo [49] argues strongly against cyclic AMP having a direct proliferogenic role in vivo as opposed to an inhibitory effect in vitro, although definite evidence in the case of the adrenal cortex is lacking.

Thus far, it has been assumed implicitly that ACTH is directly responsible for the growth of the adrenal in vivo. This assumption may have created the paradox. Some years ago it was suggested that growth of the cortex in vivo was due to the hyperemia caused by ACTH, possibly acting via prostaglandin [50] and that the effect was simply to increase the supply of blood-borne nutrients to the gland. Later, it was suggested that ACTH-activated lysosomal labilization may be the stimulus for growth [51]. Thus, an indirect role of ACTH, dependent possibly on the tissue structure and vascularization of the cortex, in stimulating adrenal growth becomes not only possible but probable, in view of the failure to resolve the paradox in any other manner. Recent reports also implicate neurotropic factors in compensatory adrenal growth [52].

The slow regenerative growth of the adrenal cortex suggests that proliferation in vivo may in fact be taking place against a substantial inhibitory influence (possibly raised cyclic AMP due to pituitary ACTH secretion). It also raises the possibility that only a small minority of the cells are involved in the response. A recent report suggests that physiologic doses of ACTH will increase to a small extent thymidine incorporation and mitoses in primary monolayer cultures of human adrenocortical cells [53]. In view of the heterogeneity of such cultures and the possible effects of ACTH acting via cyclic AMP to change nucleotide pool sizes, one cannot be certain that functioning cortical cells, as opposed to fibroblasts or other adventitious cell types, are involved in the proliferative response. Experience with similar cultures has shown that the majority of adult human cortical cells, in the presence or absence of ACTH, do not proliferate significantly, in contrast to the marked growth seen in cultures of rat adult cells and human fetal cortical cells [32, 54], possibly because the culture conditions have not been optimized for the adult human cell type.

Clearly a careful study of the precise role of ACTH in stimulating adrenal growth in vivo, together with a modification of the culture environment to permit reproducible proliferation of the adult human cells, will be necessary before monolayer cell culture systems can be used to compare growth control in benign and malignant tumors of the adrenal cortex. Whatever the ultimate success of these endeavors, however, this and similar tissue culture models of endocrine cell behavior have demonstrated the need to reevaluate critically our knowledge of the growth of endocrine tissues in vivo, and must, therefore, ultimately enlarge our knowledge of this vital aspect of cell behavior.

CONCLUSION

Certain aspects of the application of cell culture systems for the study of endocrine function in health and disease have been reviewed. Cell culture offers many approaches; none is easy and many are both time-consuming and laborious. In some respects they still represent "art forms" with a complexity that defies simple analysis. If, however, tissue culture is to achieve preeminence in experimental studies, then its days as an art rather than a science must be numbered.

Certain basic problems of methodology, however, still remain to be solved by systematic experimentation, leading ultimately to the preservation of complete structural and functional integrity of purified endocrine cells in culture under completely defined conditions. It appears likely that, for most purposes, cell culture will supersede organ culture because of its potential flexibility and versatility, particularly when and if methods permit isolation of specific cell types. Further progress in the use of tissue culture to study functional activity and growth may be considerably hampered until these requirements are fulfilled. It would be unreasonable to assume that there will be one all-encompassing ideal medium or system of culture, and conditions may have to be optimized for each individual cell type or tissue, particularly for human material. Some examples have been cited illustrating the substantial advantages to be gained by the use of existing cell culture methodologies, imperfections and all, particularly in the field of human studies. Quite apart from the basic scientific advantage of allowing repeated experiments to be carried out with the same population of cells, culture makes it possible to study in a correlated manner both the structural and functional responses of human cells or tissues under conditions unmodified by the ethical or experimental limitations that supervene in vivo. A further dimension to culture studies has been introduced with the advent of perfusion systems which allow the dynamic aspects of endocrine cell behavior to be studied with greater ease. These improvements in culture technology may lead ultimately to systems which reproduce with a greater degree of fidelity the situation of endocrine cells in vivo, which may have a significant role to play in the modulation of endocrine functions in normal and disease states.

REFERENCES

1. Stanbury JB, Wyngaarden JB, Fredrickson DS: "The Metabolic Basis of Inherited Disease," 4th Ed. New York: McGraw-Hill, 1978.
2. Childs B, Der Kaloustian VM: Genetic heterogeneity. N Engl J Med 279:1205–1212, 1267–1274, 1968.
3. Goldstein JL, Motulsky AG: Genetics and endocrinology. In Williams RH (ed): "Textbook of Endocrinology," 5th Ed. Philadelphia: WB Saunders, 1974, pp 1004–1029.
4. Rimoin DL, Schimke RN: Mechanisms of gene action in disorders of the endocrine glands. In Bergsma D (ed): Part X. "The Endocrine System." Baltimore: Williams & Wilkins for The National Foundation–March of Dimes, BD:OAS VII(6):5–11, 1971.
5. O'Hare MJ, Ellison ML, Neville AM: Tissue culture in endocrine research: Perspectives, pitfalls, and potentials. Curr Top Exp Endocrinol 3:1–56, 1978.
6. Meites J, Kahn RH, Nicoll CS: Prolactin production by rat pituitary in vitro. Proc Soc Exp Biol Med 108:440–443, 1961.
7. Schulster D, Burstein S, Cooke BA: "Molecular Endocrinology of the Steroid Hormones." London: Wiley, 1976.
8. Franks LM, Wilson PD: "Spontaneous" neoplastic transformation in vitro: The ultrastructure of the tissue culture cell. Eur J Cancer 6:517–523, 1970.
9. McKelvey JF, Sheridan M, Joseph S, Phelps CH, Perrie S: Biosynthesis of thyrotropin-releasing hormone in organ cultures of the guinea pig median eminence. Endocrinology 97:908–918, 1975.
10. Pearson D, Shainberg A, Osinchak J, Sachs H: The hypothalamoneurohypophysial complex in organ culture: Morphologic and biochemical characteristics. Endocrinology 96:982–993, 1975.
11. DeVitry F, Camier M, Czernichow P, Benda PH, Cohen P, Tixier-Vidal A: Establishment of a clone of mouse hypothalamic neurosecretory cells synthesizing neurophysin and vasopressin. Proc Natl Acad Sci USA 71:3575–3579, 1974.
12. Tixier-Vidal A, DeVitry F: Ultrastructural and cytochemical features of SV40 transformed hypothalamic cell lines. Cell Tissue Res 171:39–59, 1976.
13. Mains RE, Eipper BA, Ling N: Common precursor to corticotropins and endorphins. Proc Natl Acad Sci USA 74:3014–3018, 1977.
14. Tang LKL, Spies HG: Effects of gonadal steroids on the basal and LRF-induced gonadotropin secretion by cultures of rat pituitary. Endocrinology 96:349–355, 1975.
15. Brown M, Vale W: Growth hormone release in the rat: Effects of somatostatin and thyrotropin-releasing factor. Endocrinology 97:1151–1156, 1975.
16. Machlin LJ, Jacobs LS, Cirulis N, Kimes R, Miller R: An assay for growth hormone and prolactin-releasing activities using a bovine pituitary cell culture system. Endocrinology 95:1350–1358, 1974.
17. Yasuda M, Greer MA: Studies on the corticotrophin-releasing activity of vasopressin, using ACTH secretion by cultured rat adenohypophyseal cells. Endocrinology 98: 936–942, 1976.
18. Yasuda N, Takebe K, Greer MA: Studies on ACTH dynamics in cultured adenohypophyseal cells: Effect of adrenalectomy or dexamethasone In Vitro. Endocrinology 98:717–721, 1976.
19. Fujimoto WY, Ensinck JW, Williams RH: Somatostatin inhibits insulin and glucagon release by monolayer cell cultures of rat endocrine pancreas. Life Sci 15:1999–2004, 1974.

20. Shin SI, Baum SG, Fleischer N, Rosen OM: Retention of endocrine function by an insulin-secreting pancreatic islet cell tumour from Syrian hamster through serial transplantation in nude mice. J Cell Sci 18:199–206, 1975.
21. Braaten JT, Greider MH, McGuigan JE, Mintz DH: Gastrin in the perinatal rat pancreas and gastric antrum: Immunofluorescence localization of pancreatic gastric cells and gastrin secretion in monolayer cell cultures. Endocrinology 99:684–691, 1975.
22. Hollande E, Giron B, Lehy T, Accary JP, Rozé C: In vitro secretion of gastrin, insulin and glucagon in tissue cultures of pancreas from a child with neonatal intractable hypoglycemia. Gastroenterology 71:255–262, 1976.
23. Martin TJ, Greenberg PB, Michelangeli V: Synthesis of human parathyroid hormone by cultured cells: Evidence for release of prohormone by some adenomata. Clin Sci 44:1–8, 1973.
24. Deftos LJ, Rabson AS, Buckle RM, Aurbach GD, Potts JT Jr: Parathyroid hormone production in vitro by human parathyroid cells transformed by simina virus 40. Science 159:435–436, 1968.
25. Kerkof PR, Long PJ, Chaikoff IL: In vitro effects of thyrotropic hormone. I. On the pattern of organization of monolayer cultures of isolated sheep thyroid gland cells. Endocrinology 74:170–179, 1964.
26. Winand RJ, Kohn LD: Thyrotropin effects on thyroid cells in culture. J Biol Chem 250:6534–6540, 1975.
27. Kaneko Y: Cyclic AMP level of human thyroid cells in monolayer culture. TSH induced refractoriness to TSH action. Horm Metab Res 8:202–206, 1976.
28. Rapoport B: Dog thyroid cells in monolayer tissue culture: Adenosine 3′,5′-cyclic monophosphate response to thyrotropic hormone. Endocrinology 98:1189–1197, 1976.
29. Verrier B, Planells R, Hennen G, Lissitsky S: Chemical composition of porcine thyroid cell plasma membranes. Mol Cell Endocrinol 5:215–221, 1976.
30. Bidey SP, Marsden P, McKerron CG, Anderson J: Evidence for differential synthesis of thyroxine and triiodothyronine by cultured human thyroid cells following exposure to thyrotrophin or dibutyryl cyclic AMP. Biochem Biophys Res Commun 70:418–424, 1976.
31. O'Hare MJ, Nice EC, Magee-Brown R, Bullman H: High-pressure liquid chromatography of steroids secreted by human adrenal and testis cells in monolayer culture. J Chromatogr 125:357–367, 1976.
32. Kahri AI, Huhtaniemi I, Salmenperä M: Steroid formation and differentiation of cortical cells in tissue culture of human fetal adrenals in the presence and absence of ACTH. Endocrinology 98:33–41, 1976.
33. Khatim MS, O'Hare MJ: Testosterone and progesterone secretion by adult rat testis interstitial cells in monolayer culture. J Endocrinol 69:19P–20P, 1976.
34. O'Hare MJ, Bullman H, Nice EC: Steroid secretion by adult, prepubertal and foetal human testicular cells in monolayer culture. J Endocrinol 71:97P–98P, 1976.
35. Dorrington JH, Armstrong DT: Follicle-stimulating hormone stimulates estradiol-17β synthesis in cultured Sertoli cells. Proc Natl Acad Sci USA 72:2677–2681, 1975.
36. Fritz IB, Rommerts FG, Louis BG, Dorrington JH: Regulation by FSH and dibutyryl cyclic AMP of the formation of androgen-binding protein in Sertoli cell-enriched cultures. J Reprod Fertil 46:17–24, 1976.
37. Salomon DS, Sherman MI: Gonadotrophin stimulation of progesterone synthesis by midpregnancy mouse ovarian cells in vitro. Endocrinology 99:800–808, 1976.
38. Erickson GF, Ryan KJ: Stimulation of testosterone production in isolated rabbit thecal tissue by LH/FSH, dibutyryl cyclic AMP, PGE2alpha, and PGE2. Endocrinology 99:452–458, 1976.

39. Erickson GF, Ryan KJ: The effect of LH/FSH, dibutyryl cyclic AMP, and prostaglandins on the production of estrogens by rabbit granulosa cells in vitro. Endocrinology 97:108–113, 1975.
40. Stouffer RL, Tyrey L, Schomberg DW: Changes in ^{125}I labeled human chorionic gonadotropin (hCG) binding to porcine granulosa cells during follicle development and cell culture. Endocrinology 99:516–525, 1976.
41. Masui H, Garren LD: Inhibition of replication in functional mouse adrenal tumor cells by adrenocorticotropic hormone mediated by adenosine 3′:5′-cyclic monophosphate. Proc Natl Acad Sci USA 68:3206–3210, 1971.
42. Iglesias R, Mardones E: Influence of hormones on the growth of a transplantable supra-renal tumour. Br J Cancer 12:28–31, 1958.
43. Ramachandran J, Suyama AT: Inhibition of replication of normal adrenocortical cells in culture by adrenocorticotropin. Proc Natl Acad Sci USA 72:113–117, 1975.
44. Gospodarowicz D, Gospodarowicz F: The morphological transformation and inhibition of growth of bovine luteal cells in tissue culture induced by luteinizing hormone and dibutyryl cyclic AMP. Endocrinology 96:458–467, 1975.
45. Gospodarowicz D, Handley HH: Stimulation of division of Y_1 adrenal cells by a growth factor isolated from bovine pituitary glands. Endocrinology 97:102–107, 1975.
46. Jones KL, Gospodarowicz D: Biological activity of a growth factor for ovarian cells. Proc Natl Acad Sci USA 71:3372–3376, 1974.
47. Gospodarowicz D, Jones KL, Sato G: Purification of a growth factor for ovarian cells from bovine pituitary glands. Proc Natl Acad Sci USA 71:2295–2299, 1974.
48. Ney RL: Effects of dibutyryl cyclic AMP on adrenal growth and steroidogenic capacity. Endocrinology 84:168–170, 1969.
49. Voorhees JJ, Duell EA, Stawiski M, Harrell ER: Cyclic nucleotide metabolism in normal and proliferating epidermis. Adv Cyclic Nucleotide Res 4:117–162, 1974.
50. Maier F, Staehelin M: Adrenal hyperaemia caused by corticotrophin. Acta Endocrinol (Kbh) 58:613–618, 1968.
51. Szego CM, Rakich DR, Seeler BJ, Gross RS: Lysosomal labilization: Rapid target-specific effect of ACTH. Endocrinology 96:863–874, 1974.
52. Engeland WC, Dallman MF: Neural mediation of compensatory adrenal growth. Endocrinology 99:1659–1662, 1976.
53. Armato U, Andreis PG, Draghi E: Dose-related persistent proliferogenic action of corticotrophin 1–24 in normal adult human adrenocortical cells in primary tissue culture. J Endocrinol 72:97–98, 1977.
54. Roos BA, Bundy LL, Bailey R, Deftos LJ: Calcitonin secretion in vitro. I. Preparation of monolayer C-cell cultures. Endocrinology 95:1142–1149, 1974.

The Use of Cell and Organ Culture Methods to Study Renal Birth Defects*

Michel Bergeron, MD, Diane K. Fast, PhD, Charles R. Scriver, MD, FRSC, and Olli Simell, MD†

The embryologic origin of mammalian kidney is both interesting and complex [1]. Because many types of differentiated cells come to serve the functions of the mature organ, one perceives numerous opportunities for malformation during ontogeny to occur and mutation to be expressed then and after. Defects of renal development are said to affect about 10% of livebirths [2]. Hay and Tonascia [3] listed 109 anatomic anomalies of kidney and ureter in their classification of congenital malformations; disorders of renal function were excluded. A recent compilation of the hereditary disorders of renal transport enumerated at least 28 conditions [4]. On the other hand, classification of the important hereditary glomerulopathies and of the polycystic diseases with renal involvement has remained a challenge, probably because we know too little to classify with authority. Perhaps it is not surprising that renal birth defects have yet to earn a place of their own among the nosologic tables in McKusick's "Mendelian Inheritance in Man" [5].

Success with renal organ culture and selective culture of particular renal cell types ought to illuminate both the mechanisms of some renal malformations and how mutation can perturb a working epithelium. For the past quarter century

*Supported in part by a Canadian Medical Research Council Group Award (Genetics) [C.R.S.], an MRC operating grant [M.B.], an MRC postdoctoral fellowship [D.K.F.], and study awards from the MRC and Canada Council [O.S.]. Our interest in birth defects is also supported by the Réseau Provincial de la Médecine Génétique.

†Authors are presented in alphabetical order.

Birth Defects: Original Article Series, Volume XVI, Number 2, pages 305–314

there has been a smouldering interest in such a development but, despite an occasional exciting achievement, one cannot claim that the area has caught fire. The following is a brief appraisal of progress and strategy in the area.†

RENAL EMBRYOLOGY RELEVANT TO BIRTH DEFECTS

The mature human kidney originates in the metanephros. Nephrons differentiate from the renal blastema while the ureteral bud forms the collecting system. The scenario begins with induction of the blastema and ureteral bud by diffusable substances. Nephronogenesis, with the formation of about 800,000 nephrons follows during the interval between the 5th and 32nd week of human fetal development. During this same period, the pyriform extremity of the ureteral bud is undergoing a series of dichotomies and enlargement in 3 dimensions to form the collecting ducts and calyces. Patent unions between the nephrons and the collecting-duct extremities of ureteral bud branchings are essential if the excretory role of the kidney is to be fulfilled. Mesenchymal cells of the blastema unused to form nephrons differentiate into mesangium, juxtaglomerular apparatus, and macula densa. Fetal kidney is forming urine by the midtrimester.

Birth defects of the kidney reflect disorder in the sequence and outcome of developmental events. In broad terms, there can be: anomalies of position and number of the kidneys; failure of blastemal induction; reduction in the number of nephrons; segmental hypoplasia. These conditions are usually not hereditary. A second class of anomalies involves the formation of renal cysts either solitary or multiple; the latter are often hereditary and reflect a disturbance in the continuity of ureteral and blastemal components. Then, there are disorders of glomerular or tubular differentiation and function; such conditions, more often than not, are mendelian. Ontogeny of function in the perinatal period is the final tuning of the system after it has developed through the major stages of morphogenesis.

Perceptive, succinct reviews of renal ontogeny and differentiation were presented in the symposium on Renal Growth and Development at the VIIth International Congress of Nephrology [6-9].

THE HEREDITARY NEPHROPATHIES

Whereas many renal disorders that compromise function, and therefore have medical significance, are not hereditary, those that are [10] hold special interest because their characteristics are stable and may be susceptible to analysis in organ and cell culture systems. Mendelian nephropathies constitute about 13% of pediatric renal disease [11]. Royer et al [11] classified hereditary renal birth defects under 5 headings: 1) malformations (5% of the hereditary cases);

†Birth defects of the lower urinary tract are omitted from the discussion. A detailed survey of such anomalies is available elsewhere in the Series (see Bergsma D, Duckett JW (eds): "Urinary System Malformations in Children." New York: Alan R Liss for The National Foundation–March of Dimes, BD:OAS XIII[5], 1977).

2) nephropathies with progressive renal failure (43%); 3) nephrotic syndromes (8.5%); 4) primary tubulopathies (26.5%); 5) renal disease secondary to inborn errors of metabolism (16%).

McKusick [5] lists many of the conditions encountered by Royer and colleagues [11] ; he also lists others. The French group refers to hereditary nephropathies not listed by McKusick. These discrepancies in cataloging highlight prevailing difficulties in the nosology of hereditary renal disease [1, 7] which might eventually yield to study in culture systems. Some examples of mendelian renal disease classified according to Royer et al follow:

1) *Malformations:* infantile polycystic disease (AR, McKusick 17390*); adult-onset polycystic disease (AD, McKusick 17390 and 17400); juvenile polycystic disease (AR) with hepatic fibrosis (referred to under 26320 in McKusick); rarer conditions with renal cysts such as Meckel syndrome (AR, McKusick 24900) and cerebrohepatorenal (Zellweger) syndrome (AR, McKusick 21410).

2) *Progressive azotemic nephropathies:* Alport syndrome (AD, McKusick 10420); nephronophthisis (AR, McKusick 25610) and the variant with tapetoretinal degeneration (AR, McKusick 26690); medullary cystic disease appearing as familial juvenile nephronophthisis, inherited as an AR (McKusick 25610), or as a variant of adult–onset polycystic disease (AD, McKusick 17400).

3) *Congenital nephrosis:* Finnish type with microcystic disease (AR, McKusick 25630); infantile idiopathic nephrosis with diffuse mesangial sclerosis (probably AR, see [11] ; hereditary, late-onset nephrosis with pulmonic stenosis (AR, McKusick 26550).

4) *Hereditary tubulopathies:* primary disorders of reabsorptive or secretory transport (eg renal glycosuria, cystinuria, and distal renal tubular acidosis, see [4]).

5) *Nephropathies secondary to inborn errors of metabolism:* the infantile and juvenile forms of cystinosis (AR, McKusick 21980 and 21990); Fabry disease (XL, McKusick 30150); familial Mediterranean fever (AR, McKusick 24910), and others, see [4, 10, 11] .

Animal Models

There is only limited access to viable human renal tissue for the study of a particular disease process by culture methods in vitro. Therefore mendelian analogs, in other vertebrates, are of considerable interest for the opportunity they might provide to assist research on the human disorders of renal morphogenesis and function. Cornelius [12] , who referred to animal models as "neglected medical resources," identified 19 animal counterparts of human renal disorders, some of which are models of the various hereditary nephropathies and malformations of man. Lush [13] identified 2 biochemical genetic problems in nonhuman vertebrates. We know of other genetic models in animals and this hereditary material is compiled in Table 1.

*McKusick's catalog number is shown; AR, means autosomal recessive, etc [5] .

TABLE 1. Hereditary Human Renal Birth Defects With Possible Animal Counterparts

Human conditions	Animal counterpart	Species	Reference
1. Maldevelopment			
Polycystic kidneys	Cystic dilatation of tubules	Rat (Gunn)	[14]
Renal agenesis	Short-Danforth syndrome	Mouse	[15]
2. Maldevelopment with progressive azotemia			
Nephronophthisis and tapetoretinal degeneration	KD mutant	Mouse	[16]
3. Congenital nephrosis			
Finnish variety (or others, see [10])	Nephrosis	Mouse	[17]
4. Tubulopathies			
Diabetes insipidus	Diabetes insipidus	Mouse	[18]
X-linked hypophos-phatemia	X-linked hypophos-phatemia	Mouse	[19]
Urolithiasis	High urate excretor	Dog (Dalmatian)	[13, 20]
Cystinuria	Cystinuria and isolated cystinuria	Dog	[13, 21]
Renal aminoaciduria	Hypertaurinuria	Mouse	[22]
Hyperaminoaciduria	Proline oxidase deficiency	Mouse	[23]
Fanconi syndrome	Fanconi syndrome	Dog (Basenji)	[24]

Use of Renal Cell and Organ Culture Systems Fetal Kidney Organ Culture

Fetal Kidney Organ Culture

Grobstein and colleagues [25, 26] were the first to use organ culture to study mammalian metanephric nephrogenesis. They dissected the ureteral bud from blastema in 11-day fetal mouse kidney and separated one component from the other by a filter membrane immersed in organ culture media. Ureteric tissue acted as a transmembrane inducer of blastemal differentiation to form nephrons; other embryonic mesenchymes could also serve as inducers. Saxén and colleagues [27] used the same method to record nephrogenesis by cinematography and to document the ontogeny of tubular enzymes. Gossens and Unsworth [28] studied tubulogenesis under defined conditions and found that induction and later development were probably separate phenomena. Bernstein [7] describes the use of fetal organ culture to study glomerular differentiation and the onset of tubular functions, such as PAH transport.

Crocker et al [1] adapted Grobstein's method to study impaired nephrogenesis in fetal mouse kidney. They found that in vitro conditions equivalent to hypokalemia in the fetus interfered with nephrogenesis. Under such conditions the ureteral bud was dilated, branching was diminished, and blastemal induction was reduced. Since man resembles mouse in the normal occurrence of fetal hyperkalemia relative to the maternal serum potassium concentration [1], the line of investigation developed by Crocker, if applied to the KD mouse (Table 1), might be illuminating for interpretation of human nephronophthisis.

Little imagination is required to perceive how the fetal organ culture technique, adapted to the appropriate animal models, might serve investigators who seek interpretations of human disease counterparts. As yet there is little apparent activity in this direction.

Renal Cell Culture

Selective culture of renal cells has played several distinguished roles in medical research. Cultured monkey kidney cell lines were used early for the propagation of viral cytopathogenic agents [29]. Subsequent development of these techniques led to the production of vaccines and the elimination of poliomyelitis as a major public health problem. The Madin-Darby canine kidney (MDCK) cell line [30] was important in characterizing immunologic and cytologic effects of oncogenic viruses [31] long before this cell line was used as a model of transepithelial transport. More recently, selective culture of glomerular and epithelial cells has begun to play a role in the study of renal function and disease.

Glomerular Cell Culture

Glomerular cultures have been used in an attempt to characterize the mechanisms of glomerular diseases. The glomerular filtration apparatus has 4 major components [32]: endothelium, basement membrane, epithelium, and mesangium in the capillary loops. Three cell types grow in culture: endothelial cells which, in situ, line the capillary wall and form fenestrae (diameter 600–1,000 Å); epithelial cells with podocytes external to the capillaries in situ; mesangial cells with phagocytic and contractile properties in situ. This diversity of structure and function among the differentiated glomerular components imposes constraints on the use of culture techniques since any dedifferentiation in vitro will negate the effort to study specific cell types. Karnovsky and Kreisberg [33] used a tissue dissociation method to obtain individual cell types (epithelial, mesangial, and renin-like) from rat glomeruli which were then cloned and maintained in culture. Certain problems were encountered: the 3 types of cells did not grow equally well in culture and they did not always maintain their in vivo biochemical and antigenic properties in the in vitro system. Furthermore, a paucity of specific markers has made identification of the cell type in vitro a problem, a solution for which rests, at present, on techniques of electron microscopy and the study of functional properties such as collagen synthesis, immunofluorescence, and phagocytosis [34–39]. Success in culture has been greatest with mesangial cells, whose infrastructural and biochemical properties persist through multiple passages in culture. Since tissue obtained from young donors, in general, facilitate studies in culture, it is encouraging that investigators have succeeded in establishing cultures of glomerular elements obtained at autopsy, or from renal biopsy, of newborns and infants [35, 37]. Further development of this approach is likely to facilitate the study of specific human renal disease [40, 41].

Isolated Tubular Epithelial Cells

Outgrowth of epithelial cells from renal tissue explants would be most desirable when such cells are specifically required for certain lines of investigation. Unfortunately, overgrowth of stromal fibroblasts from the explant occurs rapidly and the goal of isolated epithelial cells in culture is soon obliterated. Gilbert and Migeon [42, 43] recognized that D-amino acid oxidase is an enzyme unique to epithelium; with this in mind, they designed a selective growth medium for culture of rat and human kidney tubular epithelial cells. Substitution of D-valine for the L-enantiomer in dialyzed nutrient medium allowed the epithelial cells to proliferate while fibroblast growth was inhibited. The selected cells possessed D-amino acid oxidase, carbonic anhydrase, alkaline phosphatase, and the renal-specific lactate dehydrogenase; accordingly, they seemed to be of tubular origin but the nephron segment of origin could not be defined. Although the surviving cells gave rise to clones, they did not survive many cell transfers; dedifferentiation may have been the cause of the declining growth potential in serial passages.

Intact Tubular Epithelium

Leighton and colleagues [44] observed that the MDCK cell line showed cellular polarity in monolayer culture with tight junction formation and transport activity. Hemicyst (dome) formation was a marker of the functional activity. A pig kidney line (LLC-Pk_1) and frog urinary bladder monolayer cultures also showed hemicyst formation. Misfeldt et al [45] and others [46–49] studied transepithelial transport of the MDCK cell line in vitro. The monolayer is an effective permeability barrier with 84–100 ohms • cm^2 resistance. It has a selective permeability for cations (P_{Na}/P_{Cl}=1.7), and in the absence of a chemical gradient can generate a transepithelial electrical potential of 1.4 mV, apical surface negative, and a net water flux of 7.3 μl cm^{-2} hr^{-1}. Ouabain [47] and iodoacetate [45] abolish asymmetry of fluxes, and the potential difference and hemicyst formation disappear. Under appropriate conditions, an ouabain-insensitive mode of Na^+ transport with electroneutral exchange can also be identified in the MDCK cell line [48]. The MDCK epithelium in culture is sensitive to cyclic AMP [46] and possesses adenylate cyclase activity responsive to vasopressin, oxytocin, prostaglandins E_1 and E_2, and glucagon [49].

Cultured epithelium, other than MDCK, has been studied. A pig kidney cell line (LLC-Pk_1) responds to ADH and salmon calcitonin, and is structurally and functionally polarized by virtue of microvilli and tight junctions [50, 51].

In situ micropuncture and perfusion studies of isolated nephron segments show that the mammalian nephron has segmental functional heterogeneity. Because the majority of human tubular birth defects are disorders of segmental functions, it would be desirable to have culture methods that allow one to study epithelium from specific segments in vitro. As yet, it has not been possible to culture either cells or epithelium from dissected segments of mammalian nephrons [52]. However, recent success with selective culture of the granular cells from toad bladder [53] may be a harbinger of things to come.

ATTEMPTS TO USE CULTURED EPITHELIUM TO STUDY INBORN ERRORS OF RENAL TRANSPORT

We have used the D-valine technique [42, 43] to culture epithelial cells from rat and mouse kidney. Our goal was to obtain an intact epithelium in vitro from 3 mouse models (Table 1: hypertaurinuria (tau^{t-}) [22]; X-linked hypophosphatemia (Hyp/Y) [19]; hyperprolinemia (PRO/Re) [23]). It was our hope that the epithelium would function as a permeability barrier with vectorial transports of taurine, phosphate, and L-proline. We were unsuccessful. Patches of epithelial cells were obtained with kidney cortex explants, but an epithelial sheet was not obtained, nor did hemicyst formation appear.

Our cultures were set up on sterilized Millipore filters, or other porous supporting materials, retained in place by a glass ring in petri dishes or wells filled with nutrient medium; $2-4 \times 10^5$ cells were plated on areas 25 mm in diameter. Epithelial cell selection was less successful with mouse kidney than with rat kidney. Since it was our intention to study transepithelial transport in the 3 mendelian mouse models, and because we could not obtain intact epithelium in vitro, the work was abandoned after 18 months.

COMMENTS

There are many birth defects that cause maldevelopment or malfunction of the kidney in man and animal. Those that mendelize are ideally suited for study in organ culture or selective cell systems. Promising beginnings have been reported with fetal organ culture, selective culture of normal glomerular components, and propagation of normal renal epithelial cells in vitro. However, little work has been done with disease models, human or otherwise. The challenge is obvious; the rewards from a successful application of somatic cell culture methods to the study of renal birth defects are great and await successful contestants.

REFERENCES

1. Crocker JFS, Brown DM, Vernier RL: Developmental defects of the kidney. A review of renal development and experimental studies of maldevelopment. Pediatr Clin North Am 18:355–376, 1971.
2. Kissane JM: Congenital malformations. In Heptinstall RH (ed): "Pathology of the Kidney." Boston: Little, Brown and Co, 1966, pp 63–117.
3. Hay S, Tonascia S: "A Classification of Congenital Malformations." San Francisco: US Dept of Health, Education & Welfare Public Health Service, Dental Health Center, 1968.
4. Scriver CR, Chesney RW, McInnes RR: Genetic aspects of renal tubular transport. Diversity and topology of carriers. Kidney Int 9:149–171, 1976.
5. McKusick VA: "Mendelian Inheritance in Man. Catalogs of Autosomal Dominant, Autosomal Recessive, and X-Linked Phenotypes," 5th Ed. Baltimore: Johns Hopkins University Press, 1978.
6. Horster M, Schmidt U, Larsson L, Olbricht C, Wisser J, Zink H: Differentiation of renal electrolyte and water transport. Studies on single nephrons in vitro and in situ. In Proc VII Int Congr Nephrol. Montreal: Les Presses de l'Univ de Montréal, and Basel: S Karger, 1978, pp 241–248.
7. Bernstein J: Morphologic development of the metanephric tubule. Ibid, pp 249–254.
8. Segal S, Roth KS: Developmental aspects of renal amino acid and sugar transport. Ibid, pp 255–262.
9. Diezi J, Michoud-Hausel P: Fetal development of renal tubular transports and ATPase activity. Ibid, pp 263–266.
10. Milne MD: Genetic aspects of renal disease. Prog Med Genet 7:112–162, 1970.
11. Royer P, Habib R, Mathieu H, Broyer M (trans.by A Walsh): Pediatric Nephrology. Major Probl Clin Pediatr XI:1–454, 1974.
12. Cornelius CE: Animal models – A neglected medical resource. N Engl J Med 281:934–944, 1969.
13. Lush IE: The biochemical genetics of vertebrates except man. Front Biol 3:1–118, 1967.
14. Lozzio BB, Chernoff AI, Machado ER, Lozzio CB: Hereditary renal disease in a mutant strain of rats. Science 156:1742–1744, 1967.
15. Russell ES: Problems and potentialities in the study of genic action in the mouse. In Burdette WJ (ed): "Methodology in Mammalian Genetics." San Francisco: Holden-Day, 1963, pp 217–232.
16. Lyon MF, Hulse EV: An inherited kidney disease of mice resembling human nephronophthisis. J Med Genet 8:41–48, 1971.
17. Hulse EV, Lyon MF, Meredith R: Research news: New Mutants. Mouse Newsletter 32:38, 1965.
18. Falconer DS, Latsyzewski M, Isaacson JH: Diabetes insipidus associated with oligosyndactyly in the mouse. Genet Res 5:473–488, 1964.
19. Eicher EM, Southard JL, Scriver CR, Glorieux FH: Hypophosphatemia: Mouse model for human familial hypophosphatemic (vitamin D-resistant) rickets. Proc Natl Acad Sci USA 73:4667–4671, 1976.
20. Harvey AM, Christensen HN: Uric acid transport system: Apparent absence in erythrocytes of the Dalmatian coach hound. Science 145:826–827, 1964.
21. Bovee KC, Thier SO, Rea C, Segal S: Renal clearance of amino acids in canine cystinuria. Metabolism 23:51–58, 1974.
22. Chesney RW, Scriver CR, Mohyuddin F: Localization of the membrane defect in transepithelial transport of taurine by parallel studies in vivo and in vitro in hypertaurinuric mice. J Clin Invest 57:183–193, 1976.

23. Scriver CR, McInnes RR, Mohyuddin F: Role of epithelial architecture and intracellular metabolism in proline uptake and transtubular reclamation in PRO/Re mouse kidney. Proc Natl Acad Sci USA 72:1431–1435, 1975.
24. Bovee KC, Joyce T, Reynolds R, Segal S: The Fanconi syndrome in Basenji dogs: A new model for renal transport defects. Science 201:1129–1131, 1978.
25. Grobstein C: Inductive epithelio-mesenchymal interaction in cultured organ rudiments of the mouse. Science 118:52–55, 1963.
26. Grobstein C: Inductive interaction in the development of the mouse metanephros. J Exp Zool 130:319–339, 1955.
27. Saxén L: Inductive interactions in kidney development. In "Control Mechanisms of Growth and Differentiation." Symposia of the Society for Exp Biol, No XXV. New York: Academic Press, 1971, pp 207–221.
28. Gossens CL, Unsworth BR: Evidence for a two-step mechanism operating during in vitro mouse kidney tubulogenesis. J Embryol Exp Morphol 28:615–631 1972.
29. Enders JF, Peebles TC: Propagation in tissue cultures of cytopathogenic agents from patients with measles. Proc Soc Exp Biol Med 86:277–286, 1954.
30. Madin SH, Darby NB Jr: Established kidney cell lines of normal adult bovine and ovine origin. Proc Soc Exp Biol Med 98:574–576, 1958.
31. Gaush CR, Hard WL, Smith TF: Characterization of an established line of canine kidney cells (MDCK). Proc Soc Exp Biol Med 122:931–935, 1966.
32. Rhodin JAG: Structure of the kidney. In Strauss MB, Welt LG (eds): "Diseases of the Kidney" Boston: Little, Brown and Co, 1971, pp 1–30.
33. Karnovsky MJ, Kreisberg JI: Isolation and characterization of rat glomerular cells in vitro. International Symposium on Correlation of Renal Ultrastructure and Function. Aarhus, August 1978, p 19.
34. Dechenne C, Foidart-Willems J, Mahieu PM: Ultrastructural studies on dog renal glomerular and tubular cells in culture. J Submicr Cytol 7:165–184, 1975.
35. Fish AJ, Michael AF, Vernier RL, Brown DM: Human glomerular cells in tissue culture. Lab Invest 33:330–341, 1975.
36. Camazine SM, Graeme BR, Unanue ER, Karnovsky MJ: Isolation of phagocytic cells from the rat renal glomerulus. Lab Invest 35:315–326, 1976.
37. Scheinman JI, Fish AJ, Brown DM, Michael AJ: Human glomerular smooth muscle (mesangial) cells in culture. Lab Invest 34:150–157, 1976.
38. Kreisberg JI, Emmett NL, Barber AC, Karnovsky MJ: Techniques for the isolation and culture of glomerular epithelial cells from rat glomeruli and their discrimination from other glomerular cell types. Supra #6, pp Z–1.
39. Mahieu P, Foidart J, Dechenne C: Isolation and cultivation of homogenous epithelial and mesangial cell lines derived from normal rat glomeruli. Supra #6, pp Z–1.
40. Atkins RC, Glasgow EF, Holdsworth SR, Mathews FE: The macrophage in human rapidly progressive glomerulonephritis. Lancet 1:830–832, 1976.
41. Sherwood JB, Goldwasser E: Erythropoietin production by human renal carcinoma cells in culture. Endocrinology 99:504–510, 1976.
42. Gilbert SF, Migeon BR: D-valine as a selective agent for normal human and rodent epithelial cells in culture. Cell 5:11–17, 1975.
43. Gilbert SF, Migeon BR: Renal enzymes in kidney cells selected by D-valine medium. J Cell Physiol 92:161–168, 1977.
44. Leighton J, Brada Z, Estes LW, Justh G: Secretory activity and oncogenicity of a cell line (MDCK) derived from canine kidney. Science 163:472–473, 1969.
45. Misfeldt DS, Hamamoto ST, Pitelka DR: Transepithelial transport in cell culture. Proc Natl Acad Sci USA 73:1212–1216, 1976.

46. Tchao R, Valentich JD, Rabito A, Leighton J: Studies on the regulation of transepithelial fluid transport by a cell line: MDCK. (Abstract) In Vitro 13:143, 1977.
47. Abaza NA, Leighton J, Schultz SG: Effects of Ouabain on the function and structure of a cell line (MDCK) derived from canine kidney. In Vitro 10:172–183, 1974.
48. Rindler MJ, Saier MH Jr: An electroneutral exchange carrier for sodium in a dog kidney epithelial cell line (MDCK). Supra #6, pp Z–2.
49. Rindler MJ, Chuman LM, Saier MH Jr: Hormone responsiveness of an established but differentiated kidney epithelial cell line (MDCK). (Abstract) Fed Proc 36:911, 1977.
50. Ausiello DA, Goldring SR, Dayer JM, Krane SM: Cultured pig kidney cells: Response to ADH and calcitonin. (Abstract) Kidney Int 12:549, 1977.
51. Ausiello DA, Hall D, Dayer JM: Activation of protein kinase by antidiuretic hormone (ADH) and calcitonin (SCT) in cultured kidney cells. Supra, pp Z–1.
52. Handler JS: Renal cells in culture. Supra #6, pp 695–699.
53. Elliott AY, Stein N, Fraley EE: Technique for cultivation of transitional epithelium from mammalian urinary bladder. In Vitro 11:251–254, 1975.

Diseases of the Retinal Pigment Epithelium*

Irene H. Maumenee, MD and Monte A. Del Monte, MD

A large number of retinal degenerative processes have their presumed origin in the pigment epithelium. These disorders may be divided into 2 major groups: 1) those in which there is primarily peripheral or central and peripheral retinal involvement – retinitis pigmentosa, rod-cone dystrophy, fundus albipunctatus, retinitis punctata albescens, choroideremia, fleck retina of Kandori, gyrate atrophy, and others, and 2) those in which there is primarily central retinal involvement as evidenced by earlier loss of central visual acuity – cone dystrophy (recessive form), cone-rod dystrophy, fundus flavimaculatus, Best disease, butterfly-shaped pigment dystrophy of the fovea, dominant drusen, reticular dystrophy, macroreticular dystrophy, and others. Much heterogeneity exists for most of these conditions. For example, in retinitis pigmentosa (RP), autosomal recessive, autosomal dominant, and X-linked inheritance have been described [1, 2], and we have observed further subdivisions in each group (Table 1). In addition variable degrees of severity as expressed by age of onset and rapidity of progression of the disease are described for each type.

Arguments for the existence of heterogeneity in autosomal recessive RP are as follows: 1) variable ages of onset with intrafamilial consistency, 2) high inbreeding coefficient in spite of high incidence, 3) increased proportion of short-range migration among parents [4], and 4) occurrence of a retinal degeneration in various systemic diseases [5]. Furthermore, retinal degenerative disorders are occasionally seen in which the primary defect seems to lie in the retinal pigment epithelium, but which are seen in isolated patients or families only. A few representative pictures are shown of various retinal degenerative disorders (Figs. 1–4). They all involve patients between the ages of 20 and 35 years. These lesions are usually quite similar among sibs although variations may be seen as well. They change considerably with age and at a late stage a differential diagnosis between the

*Supported in part by grants from the National Institutes of Health (EY 01773) and the Retinitis Pigmentosa Foundation.

Birth Defects: Original Article Series, Volume XVI, Number 2, pages 315–326

TABLE 1. Subgroups of Retinitis Pigmentosa

	Autosomal recessive	
Type I	Onset of night blindness before age 5	EOG*: flat
Type II	Onset of night blindness in teens	EOG: flat
Type III	Congenital amaurosis	
Others		
	Autosomal dominant	
Type I	Delayed onset (age 40 to 60 years)	EOG: normal
Type IIA	Early onset (before age 5 years)	EOG: normal in early stages
Type IIB	Early onset (before age 5 years)	EOG: flat
Type III	Congenital amaurosis	
Others		
	X-chromosomal retinitis pigmentosa	
Type I	X-linked RP	EOG: flat
	Carriers	EOG: normal to reduced
Type II	Choroideremia	EOG: flat
	Carriers	EOG: normal to reduced
Type III	Choroidal sclerosis**	EOG: ?
	Carriers	EOG: ?
Others		

*EOG – electrooculogram.
**The existence of choroidal sclerosis as a separate entity from choroideremia is debated by several authors [3].

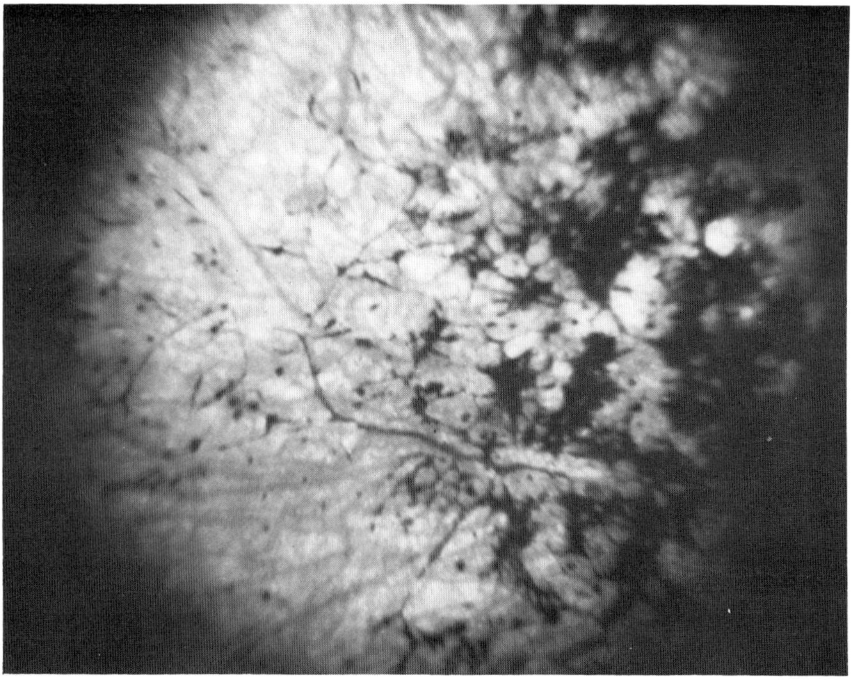

1A

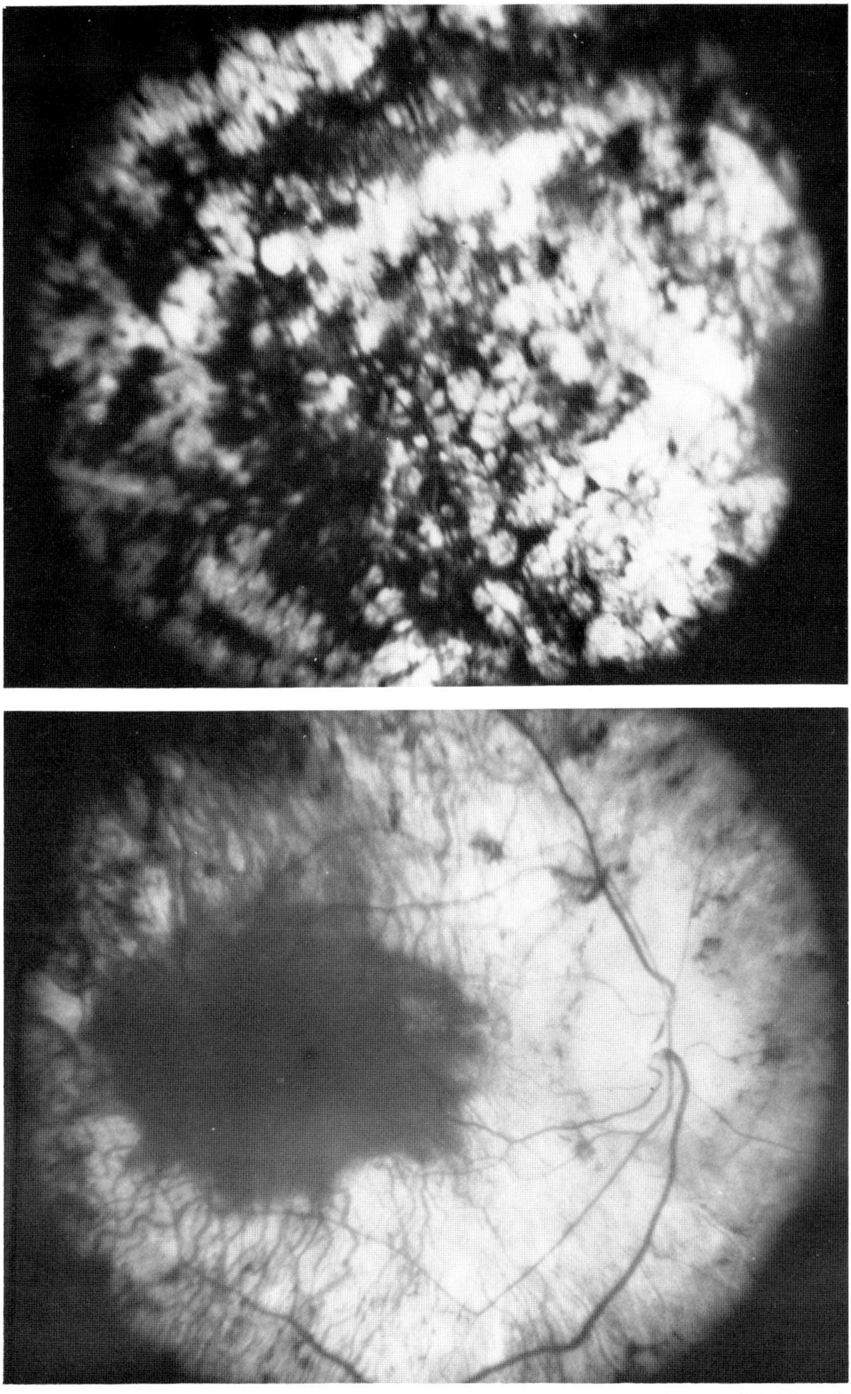

1B

1C

Fig. 1. Fundus pictures covering adjoining retinal areas of a patient with classic RP. Note the preservation of pigment in the macular area in contrast to depigmentation and hyperpigmentation in the retinal periphery.

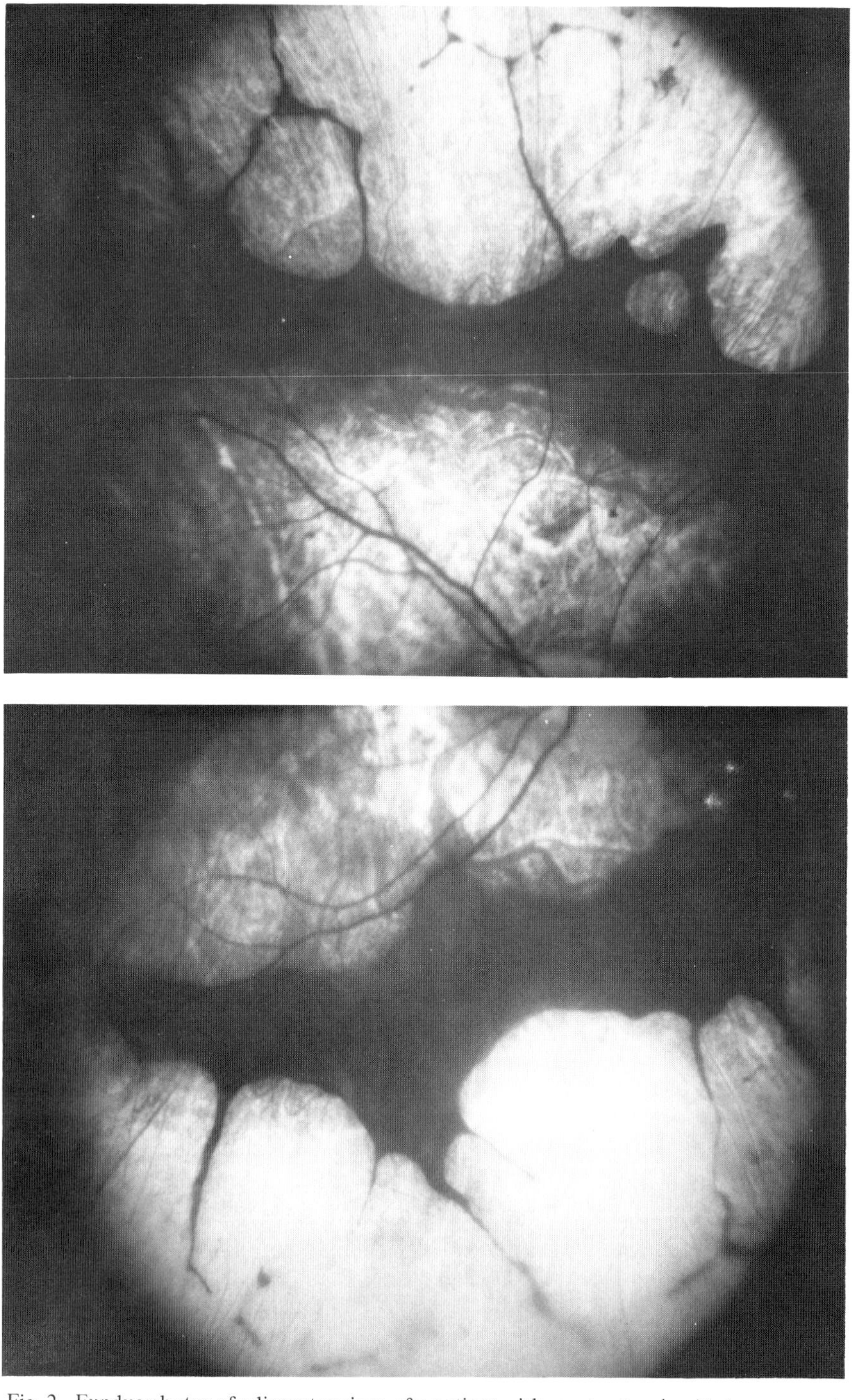

2A

2B

Fig. 2. Fundus photos of adjacent regions of a patient with gyrate atrophy. Note some persistence of normal macular pigmentation and lobulated appearance of degenerative areas, which in the end stage will leave the appearance of complete chorioretinal atrophy, visibility of bare sclera traversed by isolated narrowed retinal vessels.

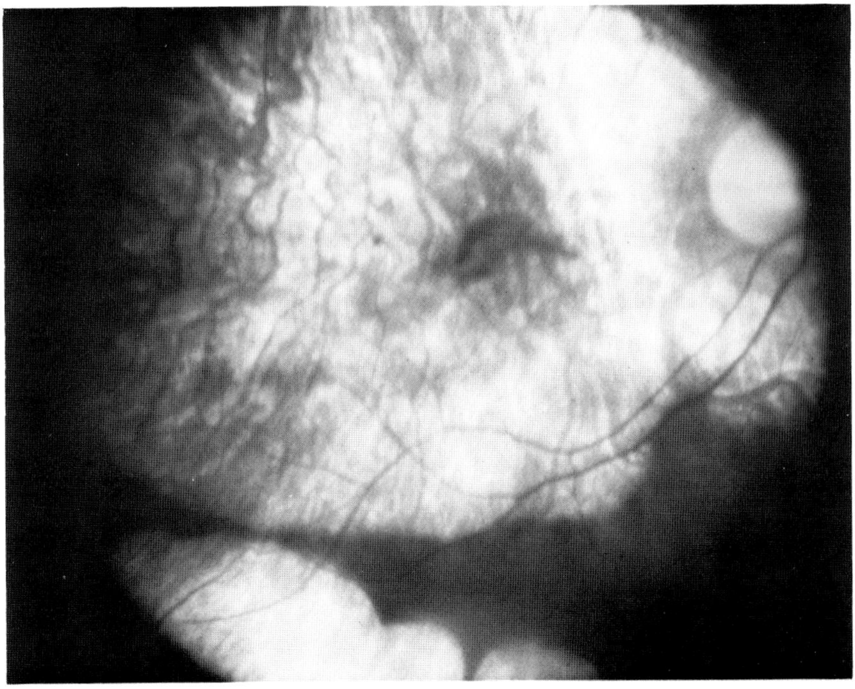

2C

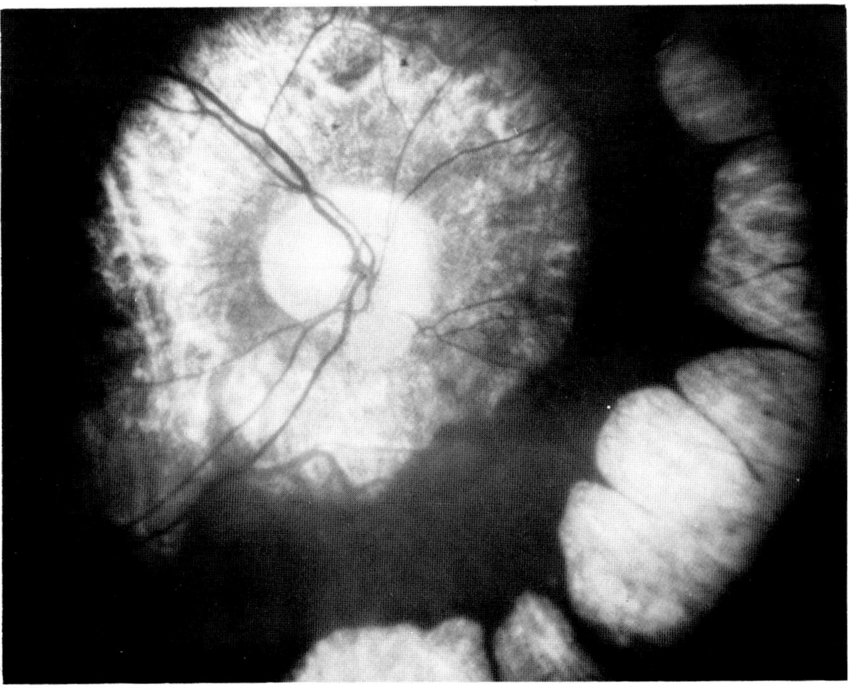

2D

2E

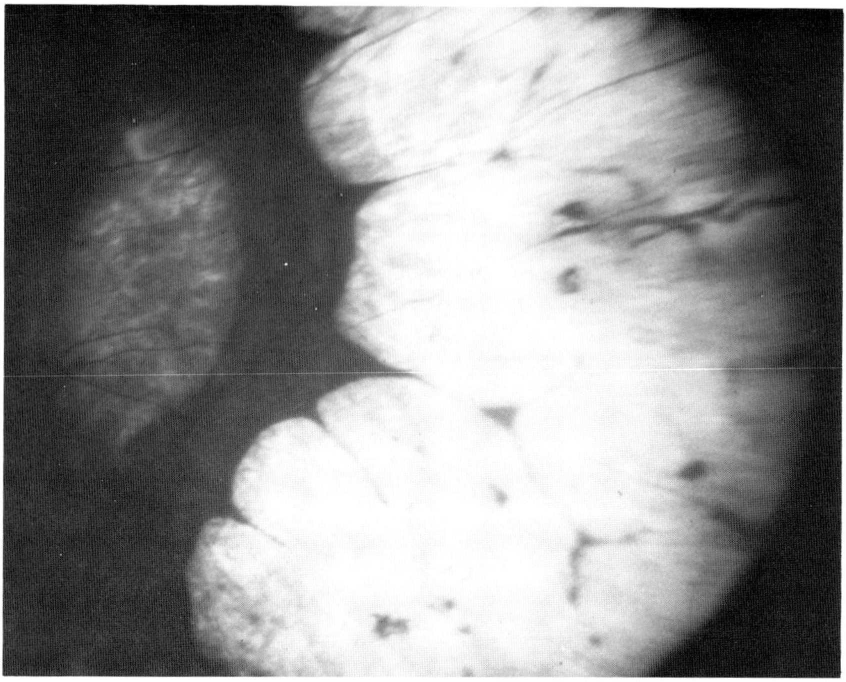

3A

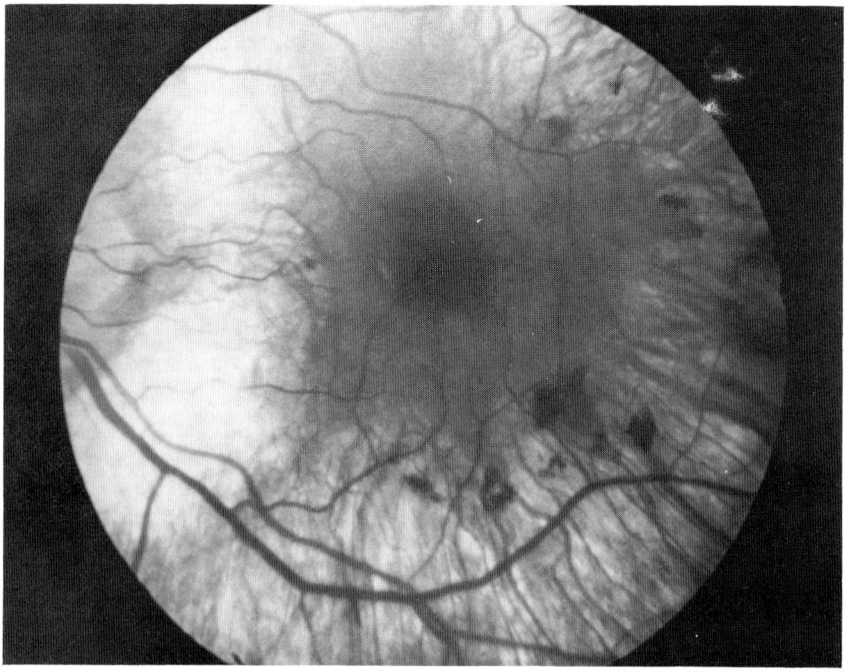

Fig. 3. A and B) Note preservation of macular area with diffuse chorioretinal atrophy and rarefication of choroidal vessels in patient with classic choroideremia. C) Mottled appearance of the fundus of the patient's sister. This mottling is characteristic for carriers, but at times the pigment mottling is much less striking.

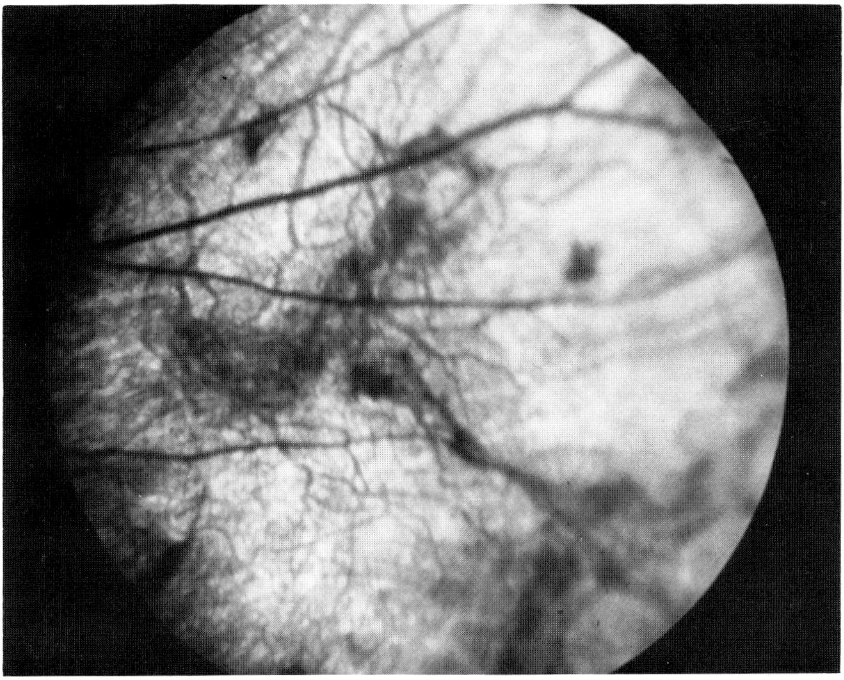

3B

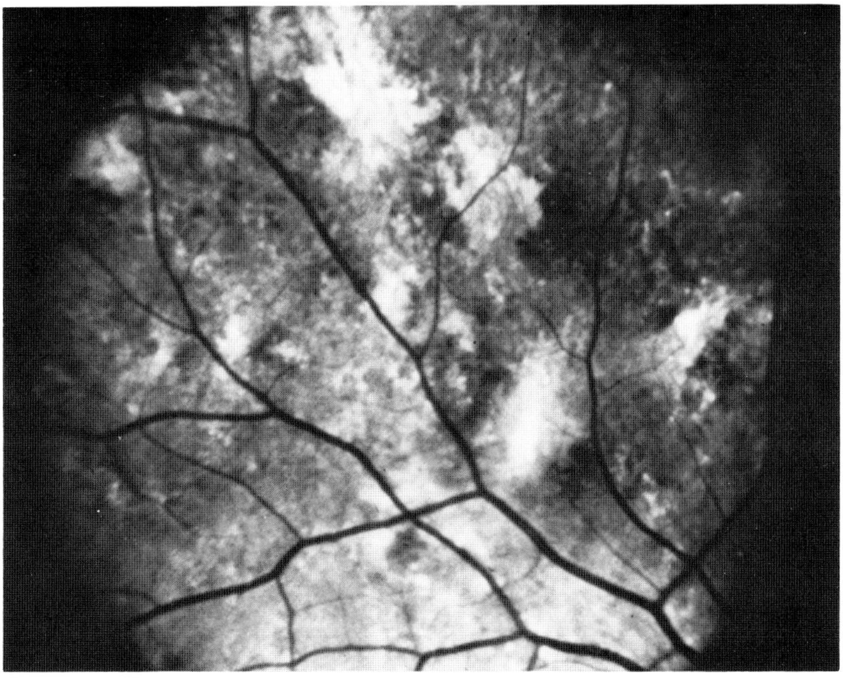

3C

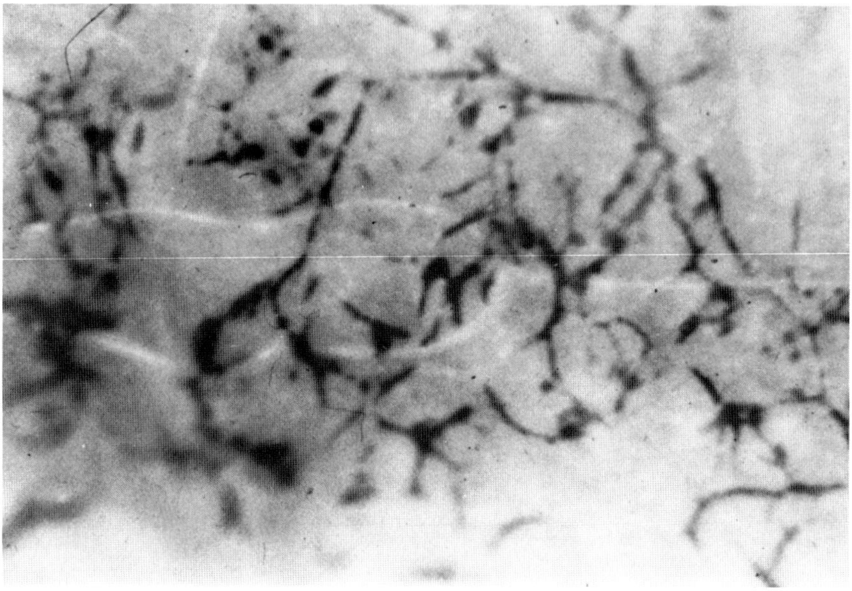

4A

Fig. 4. A–C)RP-like pigment migration at autopsy in the retina of a 20-year-old patient with Sanfilippo syndrome type A. B) Light microscopy and C) electron microscopy show massive intracellular ballooning of the retinal pigment epithelium (arrow) due to intralysosomal vacuoles. (Technical assistance, Dr. K.R. Kenyon.)

various entities is often impossible because of the widespread, nonspecific chorioretinal atrophy. Histologic observations are available on only a few of these disorders and in most of these instances on older patients only, at which point only conjectures can be made about primary and secondary changes. The evidence that these disorders are located in the retinal pigment epithelium (RPE) is circumstantial and primarily based on the observation that the electrooculogram (EOG) is abnormal in Best macular degeneration – a condition in which histologic observations are available and the pathology indicates the defect is indeed centered in the pigment epithelium. In the conditions mentioned in the first paragraph the EOG is abnormal.

The human RPE has multiple functions. It has secretory and nutritive functions of the photoreceptor cells. Through its pigmentation, it screens out stray light; it stores and converts retinol to the biologically active 11-*cis* form and thus protects the photoreceptors from excessive amounts of this necessary, but toxic compound; it phagocytoses the shedded photoreceptor outer segments; and it has

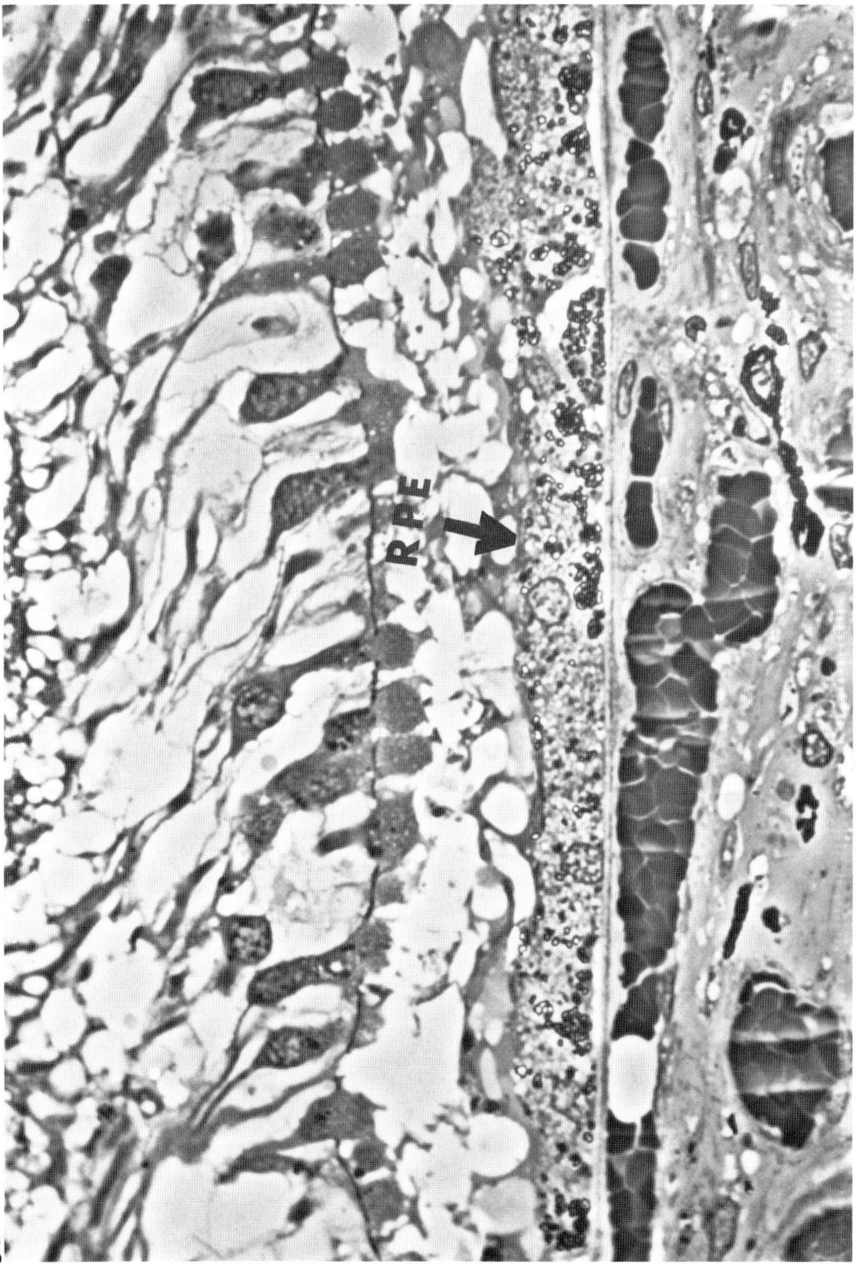

4B

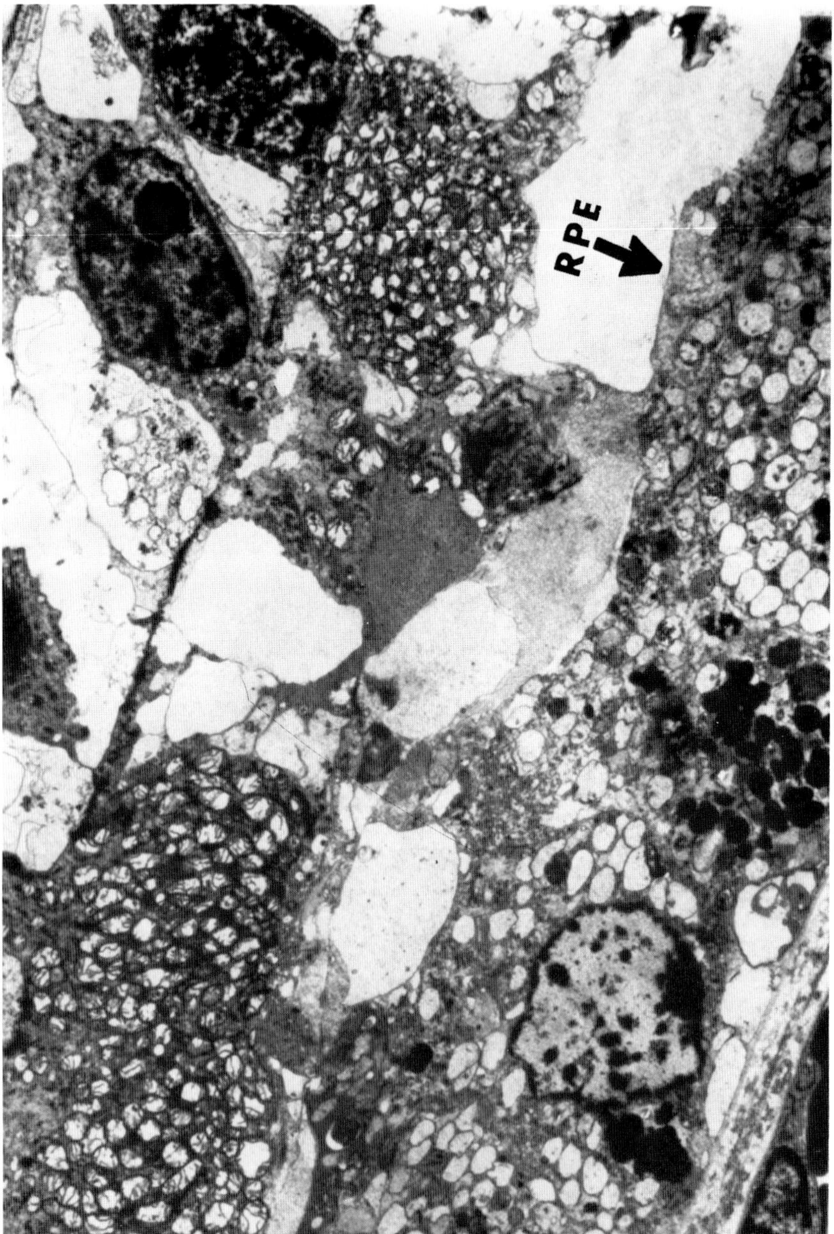

4C

an important morphogenic role in the differentiation of the rod outer segments and of the choroid. Given its multiple functions with complex biochemical activities, multiple ways of dysfunction can be postulated. They may all lead to identical clinical pictures and pathology. Inversely, an identical mutation involving the RPE may produce a different phenotype if there are variations in the genetic makeup of the photoreceptors, leading to variable expressivity among sibs even though they carry an identical genetic defect. Genocopies, on one hand, and marked clinical variability among sibs, on the other, are certainly all observed in retinal degenerations. This demonstrates the limited phenotypic responses of the retina, as well as the remoteness of the response from the gene defect. Various systemic diseases have an associated RP-like ocular complication (Table 2). In the mucopolysaccharidoses types I, II, and III, a retinal degeneration virtually indis-

TABLE 2. Extraocular Diseases Accompanied by Retinitis Pigmentosa or One of Its Variants

Metabolic diseases with retinitis pigmentosa
Mucopolysaccharidoses I, II, III
Abetalipoproteinemia
Hooft disease
Juvenile amaurotic idiocy (ceroid lipofuscinosis)
Cystinosis
Refsum disease
Gyrate atrophy
Retinitis pigmentosa and central nervous system disease
Van den Bosch syndrome
Spastic paraplegia and retinal degeneration (Laurence-Moon syndrome)
Bardet-Biedl syndrome
Olivopontocerebellar atrophy and retinal degeneration
Pelizaeus-Merzbacher disease
Pallidal degeneration with retinitis pigmentosa
Hereditary muscular atrophy with ataxia, retinitis pigmentosa, and diabetes insipidus
Syndromes combining retinitis pigmentosa and deafness
Usher syndrome
Alström syndrome
Hallgren syndrome
Alport syndrome
Flynn-Aird syndrome
Other syndromes with retinitis pigmentosa
Kearns-Sayers syndrome
Renal-retinal dysplasia (2 varieties exist)
Steinert myotonic dystrophy
Cockayne syndrome
Hypotrichosis, syndactyly and retinal dystrophy (Albrectsen-Svendsen)
Microphthalmia and retinal degeneration (autosomal dominant and autosomal recessive varieties exist)

tinguishable from classic RP progressively develops [6]. The enzyme defects for these subgroups of mucopolysaccharidoses (MPS) are well established. The defect in MPS type I (Hurler and Scheie syndromes) is an α-iduronidase deficiency. In the Hunter syndromes types A and B the defect lies in iduronide sulfate sulfatase deficiency. The defects for the Sanfilippo syndromes are heparan sulfate sulfatase deficiency in MPS type IIIA and heparan sulfate N-acetylglucosaminidase deficiency in MPS type IIIB. It can be seen from these examples that various metabolic defects can lead to similar retinal pathology. These MPS types have as common denominator the storage of heparan sulfate.

Very little is known about the biochemistry of the normal human pigment epithelium. This is in large proportion due to the fact that it is present in small quantities in each eye only. It is only one cell layer thick making acquisition of significant amounts of tissue from a single human eye difficult, and thus a biochemical study impossible. In addition, the rod outer segments and the pigment epithelium are so closely associated in vivo that specimens of one layer are invariably contaminated with the other. Thus, the biochemical study of in vitro cell cultures seems the plausible approach to biochemical study of this tissue. We therefore elected to study the tissue culture behavior of the normal human retinal pigment epithelium, to be prepared for study of eyes with true retinitis pigmentosa as they become available.

For additional information see the article by Del Monet and Maumenee, which follows in this volume.

REFERENCES

1. Hussels I: Une famille atteinte de rétinopathie pigmentaire liée au sexe, de maladie de Parkinson et d'autres troubles neuropsychiatriques. J Genet Hum 16:106–155, 1967.
2. Hussels-Maumenee I, Pierce ER, Bias WB, Schleutermann DA: Linkage studies of typical retinitis pigmentosa and common markers. Am J Hum Genet 27:505–508, 1975.
3. Krill AE: Diffuse choroidal atrophies. In Krill AE, Archer D (eds): "Krill's Hereditary Retinal and Choroidal Diseases." New York: Harper & Row, 1977, vol II, pp 979–1042.
4. Morton NE, Klein D, Hussels IE, Dodinval P, Todorov A, Lew R, Yee S: Genetic structure of Switzerland. Am J Hum Genet 25:347–361, 1973.
5. Deutman AF: Hereditary diseases and syndromes with retinal, choroidal, or optic nerve abnormalities. Supra #3, pp 1299–1338.
6. Leung L-SE, Weinstein GW, Hobson RR: Further electroretinographic studies of patients with mucopolysaccharidoses. In Bergsma D (ed): Part VIII. "Eye." Baltimore: Williams & Wilkins for The National Foundation–March of Dimes, BD:OAS VII(3):32–40, 1971.

New Techniques for In Vitro Culture of Human Retinal Pigment Epithelium*

Monte A. Del Monte, MD and Irene H. Maumenee, MD

INTRODUCTION

Study of the biochemistry of the human ocular tissues is only in its infancy. Unlike much of the remainder of the body where tissues are bulky and large biopsies are possible, the majority of important differentiated ocular tissues are epithelioid and present in small quantities of only one or several cell layers thick. This makes it difficult to acquire significant amounts of gross tissue from single human eyes for biochemical studies of uncommon disorders. In addition, many ocular tissues, notably the retinal pigment epithelium (RPE) and rod outer segments, are so closely associated in vivo that specimens of one are invariably contaminated with the other. It would seem that the biochemical study of pure in vitro cultures of many of the specialized ocular epithelia may be the only possible approach to circumvent these problems.

One of the most important of the human ocular tissues is the RPE which plays an active role in the normal functioning of the photoreceptor cells, including: 1) secretory and nutritive functions [1], 2) pigmentation, ie screening out stray light, 3) storage and conversion of retinal to the biologically active 11-*cis* form, thus protecting the photoreceptors from excessive amounts of this necessary, yet toxic, compound [2], 4) phagocytosis of shedded photoreceptor outer segments [3], and 5) important morphogenic roles in the differentiation of the rod outer segments and choroid (D. A. Newsome, personal communication).

In light of these important functions, many examples of visual failure may be secondary to dysfunction of the RPE. Unfortunately, however, the normal metabolism of human RPE is understood in fragments only, for the reasons previously mentioned. Multiple studies of the biochemistry of RPE from lower animals have been published over the last 10 years [1, 4–7], mostly as a result of the examination of pooled tissues from many animals of one species. Human RPE has been

*Supported in part by grants from the National Institutes of Health (EY 01773) and Retinitis Pigmentosa Foundation.

Birth Defects: Original Article Series, Volume XVI, Number 2, pages 327–338

much more difficult to study, both because of the difficulty in obtaining adequate quantities of fresh tissue from postmortem eyes and because it has proved to be difficult to grow RPE in culture. This study presents new techniques for the in vitro culture of human RPE, permitting production of sufficient human RPE for metabolic study.

MATERIALS AND METHODS

Preparation of Human RPE Cultures

Postmortem eyes were obtained from the Maryland Eye Bank within 96 hours of death. The anterior segment of the eye was removed by a circumferential incision 5 mm posterior to the limbus. The vitreous and neurosensory retina were then easily separated from the pigment epithelium, cut free at the optic nerve, and removed. The posterior segment of the globe was then bisected with a saggital incision posterior through the optic disk. Each hemiglobe was then filled with Earle's balanced salt solution (GIBCO) and the RPE gently vacuumed free from Bruch membrane with a fire-polished Pasteur pipette under direct observation with a dissecting microscope (Fig. 1). The explants were placed directly into culture dishes containing media consisting of Hams F12-M media supplemented with 16% fetal calf serum, 0.075% sodium bicarbonate, 0.02 mM glutamine, 100 units/ml penicillin, 100 μg/ml streptomycin, and 2 cc fetuin per 100 cc of media. Media constitutents were obtained from GIBCO, Grand Rapids, Michigan. Some cultures were also grown in the presence of 30 ng/ml epithelial growth factor (EGF) [8] obtained from Collaboration Research, Inc., Waltham, Massachusetts. All cultures were incubated at 37° in a humidified 95% air, 5% CO_2 atmosphere.

Preparation of Collagen Coated Culture Vessels

A 0.25–0.50% solution of acid soluable collagen (Sigma type III) in 0.1 N acetic acid was painted on the surface of the culture vessels with a fine brush. The thin collagen coating was then gelled by exposure to NH_3 fumes from ammonium hydroxide for 6–12 hours. The excess ammonia was then neutralized with buffered saline. Dishes were sterilized by exposure overnight to ultraviolet light. Figure 2 shows an SEM view of the finished collagen coating showing the fibrillar structure.

Growth Studies

Cell attachment (colony formation) and proliferation were measured as follows: Human RPE was freshly prepared as described, and an aliquot was removed for cell count on a hemocytometer. For measurement of colony formation, the remaining cells were distributed evenly into sterile Lab-Tek 16-well slides with or without collagen coatings and/or EGF. Thirty-two of each type were prepared for each experiment. Because of the large, pigmented nature of the growing cells, cell attachment and colony formation were easily measured by directly counting colonies of newly growing RPE cells under phase contrast microscopy. Cell proliferation was measured by distributing cells into 35-mm culture dishes. At 5, 10, 15, 20, and 30 days after culture initiation, 3 dishes of each type were trypsinized to remove cells; an aliquot of this was then directly counted using a hemocytometer. To measure plating efficiency of these subcultured cells, the trypsinized cells remaining

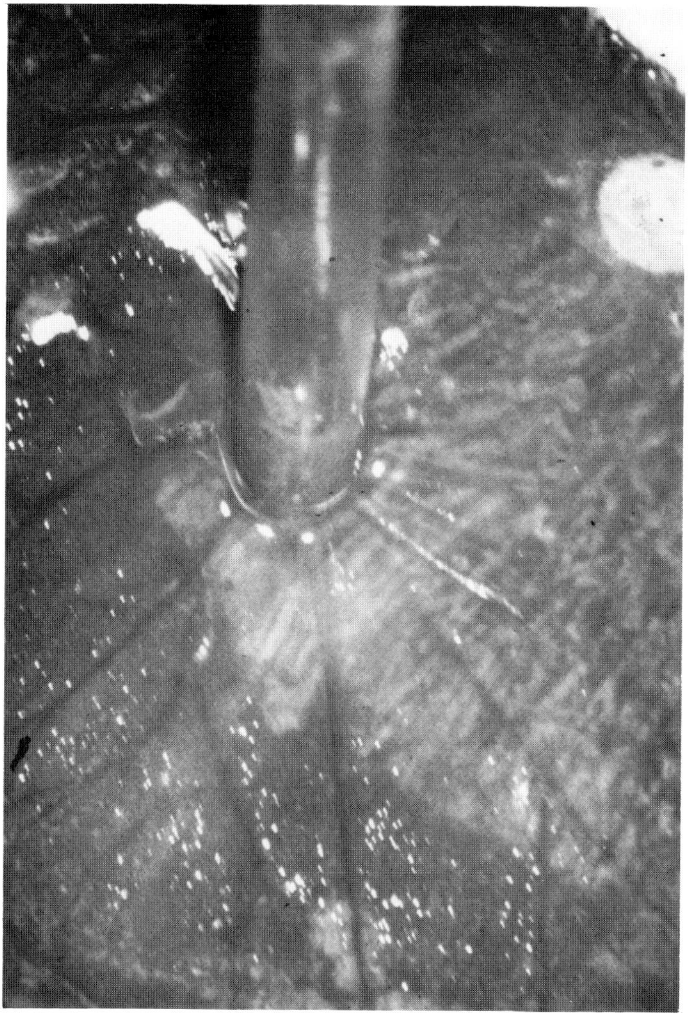

Fig. 1. Harvesting human RPE by vacuuming with a fire-polished Pasteur pipette. Velvety RPE at left is being lifted into pipette leaving shiny Bruch membrane at right.

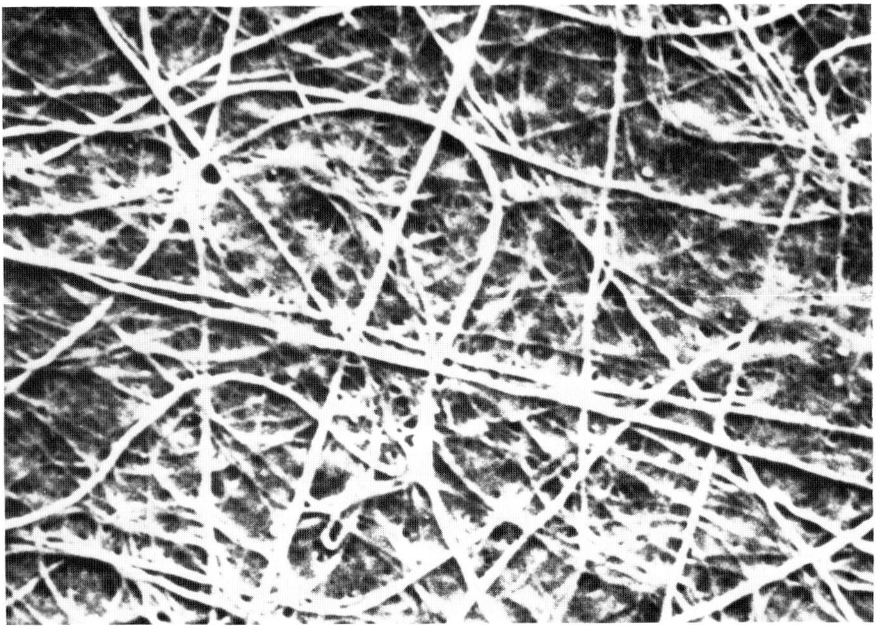

Fig. 2. Scanning electron micrograph of collagen coating on tissue culture dish (× 10,000).

after counting were replated into 35-mm culture dishes. Five days of incubation were allowed for readherence of viable cells, then all nonadherent cells were washed free with buffered saline and the remaining growing cells were trypsinized free and again counted. The plating efficiency of the subcultured cells was defined as the percentage of the subcultured cells which were adherent and viable after this 5-day period.

RESULTS

In Vitro Human RPE Culture Morphology

Figure 3 shows pigment cell explants immediately after being placed in culture. At a higher power (Fig. 4) the newly explanted cells are highly pigmented, basically hexagonal cells about 12–15 microns in diameter and found either singly or in small clusters of up to 20–25 cells. After 5 days under these culture conditions, a small percentage (0.05–0.25%) of the cells stick to the culture vessels and begin to grow as shown in Figure 5. As the cells begin to grow, they enlarge to 4–6 times their dormant (in vivo) size, producing epithelial colonies of cells with large clear nuclei and 1 or 2 prominent nucleoli. The cells remain highly pigmented with numerous pigment granules, especially in the area immediately around the nucleus, sur-

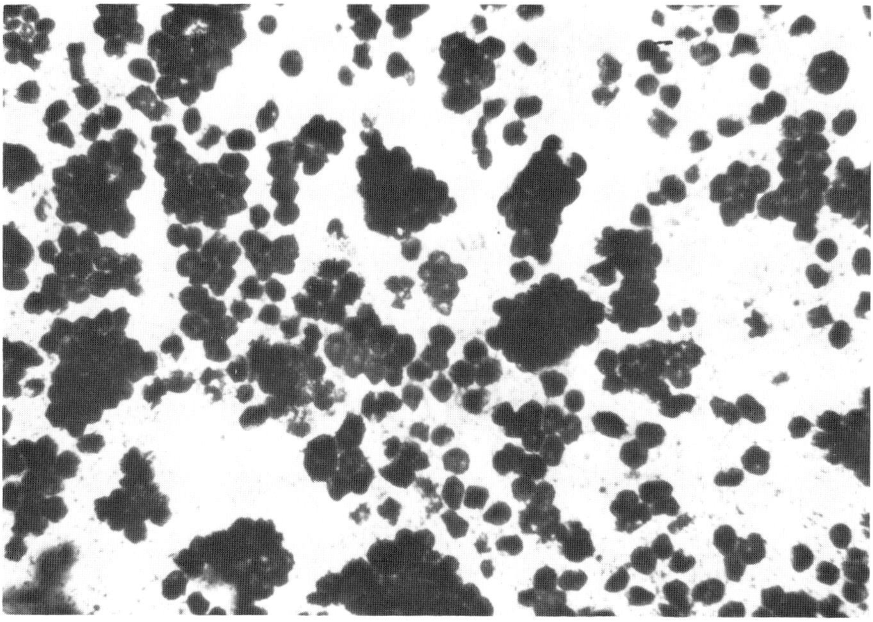

Fig. 3. Primary explants of human RPE as examined by phase contrast (× 80) immediately after harvesting.

rounded by more attenuated, clearer cytoplasm. Figure 6, taken at the growing edge of a colony after 21 days in culture, shows dividing nuclei suggestive of continued active cell proliferation. Even continued cultures as long as 120 days, as shown in Figure 7 from the edge of a colony, produced little additional morphologic change with continued granular pigmentation and epithelioid morphology in most cases. In the center of the colonies, however, as the cells reach confluence (at 33 days, Fig. 8) they became smaller and more hexagonal, but remain pigmented and epithelioid. Thus, when cultures reached confluence, the cell morphology more closely resembles the in vivo state.

Donor Factors Influencing Culture Success

Table 1 illustrates the importance of various donor characteristics in obtaining successful cultures, defined as areas of confluent growth totaling 4–5 cm^2 or the approximate size of a quarter. Of 21 consecutive pairs of eyes cultured using our most successful techniques with both collagen and EGF, the overall success rate was 76%. Successful culture was obtained in greater than 85% of patients aged < 60, with a slight drop to 75% for patients aged 60–80, and a significant fall off in the older patient. Sex of the donor made no difference. Eyes cultured within

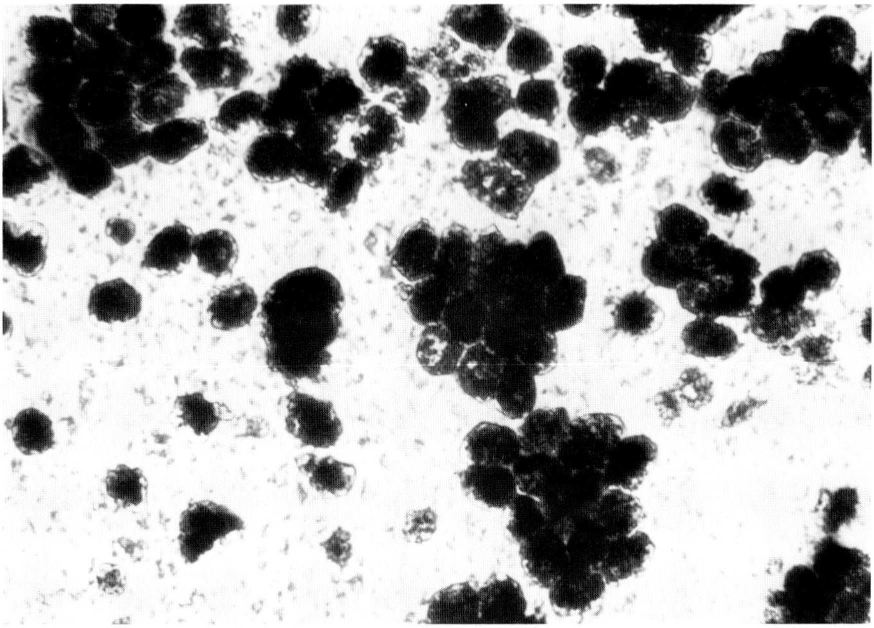

Fig. 4. Higher power phase contrast micrograph (× 200) of primary RPE explants shown in Fig. 3.

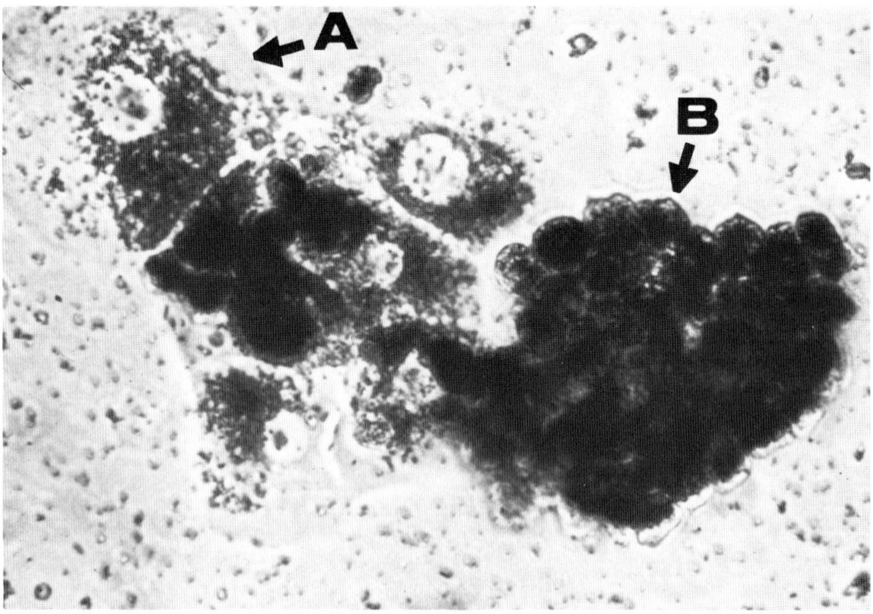

Fig. 5. Human RPE after 5 days in culture, showing A) early colony formation of proliferating cells, compared to B) dormant or nonviable explanted cells which continue to float free in the dish (× 200 phase contrast).

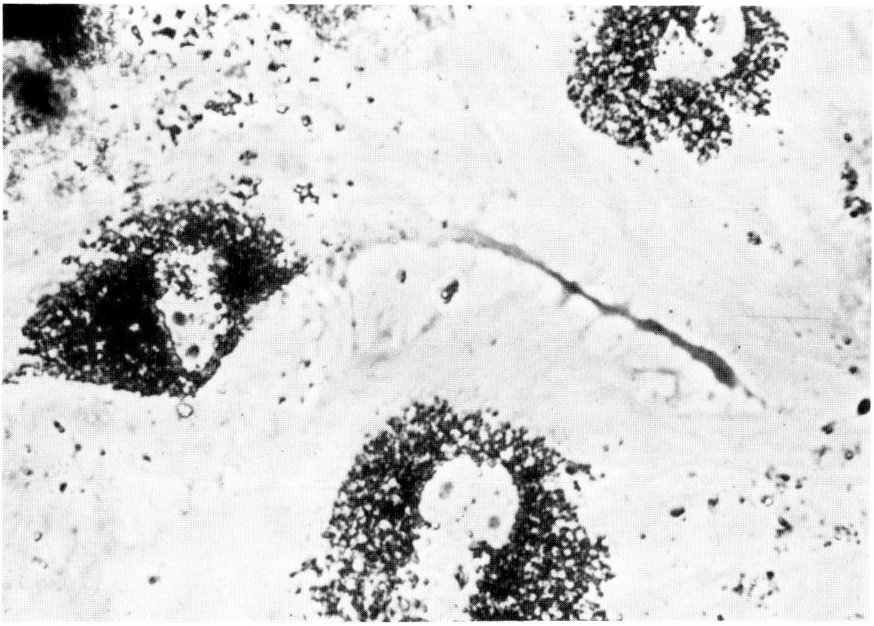

Fig. 6. Human RPE after 21 days in culture showing multiple dividing epithelioid cells (× 200 phase contrast).

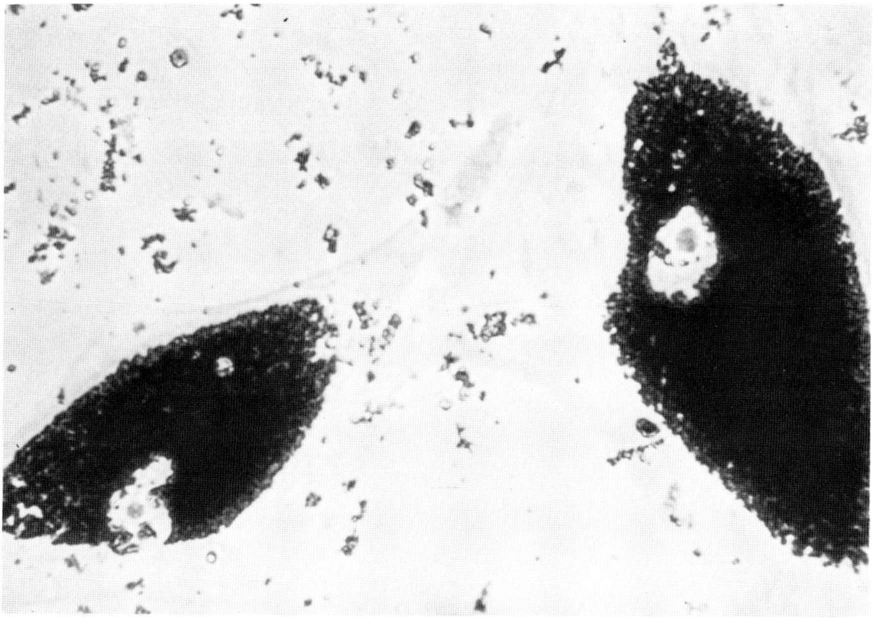

Fig. 7. Typical large epithelioid, heavily pigmented human RPE cells in continuous culture for 120 days (2nd passage) from the edge of an enlarging colony (× 200 phase contrast).

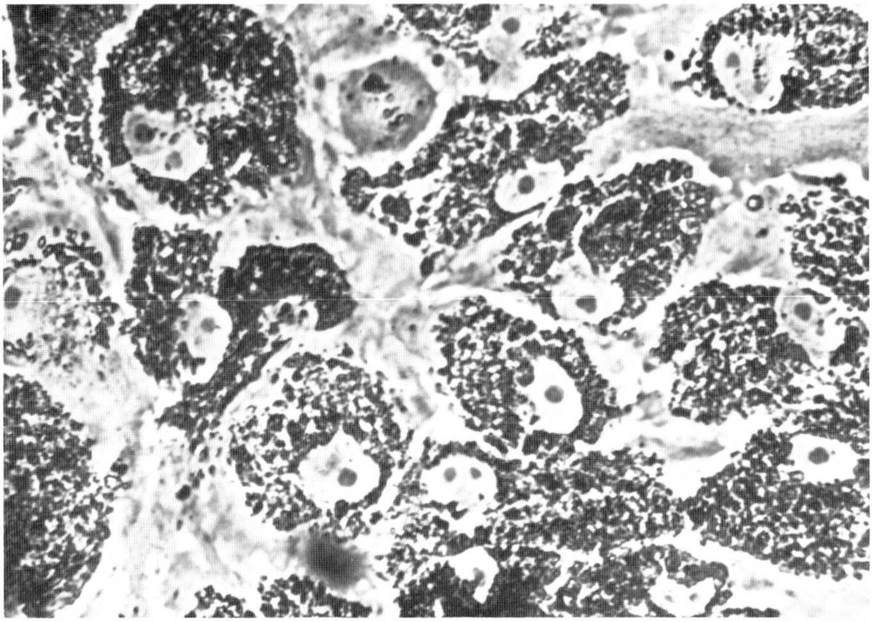

Fig. 8. Phase contrast (× 200) picture of the center of a confluent culture after 33 days in culture.

Table 1. Donor Factors Influencing Culture Success With Human RPE

	SUCCESS/ATTEMPTS	%	TOTAL
AGE OF PATIENT			
< 40	3/3	100	
40-60	6/7	85	16/21-76%
60-80	6/8	75	
> 80	1/3	33	
MALE	6/8	75	
FEMALE	10/13	77	
TIME FROM DEATH			
< 24 HR	5/5	100	
24-48 HR	9/10	90	
48-72 HR	2/4	50	
> 72 HR	0/2	0	
CAUSE OF DEATH	NO OBVIOUS RELATIONSHIP EXCEPT SEVERE JAUNDICE ASSOCIATED WITH POOR RESULT 1/4 (25%)		

48 hours of death were successful greater than 90% of the time, with 50% success between 48 and 72 hours, and no growth in eyes more than 72 hours postmortem. Cause of death was not obviously related to culture success except for jaundice. In only 1 out of 4 pairs of eyes from severely icteric patients did we obtain cell growth.

Influence of Epithelial Growth Factor and Collagen on Growth of Human RPE

There was significant improvement in culture success, as defined above, resulting from the combined use of EGF and collagen coated culture vessels. In our studies successful growth increased from 1 of 7 (14%) with no addition of either collagen or EGF, to 4 of 8 (50%) with the addition of EGF only, to 16 of 21 (76%) with the use of both EGF and collagen.

Figure 9 illustrates the importance of collagen coating and EGF for the successful growth of human RPE in culture. It shows the relationship between colony formation – that is the number of cells that stick and begin to grow – and collagen or EGF. Each point represents the mean of 5 studies with the range shown by the horizontal bars. Here we see that collagen coating greatly increases the number

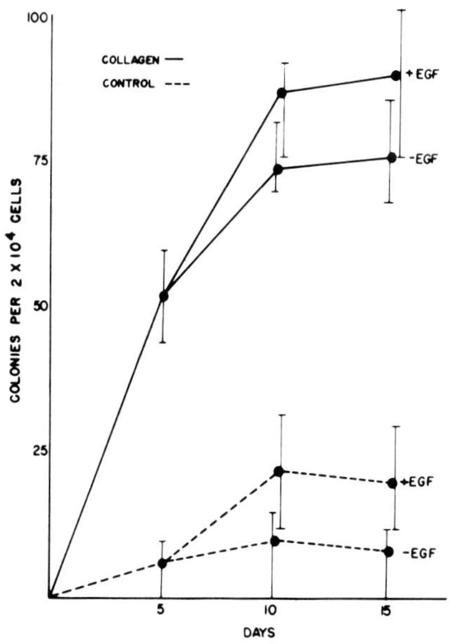

Fig. 9. Effect of EGF and collagen coating on successful colony formation. Solid lines represent collagen coated vessels, dashed lines represent controls with cultures +EGF and EGF as indicated.

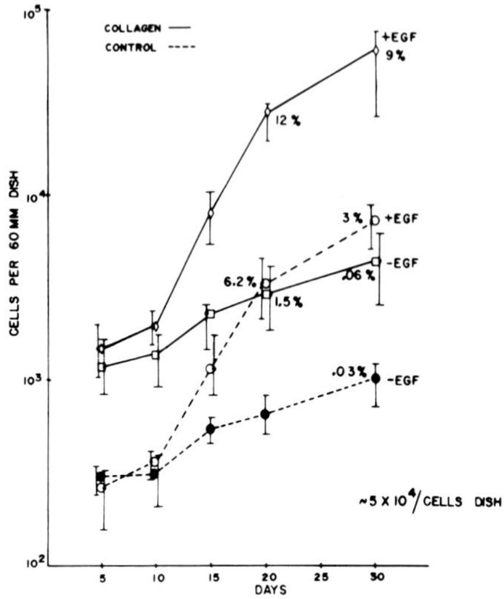

Fig. 10. Effect of EGF and collagen coating on human RPE cell proliferation and plating efficiency on subculture. Y-axis represents log-plot of cell number per dish, X-axis represents time in culture. Solid lines indicate collagen coated vessels, dashed lines indicate controls with +EGF and –EGF as shown. Initial cell density 5×10^4 cells/dish. Also shown are plating efficiency upon subculture at designated points.

of colonies formed over controls. By 10 days in culture, the use of collagen resulted in a 10-fold increase of colony formation. As can be seen, EGF has little effect on colony formation.

Figure 10 illustrates the effect of collagen coating and EGF on cell multiplication. Here we see an initial difference in the cell number on day 5, secondary to better colony formation with collagen. More interesting is the increased cell multiplication (indicated by the steep slope) in cultures with EGF, regardless of the presence or absence of collagen coating, over cultures without EGF, especially between day 10 and day 20. Also of interest is the increased log phase growth that persists longer in cultures containing EGF (from day 15 to day 20) than those without EGF in which growth begins to slow by day 15. The combination of addition of EGF and of collagen coating as shown here yielded almost 60 times more cells than obtained in controls after 30 days in culture.

In addition, from this figure we can see the positive effect of EGF alone on plating efficiency of subcultured RPE cells either with or without collagen. EGF-containing cultures showed relatively high plating efficiencies on subculture of 3–12% compared with 0.05–0.25% for primary cultures and 0.03–1.5% for subcultures of culture growing in the absence of EGF. EGF thus seems to greatly increase the overall viability of subcultured RPE cells.

DISCUSSION

There have been many studies on culture of RPE from lower animals [9–11] but only a few on successful growth of human RPE, most notably the work of Albert et al [12] and Mannagh et al [13]. Albert and colleagues noted progressive depigmentation and change from epithelioid morphology to mosaic, tubular, and spindle growth patterns. Mannagh et al had greater success with culture initiation (65% of donor eyes); however, progressive depigmentation again occurred. Clearly, new techniques for culture were needed that would produce reliable success without dedifferentiation or contamination with fibroblastic cell lines. Initial attempts at culturing human RPE by methods similar to those of Albert and colleagues were successful in only 1 of 7 pairs of eyes (14%). Failure seemed to be caused by 2 problems: 1) failure of explanted cells to adhere to plastic or glass tissue culture dishes and form colonies in significant numbers, a prerequisite for monolayer growth in mammalian cells, and 2) the tendency for the few cells that did adhere to remain dormant without multiplying.

The first of these problems has been markedly reduced by coating the base of culture dishes with acid-soluble collagen. This has increased the number of colony-forming units from $6\text{–}8/2\times10^4$ cells plated to $74\text{–}76/2\times10^4$ cells plated – a 10-fold increase. In addition, to stimulate cell multiplication and maintain a differentiated state, many growth conditions were tested – including different concentrations and types of sera, supplementary amino acids and growth factors, including chick embryo extract, fetuin, and most importantly EGF. While the majority of these conditions had no significant effect on growth, EGF (although having no effect on colony formation) caused marked increase in cell proliferation in our system. When EGF is used, cell doubling time is shortened and cells remain in log-phase growth longer, resulting in 10 times more cells after 30 days in culture. Also, cells subcultured from EGF-containing cultures grow much more readily after passage. The combination of collagen-coated dishes and EGF increases cell yield after 30 days by 58–60-fold over controls. Also, cell morphology remains epithelioid and well pigmented after at least 4 months in culture.

Using these techniques, it is now possible to obtain adequate quantities of human RPE cells from single pairs of normal or pathologic eyes for not only histologic, but also, for the first time, biochemical and metabolic studies of this important cell line.

SUMMARY

The proper functioning of the many types of ocular epithelium, most notably the RPE, is critical to the sensory functions of the human eye. We have developed new techniques for the in vitro culture of human RPE using collagen coated vessels and EGF. These techniques increased culture success from 14% to 76% of pairs of eyes. Human RPE has been cultured for up to 4 months while retaining marked pigmentation and epithelioid characteristics. Use of pure cultures of human RPE will allow biochemical study of this important tissue.

REFERENCES

1. Berman ER: Acid hydrolases of the retinal pigment epithelium. Invest Ophthalmol 10:64–68, 1971.
2. Krinsky NI: The enzymatic esterfication of vitamin A. J Biol Chem 232:881–894, 1958.
3. Herron WL, Riegel BW, Myers OE, Rubin ML: Retinal dystrophy in the rat. A pigment epithelial disease. Invest Ophthalmol 8:595–604, 1969.
4. Anderson RE, Lissandrello PM, Maude MB, Matthes MT: Lipids of bovine retinal pigment epithelium Exp Eye Res 23:149–157, 1976.
5. Bach G, Berman ER: Characterization of a sialoglycan isolated from cattle retina. Ophthalmol Res 1:257–272, 1970.
6. Berman ER, Schwell H, Feeney L: The retinal pigment epithelium, chemical composition and structure. Invest Ophthalmol 13:675–687, 1974.
7. Hayasaka S, Hara S, Mizuno K: Distribution and some properties of cathepsin D in the retinal pigment epithelium. Exp Eye Res 21:307–313, 1975.
8. Savage CR, Inagami T, Cohen S: The primary structure of epidermal growth factor. J Biol Chem 247:7612–7621, 1972.
9. Chader GJ, Newsome DA, Bensinger RE, Fletcher RT: Studies on the differentiation of retinal pigmented epithelium cells in culture. Invest Ophthalmol 14:108–113, 1975.
10. Edwards RB, Szamier RB: Defective phagocytosis of isolated rod outer segments by RCS rat retinal pigment epithelium in culture. Science 197:1001–1003, 1977.
11. Middleton CA, Pegrum SM: Contacts between pigmented retina epithelial cells in culture. J Cell Sci 22:371–383, 1976.
12. Albert DM, Tso MOM, Rabson AS: In vitro growth of pure cultures of retinal pigment epithelium. Arch Ophthalmol 88:63–69, 1972.
13. Mannagh J, Arya DV, Irvine AR Jr: Tissue culture of human retinal pigment epithelium. Invest Ophthalmol 12:52–64, 1973.

ABH Blood Group Antigens on Cultured Epithelial Cells

Stephanie Phillips, PhD, Orlando J. Miller, MD, and Elvin A. Kabat, PhD

Cell surface expression of human ABH blood group antigens in the adult is limited to red blood cells and epithelial derivatives. These antigens are not detectable during the first month of embryonic life despite the presence of tissues which will later express them. Surface A, B, or H antigens appear at about the fifth week, at first only on endothelial cells [1, 2]. In slightly older embryos, the meconium and the surface epithelium of stomach and small intestine become positive. By 7–8 weeks, the outer layers of skin and epithelium lining the oral cavity express A, B, or H, and erythrocytes show a positive reaction for the first time. Over the next few weeks, selected epithelial cell types lining the digestive tract become antigen positive in the majority of fetuses, thought to be genetic secretors. As development proceeds, localized ABH expression occurs: liver remains negative while the columnar epithelium of the gallbladder becomes positive; in the lung, luminal surfaces of bronchi and alveoli become positive before those of the trachea; in the male reproductive tract, only the epithelial lining of seminal vesicles is positive; in the female genital system, the columnar epithelium of the fallopian tubes becomes positive while the ovaries are negative. In some tissues the appearance of the epithelial antigens is transient [3]. By 12 weeks' gestation, all tissues destined to be positive in the adult are expressing ABH [1]. From these observations, it is apparent that the ABH antigens are synthesized only in certain cell types at set stages in development. One can conclude that the series of enzymes in the biosynthetic pathway leading to the synthesis of these complex carbohydrate antigens is strictly regulated.

When epithelial cultures are derived from tissues in which ABH expression occurs, the cultures frequently contain a variable proportion of cells positive for the blood group antigen of the donor. From less than 1% to as many as 75% of cells may express surface ABH in cultures from human amniotic fluid [4–6], human umbilical vein endothelium [7], fetal kidney [8], lung [8, 9], semen [10], testis tubules and prostate (unpublished observations). These antigens are not present on fibroblasts derived from the same tissues. Cells possessing blood group anti-

Birth Defects: Original Article Series, Volume XVI, Number 2, pages 339–344

genic determinants have been shown to arise from antigen-negative cells in a rabbit epithelial line [11] and in HeLa cells [12]. Recent evidence suggests that the expression of H as a surface antigen in HeLa cells may be cell cycle dependent, being highest around the time of mitosis and G1 [13].

The carbohydrate moiety of the blood group glycoproteins or glycolipids is thought to be synthesized by the sequential action of a series of glycosyltransferases [14]. The group A individual has an N-acetyl-galactosaminyltransferase capable of linking N-acetyl-D-galactosamine $\alpha 1 \rightarrow 3$ to the terminal galactose of the H substance of the O red cell, while the group B individual has instead a transferase which exclusively adds D-galactose $\alpha 1 \rightarrow 3$ to the same acceptor sites on H substance. The group O person lacks the ability to add sugar to H substance. H activity itself is a product of a reaction in which an $\alpha 1,2$-fucosyltransferase transfers L-fucose to a precursor carbohydrate chain. This activity is found in all but rare individuals. The function of the blood group complex carbohydrates is not known, nor is it understood how their synthesis is regulated.

One could study the genetics and the regulation of the synthesis of these antigens of differentiated epithelial cells better if one could isolate pure populations of antigen-positive cells and if such cells could be grown for reasonable lengths of time in culture. We are trying to deal with both of these problems in our laboratory.

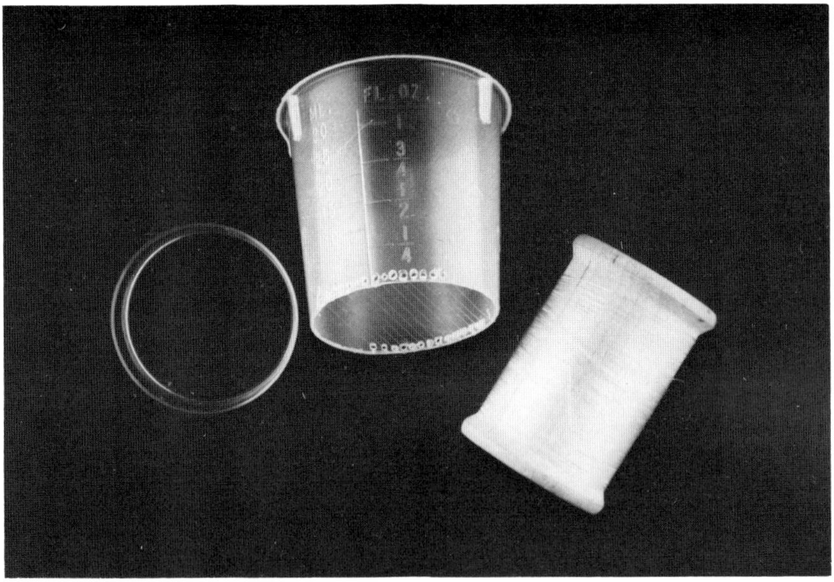

Fig. 1. Equipment for affinity separation on nylon fibers. Nylon sewing thread (right) is strung through holes in truncated disposable beaker to form harp (center), which fits snugly into 33-mm plastic Petri dish (left).

For the isolation of blood group antigen-positive cells, we have adapted the nylon fiber affinity technique of Edelman and Rutishauser [15]. We take advantage of 2 lectins which bind particular blood group substances. These are Helix pomatia lectin, which binds to group A antigen by virtue of its specificity for N-acetyl-D-galactosamine [16], and Ulex europeus lectin I which binds to H substance by virtue of its specificity for L-fucose [17, 18]. Both these lectins are powerful hemagglutinins when combined with the appropriate type of human red blood cells. We absorb purified lectin to nylon thread strung so as to form a "harp" (Fig. 1). The lectin-coated threads are then used to fish out blood-group-positive cells from a mixed suspension of positive and negative cells [19]. Cell suspensions from cultures of human fetal kidney or amniotic fluid of which a proportion of cells are positive for surface A or H antigens are allowed to bind specifically to lectin-coated nylon fibers (Fig. 2). These bound cells are then physically removed by plucking the fibers. In 8 such experiments, the bound cells exhibited no further growth, though unbound cells continued to proliferate. In other experiments, fiber-bound cells from established cell lines showed unimpaired colony-forming ability after being removed by plucking. This suggests that antigen-positive cells in these cultures might be terminally differentiated. However, the generally poor growth potential of these epithelial cultures, especially after subculture, makes it difficult to draw such a conclusion without additional evidence.

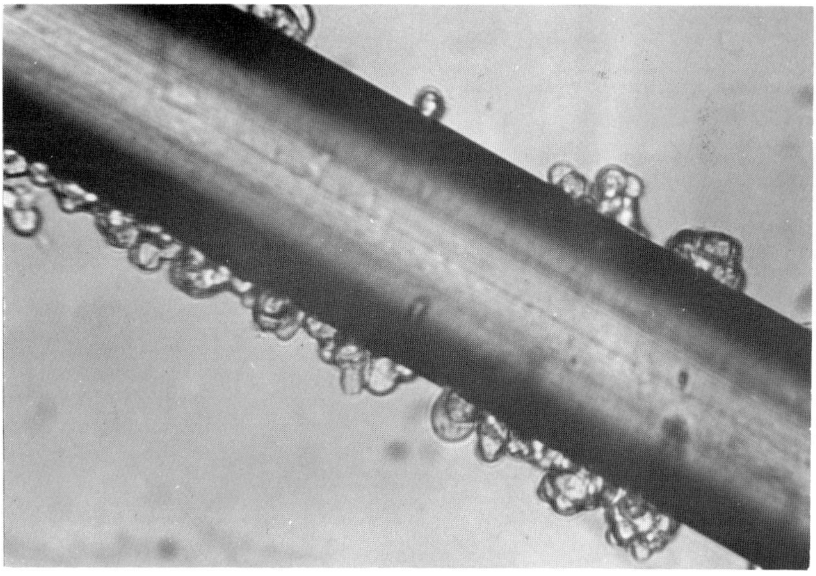

Fig. 2. Cells from a blood group AB fetal kidney culture bound to nylon fibers coated with Helix pomatia lectin (× 225).

Lacking long-term diploid human epithelial cultures, we have tried to generate, by somatic cell hybridization, permanent lines of cells expressing the human blood group antigens. Human epithelial cells derived from semen or from umbilical vein endothelium are fused to cells from established epithelioid rodent cell lines RAG (mouse) or CHO (Chinese hamster) which are deficient in the enzyme hypoxanthine-guanine-phosphoribosyltransferase (HPRT). A variable percentage of the resultant hybrid cells, selected in HAT medium [20], continues to express the ABH antigen of the human line on the cell surface, suggesting that extinction does not take place in the hybrids and that regulation of antigen expression might be occurring as it does in short-term diploid cell cultures. Efforts to obtain pure populations of antigen-positive hybrid cells by cloning have been unsuccessful; presumptive antigen-positive cells were selected on lectin-coated nylon fibers, recovered by plucking, and (unlike the diploid cells) propagated. Clones derived from these selected cells had varying percentages of positive cells, as did the original hybrids [19], indicating that cloned cells in an established hybrid cell line may give rise to mixed populations of positive and negative cells. Such populations, derived from cells presumed to carry the genes for the synthesis of the blood group antigens, could be used for chromosome analysis to correlate the presence of blood group antigens with specific chromosome(s).

We envision that mapping of blood group genes will proceed as follows: Hybrids will be made between human epithelial cell strains, in which ABH expression occurs, and HPRT-deficient rodent epithelial cell lines. After selection in HAT medium to eliminate rodent parental cells, fresh hybrids containing some percentage of blood-group-positive cells will be subjected to selection on lectin-coated fibers. The fiber-bound antigen-positive cells which presumably carry the blood group genes will be released from the fibers, grown, and karyotyped. If sufficient numbers of cells are bound, we find that it is even possible to karyotype cells directly upon removal from the fibers. The chromosome(s) found to be retained by most cells will be candidates for carrying blood group genes. Correct assignment of the genes for A and B, already shown to be on chromosome 9 [21], will serve to verify the validity of this approach to mapping surface antigens expressed as differentiated functions of selected cell types.

The above method for mapping specialized cell surface antigens may be limited by several factors. For it to work, it is essential that the cells bearing the antigens be capable of entering mitosis and, preferably, of continuing proliferation. In addition, the human antigens to be mapped must not share cross-reacting determinants with surface antigens of the rodent cell parent of the hybrid nor should the hybrid be induced to synthesize antigens coded for by the rodent genome which share determinants with the human antigens. The affinity selection technique must be highly specific, admitting very few contaminating antigen-negative cells since these might subsequently overgrow the positive cells. We think that we are on our way to dealing with these problems.

We began with the last problem, that of specificity, since it is easiest to handle experimentally. We used human red blood cells as model antigen-positive cell types to establish optimal conditions for specific binding to lectin-coated fibers. We found that cell binding to the fibers was proportional to lectin concentration in the solution used to absorb lectin to the fibers. It was also proportional to the number of cells in the suspension allowed to interact with the lectin-coated fibers. Most binding occurred within 15 minutes. If an appropriate hapten was added to the cell suspension, adsorption did not occur. Using antigen-negative Chinese hamster cells with high plating efficiency, we found that the number of cells carried nonspecifically through the selection process was in the range of 10^{-4} to 10^{-5} of input cells. Thus, the specificity seemed quite good.

The problem whether antigen-positive cells will continue to proliferate is worrisome. In vivo, ABH-positive cells often occur in locations such as in the spiny layer of epidermis [22], in which it is apparent that no further cell division will take place. Since normal epithelial cells in culture grow poorly, nonproliferation of antigen-positive cells from this source may not be significant. Carcinomas of blood-group-positive tissues tend to show a loss or a decrease in ABH antigens [23], but there are exceptions to this. We would like to investigate whether cells which express the ABH antigens in tumor lines have further growth potential.

The problem of possible cross-reaction of human blood group antigens with rodent cell surface antigens is still to be considered. We know that the mouse and Chinese hamster lines used as parents for somatic cell hybrids do not bear detectable ABH antigens. However, it is possible that synthesis of such antigens or cross-reacting antigens coded for by mouse genes may be induced by fusion to the human cells. There is precedent for this kind of induction in the case of albumin synthesis in rat-human hybrids [24].

Another unknown factor is whether the complex carbohydrate precursor molecules for the ABH antigens are coded for by the rodent genome. This will determine how many human genes will be required to maintain the synthesis of the ABH antigens. Such problems may have to be considered in the genetic analysis and mapping of other differentiated (or nonconstitutive) cell functions.

REFERENCES

1. Stejskal R, Lill PH, Davidsohn I: A, B, and H isoantigens in the human fetus. Dev Biol 34:274–281, 1973.
2. Szulman AE: The histological distribution of the blood group substances in man as disclosed by immunofluorescence III. The A, B, and H antigens in embryos and fetuses from 18 mm in length. J Exp Med 119:503–516, 1964.
3. Szulman AE: The ABH antigens in human tissues and secretions during embryonal development. J Histochem Cytochem 13:752–754, 1965.
4. Chessin LN, Bramson S, Kuhns WJ, Hirschhorn K: Studies on the A, B, O (H) blood groups on human cells in culture. Blood 25:944–953, 1965.

5. Friedhoff F, Kuhns WJ: Detection and characterization of blood group antigens on untransformed human amnion cells. Transfusion 8:244–249, 1968.
6. Kuhns WJ: Faur Y, Bramson S, Friedhoff F: Studies on the variability of ABH blood group antigens on cells in primary culture. Proc Soc Exp Biol Med 131:67–70, 1969.
7. Jaffe EA, Nachman RL, Becker CG, Minick CR: Culture of human endothelial cells derived from umbilical veins. J Clin Invest 52:2745–2756, 1973.
8. Högman CF: Blood group antigens on human cells in tissue culture. The effect of prolonged cultivation. Exp Cell Res 21:137–143, 1960.
9. Katoh Y, Stoner GD, McIntire KR, Hill TA, Anthony R, McDowell EM, Trump BF, Harris CC: Immunological markers of human bronchial epithelial cells in vivo and in vitro. J Natl Cancer Inst 62:1177–1182, 1979.
10. Phillips SG, Phillips DM, Kabat EA, Miller OJ: Human semen as a source of epithelial cells for culture. In Vitro 14:639–650, 1978.
11. Franks D, Dawson A: Variation in the expression of blood group antigen A in clonal cultures of rabbit cells. Exp Cell Res 42:543–561, 1966.
12. Kuhns WJ, Pann C: Growth kinetics in cultured epithelioid cells and phenotypic expression of blood group H. Nature [New Biol] 245:217–219, 1973.
13. Kuhns WJ: Biosynthesis of blood group H gene-associated α-2-L-fucosyltransferase during the cell cycle. (Abstract) J Cell Biol 79:10a, 1978.
14. Watkins WM, Morgan WTJ: Possible genetical pathways for the biosynthesis of blood group mucopolysaccharides. Vox Sang 4:97–119, 1959.
15. Edelman GM, Rutishauser U, Millette CF: Cell fractionation and arrangement on fibers, beads, and surfaces. Proc Natl Acad Sci USA 68:2153–2157, 1971.
16. Hammarström S, Kabat EA: Purification and characterization of a blood-group A reactive hemagglutinin from the snail Helix pomatia and a study of its combining site. Biochemistry 8:2696–2705, 1969.
17. Matsumoto I, Osawa T: Purification and characterization of a Cytisus-type anti-H(O) phytohemagglutinin from Ulex europeus seeds. Arch Biochem Biophys 140:484–491, 1970.
18. Pereira MEA, Kisailus EC, Gruezo F, Kabat EA: Immunochemical studies on the combining site of the blood group H-specific lectin I from Ulex europeus seeds. Arch Biochem Biophys 185:108–115, 1978.
19. Phillips SG, Kabat EA, Miller OJ: Nylon-fiber affinity selection of red blood cells and tissue culture cells on the basis of cell surface determinants. (Submitted for publication.)
20. Szybalska EH, Szybalski W: Genetics of human cell lines. IV. DNA-mediated heritable transformation of a biochemical trait. Proc Natl Acad Sci USA 48:2026–2034, 1962.
21. Westerveld A, Jongsma APM, Khan PM, van Someren H, Bootsma D: Assignment of the AK_1:Np:ABO linkage group to human chromosome 9. Proc Natl Acad Sci USA 73: 895–899, 1976.
22. Holborow EJ, Brown PC, Glynn LE, Hawes MD, Gresham GA, O'Brien TF, Coombs RRA: The distribution of the blood group A antigen in human tissues. Br J Exp Pathol 41:430–437, 1960.
23. Kovarik S, Davidsohn I, Stejskal R: ABO antigens in cancer. Arch Pathol 86:12–21, 1968.
24. Darlington GJ, Bernhard HP, Ruddle FH: Human serum albumin phenotype activation in mouse hepatoma-human leukocyte cell hybrids. Science 185:859–861, 1974.

Epithelial Cultures and Birth Defects

Robert J. Gorlin, DDS, MS

My assigned task is formidable – that of being sufficiently prescient to predict what the future holds in the culturing of epithelial cells to solve problems of "birth anomalies." I realize fully that even the title of this discussion is less than accurate, for it is too restrictive. I believe that the Editors of this volume would wish me to consider not only those anomalies which are congenital, ie present at birth, but rather "developmental anomalies" in the broader sense of presenting at any time from the moment of conception to death. These will range from those having single gene inheritance and being influenced little by environment to those having polygenic inheritance with considerable environmental interaction. In a few words, I am being asked, "What is most likely to pay off?"

The question posed is "Where will the breakthroughs occur in the next decade?" While 1984 has not yet arrived, its proximity would suggest that George Orwell's prognostications are not likely to occur – or at least within his timetable. Who among us can state that s/he foresaw even as late as 1955 the "chromosomal revolution"? Can one then predict with any degree of certainty which "chromosomal revolution"? Can one then predict with any degree of certainty which epithelial cells of which organs will yield the greatest information per unit time? As I perceive the acquisition of knowledge, it is by no means a continuum. Quite the contrary, it is a never ending series of quantum jumps. I suspect that we are on the verge of such an energy release.

Looking through the hazy crystal ball to a decade hence, with all of the limitations described in the preceding paragraphs, there should be considerable advance made in our understanding of diseases. The most obvious paradigm would be a metabolic disorder which would be tissue (organ) specific and which would require epithelial culture of functional cells from that tissue (organ).

Until now, cell culture has essentially been limited to fibroblasts and transformed cell lines. The art of cultured epithelial cell study will help define defects that are intrinsic to the epithelial cell versus those that are brought about by abnormalities in the cell's environment. A second, but by no means secondary,

Birth Defects: Original Article Series, Volume XVI, Number 2, pages 345–350

quantum of knowledge would be that increment manifested by new information concerning cell-cell interactions, especially regarding cell-to-cell messengers, ie chemical cytotelegraphy, if I may be permitted to coin a term; perhaps in less general terms, cell membrane properties including hormonal and polypeptide responses. For example, we know a reasonable amount about the hypothalamic messenger system, but little, in comparison, about the APUD (amine precursor uptake and decarboxylation) system of neural crest derivatives and of the myriad tumors that arise from neural crest cells (APUDomas). The hypoxia-sensitive Kulchitsky cells of the lung, for example, are probably responsible for local perfusion and ventilation and may play a significant role in sudden death syndrome and apnea of prematurity. It is probably all too evident to state that culture of a pure cell population of any endocrine tissue should greatly facilitate investigation of its physiology.

Possibilities abound, being limited only by one's interests: specific rate-limiting regulatory steps in the synthesis and secretion of various structural proteins, cell/virus interaction, cell/antigen interaction, factors controlling cell differentiation, cellular nutritional requirements, metabolic disorders involving enzyme systems limited to epithelial cells. Several questions arise immediately. Is a cell removed from its "organ unit" going to exhibit normal properties when placed in culture? I ask this because the organ unit is often a sick or dying system. For example, sick cells are very difficult to transform by chemical carcinogens, perhaps because a "lesion" during DNA synthesis is required. Does a cell require cells which are normally adjacent to it to carry out normal function? For example, ameloblasts do not lay down enamel protein unless they are proximate to dentin. Within this simple sounding statement lies a plethora of questions raised in part by Slavkin in his cogent review of this subject in this volume. He and others have definitely shown that there must be direct intercellular contact between epithelium and ectomesenchyme to effect differentiation, histogenesis, and morphogenesis. It is not a small molecule that can diffuse through a millipore filter separating the heterologous tissues that effects these changes. Further, it has been demonstrated that it is the dental papilla ectomesenchyme that gives the order to the epithelium (from whatever source) to become ameloblasts, ie it is organ specific and may even operate across species. In addition, one might ask whether the cells of the ectomesenchyme adjacent to the inner enamel epithelial cells differentiate to become odontoblasts only because of cell-cell interaction or were they destined to become odontoblasts upon leaving the neural crest? Would a "gemisch" of dental papilla ectomesenchyme when placed adjacent to inner enamel epithelium behave the same way?

For the sake of discussion, let us hypothesize that we possess a technique to easily isolate a nephron (renal corpuscle, proximal convoluted tubule, loop of

Henle, distal convoluted tubule) without danger to its component cells. We know, for example, that cells in proximal convoluted tubules are intimately involved in resorption. While surface area is a factor, there is a plethora of others: types of enzymes at cell membranes as well as within the cells, arrangement and complexity of mitochondria, unfolding at basal ends of cells, the relation of the resorbing cells to the capillaries, the osmotic pressures within the peritubular connective tissue, the presence of certain hormones within the blood, and the concentration of the substance in question within the blood plasma, among others. For example, glucose is completely resorbed, and sodium is resorbed extensively. Under normal conditions, urea is completely eliminated. In the distal convoluted tubule, there is further resorption of sodium accompanied by water. The permeability is controlled by an antidiuretic hormone.

Are any or all of the properties exhibited by each of these cells a function of their position? If so, which ones? If we were to isolate a pure culture of proximal convoluted tubular cells, and another of distal convoluted tubular cells, would their study be of value? Would the isolated cell maintain its properties? Is the sum greater than the parts?

This discussion is, however, entirely in the realm of the hypothetical. The breakthrough is not about to occur. Some success has been achieved in growth of the mesangial cell of the glomerular apparatus of the fetus and newborn and its biochemical properties and ultrastructure have been maintained through several passages. However other cell types of the glomerulus (endothelial, epithelial) have not grown well in culture, have lost their biochemical and antigenic properties, and are hard to identify. Even less success has been attained in attempts at isolated tubular epithelial cell growth. While stromal fibroblast overgrowth has been overcome (Migeon, this volume), the tubular site of origin of the epithelial cells could not be ascertained and they did not survive many transfers (Bergeron et al, this volume).

Unless considerable progress is made in this area, segmental tubular dysfunctions cannot be studied by epithelial cell culture. As pointed out by Bergeron and confreres, perhaps the host of available animal models, largely uninvestigated in depth, will serve an interim function.

Are the principles adumbrated above true for all organ (cell) systems? For example, retinal epithelium provides the metabolism for the neurosensory retina. There is no other approach to study retinal biochemistry. Lens epithelium and its biochemistry should yield a ripe harvest of information. The studies reported in this volume by McAteer and Douglas, and Tanswell and Smith on interactions between alveolar epithelial cells and fibroblasts during exposure to steroids were convincing regarding the necessity for obtaining pure epithelial cell cultures. I candidly admit, in spite of the distance of culture of alveolar Type II cells from that of my personal interest in dysmorphic syndromes, that it seemed burgeoning with promise. It may be a more visceral than cerebral impression, but I believe that the lung will reveal many of its secrets within the decade, employing the methods outlined in the papers of McAteer and Douglas, and Tanswell and Smith.

I believe that a relatively intact "organ system" is going to be required for dental, oral, and intestinal mucosa. The normal behavior of a highly polarized or differentiated epithelial cell seems to be a function of adjacent epithelial cell interactions which involve gap junctions and occluding functions. This has been discussed by Witkop (this volume) utilizing 1) mucoepithelial dysplasia, a disorder described by him and his co-workers and 2) amelogenesis imperfecta (a plethora of different disorders subsumed under the same name). That gap junctions play the *sole* role in the various disorders of defective enamel formation is by no means implied or even suggested. Only within the past half dozen years are the skein of complexities of epithelial-ectomesenchymal interactions being truly appreciated as discussed above. Secretion and transportation of epithelial products cannot be carried out without occluding junctions and in the absence of an organized layer of subepithelial fibroblasts. While this fibroblast-epithelial cell contact may be transient in nature, it is nevertheless necessary. This also was demonstrated in the case of Type II alveolar cells of the lung. While one may argue that this is not a "pure" system, at least it removes humoral and probably most autonomic factors and allows examination of the direct effects of neurotransmitters, various hormones, and other factors on the metabolism of the epithelial cells. Yet one cannot dismiss the arguments that epithelial-mesenchymal interactions, epithelial cytotelegraphy, immunologically competent cells in the adjacent lamina propria, and residual nerve terminals are not in some small or large way affecting experimental results. If hyper- or hyposecretion occurs, is this due to intrinsic factors, or to extracellular factors? Does the defect rest in a faulty regulatory mechanism, abnormal secretory membranes, or in altered intracellular enzyme systems? Perhaps some of these questions may be answered by organ culture, but limitations are severe. Time is of the essence, for many organ systems are "healthy" for at most a day or more. After that time, we are dealing with sick cells and questions concerning cell migration, and turnover cannot be answered by these methods. Better maintenance methods must be developed. I feel far more sanguine about human skin epithelium growth on sterile dead pigskin as described by Freeman and his colleagues (this volume). While, to date, their technique for producing organotypic cultures has had somewhat limited experimental investigation, I perceive it as a puissant one for examination of numerous cutaneous or oral mucosal disorders. Could one modify this technique to grow epithelial cells from an amniocentesis specimen "mix"?

The 3T3 feeder-technique described in this volume by Baden and Kubilus would appear to be less informative, since the epithelial cells lose enzyme activity (histidase and arginine-to-citrulline-converting enzyme among others), retain nuclei, and fail to manifest lipid in contrast with their behavior on killed pigskin.

In the area of chemical carcinogenesis, quantification of the effects of chemicals on human epithelial cells can be effected with a far greater degree of accuracy than with explants. The epithelial cells can be handled most like bacteria and therefore more easily quantitated. Especially valuable will be the ability to investigate the relationship between somatic mutation and in vitro cell transformation.

In the area of prenatal diagnosis, application of epithelial cell cultures obtained through amniocentesis should demonstrate metabolic differences between (among) epithelial cell types. The epithelial cells are shed from the skin and oral, nasal, bladder, and gastrointestinal mucosae. Perhaps I fell less sanguine about this area than I should.

The demonstration that fetal lung fibroblasts in response to glucocorticoids produce a low molecular weight polypeptide which enhances production of surfactant by Type II cells is important. A similar relationship between fibroblasts and airway epithelium may be valid. Whether the mucus-producing cell in this culture system will be superior to that of the goblet cell of the rectal mucosa for study of cystic fibrosis remains to be seen, but I believe that I would put my wager on airway cell culture. If the ciliated cell can be maintained in culture without dedifferentiation, then our understanding of the defects in the autosomal recessive Kartagener syndrome will be significantly enhanced.

No less exciting is the nylon harp-lectin binding of blood group antigen positive cells described in this volume by Phillips and co-workers. However, this ingenious technique of plucking the fibers seems to have applicability limited to mapping of blood group genes. Their methods appear to be eminently reasonable, but may be limited by several "if's." For example, if the antigen-bearing cells are not prone to enter mitosis and to continuously proliferate, all is lost.

SUMMARY

To summarize my impressions is perhaps the most difficult aspect to this task. While in select examples cultured epithelial cells may provide answers to several important questions concerning specific birth defects; in general, I find it hard to believe that even when better methods of cell culture are developed, that it will be other than another tool which may be invaluable, but only in certain cases.

The complex interaction of heterotypic cells in many instances defeats the purpose of study of cultured epithelium as an isolated unit. Let us posit that we are investigating a possible defect in regulation of a protein secreted by epithelial cells. One must first isolate the specific cell type which synthesizes, secretes, and regulates that protein. In the case of the lung and surfactant, isolated epithelial cell culture may well tell us a lot. In the case of inherited tooth defects, tissue (primary explants of isolated secretory ameloblasts) rather than cells should be more helpful. In short, I do not view epithelial cell culture as the answer to *all* our problems any more than I see cultured fibroblasts telling us all the answers. Rather it is the nature of the questions that we ask that will be the key to unlock several but not all doors.

PART III: Overview of the Future for Studying Human Birth Defects Expressed in Epithelium in Tissue Culture

A Genetic Social Worker's Brief Comments on the Continued Participation of Families in Birth Defect Research

Anne J. Krush, MS

When one has been associated with only one small facet of a subject as broad (and yet as narrow) as cultured epithelium, it is like exploring a new country or learning a new language; and it is awesome. The objectives in cell and organ culture studies are to increase understanding of the nosology of birth defects and to provide more exact information concerning human inheritance patterns.

How can one interpret the relationship between studies of cultured epithelium and birth defects to a family in which there is grave concern and fear because of the occurrence in their family of a birth defect, whether severe or mild? First, the family needs to know that work is constantly going on to improve methods and techniques of tissue culture and that much still needs to be learned. It is an exciting science that is in its early growing period. Although the studies may not reveal the exact nature or cause of a disease, they may show a relationship between the disease in the person under study to a known disease. From this, information can be obtained concerning treatment which may or may not be available.

Families need to know why the obtaining of a biopsy of skin or some other tissue, samples of blood or other body fluids, are necessary, and in case of death, why autopsy material is important. One can explain the difference between in vivo and in vitro studies. It may even be expedient to have one or more family members visit the laboratory where tissue culture studies are carried out. There, they may have an opportunity to see their own cells growing in tissue culture and to observe cells under the microscope.

It is certainly not necessary to explain to families the exact mechanisms and terminology used in tissue culture studies. It is important for them to understand that 1) each study takes a great deal of time and 2) it may be necessary to repeat the study as the methodologies are being developed.

Birth Defects: Original Article Series, Volume XVI, Number 2, pages 353–354

Some families may wonder why, with the availability of amniocentesis, more cannot be learned about birth defects before birth. As demonstrated in this volume, much work is going on at the present time on the problem of lack of epithelial growth in specimens of amniotic fluid.

It will behoove those of us who counsel patients and their families to have an idea of the number of tissue and organ systems and diseases stemming from the systems which are already under study for pathogenesis by means of in vitro tissue culture studies, so that families may be referred for studies if they are willing. Interpretation of the need for such studies can be given to the family.

Overall Genetic Significance of the Use of Epithelial Cultures in Studying Human Birth Defects Expressed in Epithelium*

Edmond A. Murphy, MD

One of the most penetrating statements in this volume is the following: "It represents but part of the classic biologic approach of parsing complex systems into their component parts followed by controlled reassembly" (Tanswell and Smith). It is not merely that I am delighted by the apt nicety of the word "parsing" with its connotations of taking things apart like a watchmaker rather than grinding them up like a miller; or the perceptive wisdom of the phrase *controlled* reassembly; but the whole idea of conceiving the plan of campaign in these terms embodies what has been so often and so grievously overlooked in the biology of recent years. Granted that the title of this volume is not merely a marriage of convenience, we must be concerned in relating the techniques for culturing epithelium to the study of human birth defects.

There are two extreme viewpoints about the genetics of congenital malformations. The reductionistic extreme is that the beginning and end of the problem reside in identifying a faulty protein or a deficient enzyme, and that thereafter the cure and prevention of the disorder are mere technical exercises. The mystical extreme is that we are not concerned with some individual mechanism of disease, but with a whole patient in a complex environment, and that all simplification is falsification. These extreme regions are, I trust, uninhabited; but a wide range of intermediate positions are densely occupied. It can be argued that this is as it should be; that competent analysis at a variety of levels of organization makes for a healthy ecology of inquiry, so long as no group deludes itself that it is self-sufficient. We must hope that every member is on speaking terms with both of his neighbors on the long and fragile chain from the crib to the quark and back. In general, the higher the resolving power, the greater the risk that clinical relevancy has been "purified out" of the inquiry and the more likely we are to find a precise answer to a nonproblem. Conversely, the greater the relevancy the more likely that the resolving power will, to a scientist, be unacceptably low.

*Supported by grant #5R01 GM 24736 from the National Institutes of Health.

Birth Defects: Original Article Series, Volume XVI, Number 2, pages 355–359

This volume certainly contains expert and stimulating presentations at many levels – from heavily clinical topics, through refined pathology, organ culture, histology, differentiation, cytology, fine-structure electron microscopy, down to immunology and the edges of biochemistry. Let us first look at this problem from the clinical end. A malformation which has no other serious pleiotropic effects may yet have a highly complex pathogenesis. From two points at least the gravamen of the condition resides in the malformation itself: the patient's burden and the force of selection. The patient is overwhelmingly concerned with what the condition is, much less with how it is produced, what it is a mild form of, or what it is called. A *forme* sufficiently *fruste* may not engage the patient's interest at all. In the same way, genetic selection operates not on genotypes but on phenotypes. A patient who was within a hairbreadth of having a patent interatrial septum is in no worse a state than those who had been nowhere near this risk. Of course there may be more remote consequences both to the clinical burden and to the force of selection if this might-have-been condition becomes overt in a descendant. Viewed under these aspects, the inner workings are germane only insofar as they have overt expression. Two individually harmful traits occurring together may cancel each other out and the patient be none the worse. Failure to grasp this divergence between the concerns of the clinical geneticist on the one hand and the basic, or the *soi-disant* human, geneticist on the other have done nothing to foster sympathetic or fruitful relations between them.

None of this broad comment must be construed to mean that the clinical geneticist can be excused from serious strategic interest in the activities of the experimentalist. I can think of three powerful arguments to the contrary.

First, if he is to aim for any more constructive approach to prevention than genetic counseling of rather negative cast, he must devise means of offsetting the effects of disorderly gene action by reconstruction or, failing that, compensation. He may find such a means by lucky accident. However, a more rational and efficient approach is to try to understand basic mechanisms by systematic study.

Second, both sound and sensitive indexes for studies on the etiology and the optimal means of prognosis draw warrant from rational, if simplified, representations of the basic mechanism from so-called models. (The latter word is much abused by all: the mathematician uses it to emancipate himself from distasteful, though often important, biologic detail; the biologist to impart elegance to his speculations but without the irksome trammels of rigor. I would hold no brief for models which do not respect the virtues of both fact and rigor.)

Finally, what we cannot formulate, we cannot optimize. A "holding operation," a patching up of leaky health, may be a wholly inadequate counter to the birth defect. It is arguable that not all birth defects are floridly congenital, that coronary disease is as much a birth defect as cleft palate, and that we have had a quite unwarranted complacency about ineluctable senescence, and so-called degenerative disease. A prudent concern with pathogenesis may show how shallow our security is.

There are four traditional responsibilities in clinical practice: prevention, diagnosis, prognosis, and treatment. While the papers in this volume illustrate these topics bountifully, the comments which follow apply, at least by analogy, to tissues other than epithelium.

Prevention. This need not rest wholly on rational insight, as we will likely eliminate smallpox entirely before we understand it. Nevertheless, premature success with "black-box" prevention may be a Pyrrhic victory. Discoveries by this means are apt to be coarse-grained. So the preventive methods may contain much detail that is irrelevant but that we do not *know* is irrelevant and that we are there-
nobody follows them; and experts have learned from bitter experience the need to make their means of prevention as little disruptive as possible.
fore loath to abandon. But preventive measures, however secure, are void if

Culture of epithelial cells lends itself to preventive measures of two types. First it may provide an assay system in vitro for the study of etiologic factors which will have obvious advantages over current epidemiologic and experimental approaches. The conditions of experiment can be standardized; time scales can be shortened; a maze of ethical problems can be avoided.

More immediately, epithelial culture has implications for prevention at the level of public health. Here there are three obstacles. First, cost. No doubt in time a reasonable technology will emerge. But at present, it seems totally unlikely that even if the necessary support for widespread screening were forthcoming, there would be enough skilled people to carry it out. Second, time. Epithelial growth seems to be uncomfortably slow even compared with that of fibroblasts; and especially in amniocentesis, where prompt answers are called for, there seems to be a major obstacle until the whole process can be accelerated. Finally, the issues of sensitivity and specificity which become more and more burdensome as the number of tests increases. I hope beyond hope that the enthusiast will have acquired a little wisdom from the deplorable neglect of these fundamental ideas, neglect which has done so much harm to earlier screening devices. Perhaps my brevity will make for emphasis.

Diagnosis. Here the uses and the problems will be closely allied. We have heard much today on the use of identifying characteristics of various types of cells. We may expect the results of such studies to be much in demand, for instance in tumor pathology, in transplant studies, and at a somewhat more basic level, in linkage studies as Dr. McKusick has suggested. We do well to remember that the more we know about diagnosis, the more we learn about heterogeneity on the one hand and occult homogeneity on the other. Thus, it is not only our diagnostic acumen that is affected, but nosology, and the very meaning of disease as well. One merely has to reflect how electrophoresis of hemoglobin has changed the face of hematology, producing a momentary unification, then a prodigious diversification, and finally a complete regrouping of many thitherto unrelated diseases. Scriver gave us a telegrammatic glimpse of this process at work in his comments on polycystic disease of the kidney.

Prognosis. Of this topic I shall say little, not for lack of material, but because the issues are so massive and so obvious. What we call genetic counseling is merely a special form of prognosis. It rests heavily on accurate diagnosis especially in utero. One of the major deficiencies in antenatal diagnosis lies in disorders of the skin and its appendages.

Treatment. I see the greatest potential for treatment in those areas in which incompatibility of tissues is at present the major problem. It seems preposterous that burns are still an injury which threatens life, not because of the wholesale destruction of tissues, but simply because of the extent of surface involved. Skin to effect plastic restoration of surface is scarce. Skin from donors is of highly limited value because of the problems of matching. In principle, skin for repair in any desired quantity can be grown in tissue culture. We have heard today that experiments along these lines have so far met with only small success. However, I do not imagine that anybody will be unduly depressed simply because perfect success has not been attained at the first try. I have no doubt that there is still much to learn in the way of refinements of techniques.

Again hemophilia must rely at the present time, to a distressing extent, on laboriously refined products of blood fractionation. We must suppose that a highly efficient system of synthesis of antihemophilic globulin should be possible as a result of tissue culture of liver cells. It might be hoped that one could thus obviate not only the problems of finding suitable donors and keeping perpetual vigilance on their own infections, but also obtaining large amounts of blood and fractionating them. I have the impression that the main problems here are technical. Once one entertains the possibility of high-resolution engineering in tissue culture, a massive panorama of benefits comes into view, more akin to science fiction than to sober discussion at an orderly meeting. Is it too much to hope for that Dr. Slavkin's beautiful tissue studies will offer something, not only for the more florid dysplasias of teeth, but perhaps even for restorative dentistry?

I am obliged here to be everybody's champion, and while I may not give equal time to the basic aspect of this intricate relationship, I must at least speak to its importance. It would be trivial and venal to engage in partisan claims about whether the laboratory scientist is more or less important than the clinician. The relationship between them is such that equality is a meaningless term. But the *symmetry* of the relationship does not end with administrative recognition or support. There is a sense in which the final court of appeal in this endeavor is clinical; but that does not mean that this court of appeal can afford to be arbitrary or to leave the basic scientist dissatisfied.

Yet once again, I find myself preaching a gospel of reconcilation (in its aboriginal sense). While the clinician is mostly concerned with what is clearly evident to the world, with what ought to be done, and with the delicate wisdom of making decisions, the basic scientist is concerned with the inner reality and the art of the possible. Clearly both viewpoints are proper, and both constrain the approach to those topics found in this volume. The clinician may, perhaps, lay out the problem to be attacked, but he must surrender the paradigmatic aspects of the problem to the basic scientist. The dermatologist must look with pleasant expectations on the prospects of epithelial culture as means of elucidating skin disease. But six months from now the experimentor may tell him that there is no such condition as psoriasis or eczema and that rational classification cuts right across traditional dermatologic nosology. It would not be the first time that a detailed examination of inner mechanisms has had such a disruptive effect. The discovery of the tubercle bacillus, for instance, produced a fundamental regrouping of diseases – phthisis, Pott disease of the spine, lupus vulgaris, and one type of chronic salpingitis emerging as pleomorphic manifestations from a single disorder; while disorders, apparently similar in location and in manifestations – chronic bronchitis, rickets, lupus erythematosis – were proved quite distinct. Of course this conclusion does not imply that rational pathologic classification has completely demolished the clinical approach. Orthopedic management of bowed legs from a score of different causes still calls for broad general principles which are clinical in their warrant; the same would be true of dementias, destructive lung disease, or severe itching. There is here no room for triumphalism. The interaction between clinical and laboratory science should be dialectical rather than adversary.

Into the interaction (not always constructive) between the pathologist and the clinician, tissue culture comes as an angel of enlightenment and peace. It partakes of the dynamism of clinical observation on the one hand and the detail and the unconstrained exploration characteristic of pathology on the other. It is not the answer to everything. But we have every reason to believe that it will be an important new building block in our pursuit of the truth about birth defects.

Overview—"State of the Art" and its Potential

Rody P. Cox, MD

Presentations in this volume describe the current "state of the art" of epithelial cell cultures and provide an exciting glimpse into the future. It is clear that studies on epithelial cell cultures are contributing to our understanding of many basic biologic problems, as well as permitting investigation of the etiologies of inherited diseases that are expressed in cells of epithelial origin. In particular those articles dealing with skin and teeth provide models for future studies of morphogenesis and biosynthetic capabilities of epithelial cells. Culturing of epithelial cells is enhanced by modifications of the methods of culture developed for optimal growth of fibroblasts. These include: 1) feeder layers and special substrata for cell attachment (pigskin, collagen, and artificial matrices), 2) primary organ and tissue fractionation procedures, and 3) the use of epidermal growth factors and media or selective systems designed to foster the multiplication of epithelial cells and retard or eliminate contaminating fibroblasts. These advances in tissue culture methodology have made it possible to obtain epithelial cell isolates of high purity. The availability of such cell systems may be crucial to the study of inherited diseases of epithelium.

Several of the presentations suggest that multiplication of some types of epithelial cells is accompanied by loss or reduction of special proteins or enzymes that are normally constitutive in the epithelial or parenchymal cells of the tissues from which the cultures were derived. For example, Migeon has shown that carbonic anhydrase activity declines with replication of renal tubule cells. The alterations in enzymic composition and metabolite pools that occur in cultured epithelium may limit the use of epithelial cultures for certain studies. Moreover, Bissell and Bearn have shown that the activity of the P-450 dependent aryl hydrocarbon hydroxylase decreases in liver cell culture, producing an expansion of the heme pool. The interrelationship of increased heme levels and suppression of δ-aminolevulinic acid synthetase activity may interfere with

Birth Defects: Original Article Series, Volume XVI, Number 2, pages 361–364

studies of porphyrin metabolism in cell culture. These alterations also may limit the usefulness of liver cell culture for studying diseases of porphyrin metabolism such as acute intermittent porphyria.

In embryonic development it is well known that the expression of differentiated function may be coupled to a cessation of cell replication. It is not unexpected that some properties associated with epithelial cells of a particular type may be lost when these cells are placed in culture and stimulated to multiply. Some epithelial cell types may be terminally differentiated and therefore unable to replicate. Selection of progenitors of these differentiated cells may occur in culture accounting for apparent loss of epithelial cell markers or proteins. Investigations that require parenchymal cells which retain the enzymatic composition of cells of the original tissue might be carried out using nonreplicating epithelial cells in monolayer culture. Such parenchymal cell cultures could be prepared by fractionating the cells present in the original tissue and isolating the revelant cell type as described in the papers by Bissell, McAteer, Pretlow, Tanswell, Del Monte, and their associates. In some cases cell-cell interactions may be necessary for retention of the differentiated phenotype as shown by Slavkin et al in studies on tooth formation. Coculturing different cells isolated from tissue may allow expression of differentiated function and permit the investigation of the mechanisms responsible for cell interactions, as shown by Tanswell and Smith in reconstituted lung cultures. In other instances organ culture systems may be needed to retain cell polarity and organization required to investigate cellular physiology and/or heritable disorders of particular organs. Neutra has used organ culture of intestine for her studies on cystic fibrosis. Bergeron and co-workers have pointed out the difficulties in studying renal transport mechanism with cultured tubular cells since tight cell junctions and cellular polarity are essential for investigating transport. Here again organ culture systems may be needed.

Certain of the limitations in phenotypes observed in epithelial cell culture may be overcome by special conditions. Moreover elucidation of the mechanisms responsible for selective gene expression may contribute important new information on cell regulation and maintenance of differentiation. Fallon et al described the coordinate induction of glycopeptide hormones and the accompanying ultrastructural modulations of HeLa cells induced by sodium butyrate. These effects are also observed with other inhibitors of DNA synthesis that focus the cell population at the G_1-S transition site of the cell cycle. The point of arrest in the cell cycle may be of importance in determining gene expression. The studies reported by Fallon and his associates may have application to maintaining differentiated phenotypes in primary and secondary epithelial cell cultures. Benke reported that modulation of cyclic AMP levels in amniotic cells may activate gene loci which are usually expressed only in liver or kidney cells (glucose–6–phosphatase production). Bissell and Bearn's review of activation of selected human genes by hybridizing human fibroblast to rat minimal deviation hepatoma that express liver-specific functions is another approach to understanding cell regulation and determination of cell phenotypes. Assigment of genetic loci that determine epithelial cell traits to a particular human chromosome also can be carried out using cell fusion as described by Phillips and co-workers. Nitowsky's contribution to this volume clearly demonstrates the importance of recent advances in molecular biology in providing tools for dissecting the details of specific protein synthesis in epithelial cells of endocrine origin.

In view of the startling recent advances in epithelial cell culture reported in this volume, one can be optimistic about the future. However, it is difficult to predict where the most rapid advances will occur. From a historical perspective the results of studies of diploid human fibroblast cultures from patients with inherited diseases have been responsible for an explosive increase in our knowledge of human biochemical genetics. The demonstration by Krooth and co-workers that human skin fibroblasts derived from patients with inborn errors of metabolism exhibited in culture the enzyme deficiency associated with certain of these disorders provided easily obtainable material for diagnosing the diseases and for isolating and characterizing mutant proteins [1, 2]. The enzymatic defect responsible for familial hyperlysinemia was first discovered in fibroblast cultures [3]. Recent evidence indicates that several enzymes that carry out sequential reactions in lysine degradation are deficient in this disease and the mutation has characteristics suggesting a polarity effect on linked loci [4, 5]. Studies on enzyme deficiencies in intact human cells in culture have provided new insights into the regulation of metabolic pathways and the perturbations in metabolite utilization which occur as a result of an inherited metabolic disease [6, 7]. Fibroblasts from some patients with overproduction gout show purine excretory activity that resembles that observed in urine [8]. Thus the pathogenesis of phenotypic effects of enzyme deficiences can be studied at the cellular level in fibroblast culture. The availability of epithelial cells from patients with diseases that are expressed predominantly in epithelium may also elucidate the basis of these defects. The optimism expressed must be tempered with the realization that many problems remain to be solved. However, the solution to these problems – which include the maintenance of differentiated function in culture, the relationships between cell multiplication and gene expression, and the study of interactions and communication between cells of different origins – will provide important new insights into cell regulation, embryonic development, and perhaps the failure of control associated with neoplasm.

REFERENCES

1. Krooth RS, Weinberg AN: Properties of galactosemic cells in culture. Biochem Biophys Res Commun 3:518–524, 1960.
2. Krooth RS, Howell RR, Hamilton HB: Properties of acatalasic cells growing in vitro. J Exp Med 115:313–328, 1962.
3. Dancis J, Hutzler J, Cox RP, Woody NC: Familial hyperlysinemia with lysine-ketoglutarate reductase insufficiency. J Clin Invest 48:1447–1452, 1969.
4. Dancis J, Hutzler J, Woody NC, Cox RP: Multiple enzyme defects in familial hyperlysinemia. Pediatr Res 10:686–691, 1976.
5. Dancis J, Hutzler J, Cox RP: Familial hyperlysinemia: Enzyme studies, diagnostic methods, comments on terminology. Am J Hum Genet 31:290–299, 1979.
6. Holland MJC, DiLorenzo AM, Dancis J, Balis ME, Yü TF, Cox RP: Hypoxanthine phosphoribosyltransferase activity in intact fibroblasts from patients with X-linked hyperuricemia. J Clin Invest 57:1600–1605, 1976.
7. Holland MJC, Klein NC, Cox RP: Experimental modulation of PRPP availability for ribonucleotide synthesis from hypoxanthine in human skin fibroblast cultures. Exp Cell Res 111:237–243, 1978.
8. Holland MJC, Klein NC, Cox RP, Dancis J, Yü TF, Salser JS, Balis ME: Purine excretion by cultured skin fibroblasts from patients with abnormal purine metabolism. Res Commun Chem Pathol Pharmacol 14:331–342, 1976.

Views on the Future for In Vitro Epithelial Studies on Human Birth Defects Expressed in Epithelium

This volume is the product of a one-day workshop convened to discuss the feasibility of in vitro studies on human birth defects expressed in vivo in epithelium.

In the last decade cultured skin fibroblasts have been successfully used to study birth defects expressed in vivo in connective tissue. Those studies done on inborn errors of metabolism are examples of such in vitro studies and have proven to be informative as to: 1) identification of basic defects, 2) classification within clinical groups, 3) demonstration of genetic principles established in other species, 4) identification of previously unrecognized syndromes and heterogeneity within known syndromes, and 5) importance of cellular interactions. All of this has been made possible because the fibroblast, in particular that from the dermis, is readily cultured and maintains its in vivo functions in vitro.

In the next decade it is hoped that in vitro studies will yield the same results concerning birth defects involving epithelial structures.

The aims of Part I of this volume are threefold: 1) to review the methodologies used in the past (including their observations and technical limitations), as none has led to a single established strain* of normal human epithelium, 2) to explore the "state of the art" today emphasizing promising technical approaches, and 3) to share ideas for modifying the past and present methodologies to be able to establish human epithelial strains easily.

Although there are technical problems to be overcome, they appear to be surmountable. It is obvious that the techniques established and used in the past have told us a great deal about the epithelial cell. It is apparent that methodologies being developed are based on these early studies. However, establishment of epithelial strains showing structure/function of epithelium from each epithelial-containing tissue may take a modification of old techniques or an entirely new approach. Establishment of different types of epithelium from different organ systems will probably involve its own individualistic culture environment.

*The Terminology Committee of the Tissue Culture Association adopted the following definitions: "a *cell strain* is derived either from a primary culture or a cell line by the selection . . . of cells having specific properties or markers"; "a *cell line* arises from a primary culture at the time of the first subculture" and "consists of numerous lineages of cells originally present in the primary culture." (Schaeffer WI: Proposed usage of animal tissue culture terms, revised 1978. Tissue Culture Association (TCA) Manual 4:779–792, 1978.)

Birth Defects: Original Article Series, Volume XVI, Number 2, pages 365–366

At present there is no strain of normal human epithelium available for studies on birth defects expressed in the different organ systems discussed in Part II. Although the lack of epithelial strains is recognized by all contributors to Part II, the involvement of epithelium in pathology (morphologic or structural) producing human birth defects in each organ system is presented and discussed. It is apparent that many questions cannot be answered until epithelial strains of specific types from different organs are available. It is equally evident that research is in progress or contemplated using either mixed cell cultures (containing both fibroblasts and epithelial cells) or fibroblast lines. The rationale for the use of the latter being that there will be gene expression of a mutation in any somatic cell with the mutation in its genome, irrespective of its involvement in in vivo pathology.

It is hoped that the research, thoughts, ideas, and opinions presented in this volume will inspire investigators interested in studying human birth defects expressed in epithelium to broaden their horizons to include in vitro methodologies in their attempts to understand the underlying etiologies of such birth defects to ultimately assist the involved individuals in happy, creative, and productive lives.

B. Shannon Danes, MD, PhD

Index

BOOKS PUBLISHED BY ALAN R. LISS, INC.
FOR THE NATIONAL FOUNDATION

BIRTH DEFECTS: ORIGINAL ARTICLE SERIES

1975 – Volume XI

No. 7 **Morphogenesis and Malformation of Face and Brain**, Daniel Bergsma and Jan Langman, *Editors*

1976 – Volume XII

No. 1 **Cancer and Genetics**, Daniel Bergsma, R. Neil Schimke, Robert L. Summitt, and David J. Harris, *Editors*

No. 3 **The Eye and Inborn Errors of Metabolism**, Daniel Bergsma, Anthony J. Bron and Edward Cotlier, *Editors*

No. 4 **Developmental Disabilities: Psychologic and Social Implications**, Daniel Bergsma and Ann E. Pulver, *Editors*

No. 5 **Cytogenetics, Environment and Malformation Syndromes**, Daniel Bergsma and R. Neil Schimke, *Editors*

No. 6 **Growth Problems and Clinical Advances**, Daniel Bergsma and R. Neil Schimke, *Editors*

No. 8 **Iron Metabolism and Thalassemia**, Daniel Bergsma, Anthony Cerami, Charles M. Peterson, and Joseph H. Graziano, *Editors*

1977 – Volume XIII

No. 1 **Morphogenesis and Malformation of the Limb**, Daniel Bergsma and Widukind Lenz, *Editors*

No. 2 **Morphogenesis and Malformation of the Genital System**, Richard J. Blandau and Daniel Bergsma, *Editors*

No. 3 **Annual Review of Birth Defects, 1976**, Daniel Bergsma and R. Brian Lowry, *Editors*
Proceedings of the 1976 Vancouver Birth Defects Conference.
Published in 4 volumes:
- 3A **Numerical Taxonomy of Birth Defects** *and* **Polygenic Disorders**
- 3B **New Syndromes**
- 3C **Natural History of Specific Birth Defects**
- 3D **Embryology and Pathogenesis** *and* **Prenatal Diagnosis**

No. 5 **Urinary System Malformations in Children**, Daniel Bergsma and John W. Duckett, *Editors*

No. 6 **Trends and Teaching in Clinical Genetics**, Daniel Bergsma, Frederick Hecht, Gerald H. Prescott, and Joan H. Marks, *Editors*

1978 – Volume XIV

No. 1 **Genetic Effects on Aging**, Daniel Bergsma and David E. Harrison, *Editors*

No. 2 **The Molecular Basis of Cell-Cell Interaction**, Richard A. Lerner and Daniel Bergsma, *Editors*

No. 3 **The Genetics of Hand Malformations,** *by* Samia A. Temtamy and Victor A. McKusick

No. 5 **Neurochemical and Immunologic Components in Schizophrenia,** Daniel Bergsma and Allan L. Goldstein, *Editors*

No. 6 **Annual Review of Birth Defects, 1977,** Robert L. Summitt and Daniel Bergsma, *Editors*
Proceedings of the 1977 Memphis Birth Defects Conference.
Published in 3 volumes:
- 6A **Cell Surface Factors, Immune Deficiencies, Twin Studies**
- 6B **Recent Advances** *and* **New Syndromes**
- 6C **Sex Differentiation** *and* **Chromosomal Abnormalities**

No. 7 **Morphogenesis and Malformation of the Cardiovascular System,** Glenn C. Rosenquist and Daniel Bergsma, *Editors*

1979 – Volume XV

No. 1 **Sex Chromosome Aneuploidy: Prospective Studies on Children,** Arthur Robinson, Herbert A. Lubs, and Daniel Bergsma, *Editors*

No. 2 **Genetic Counseling: Facts, Values, and Norms,** Alexander M. Capron, Marc Lappé, Robert F. Murray, Jr., Tabitha M. Powledge, Sumner B. Twiss, and Daniel Bergsma, *Editors*

No. 3 **Recent Advances in the Developmental Biology of Central Nervous System Malformation,** Ntinos C. Myrianthopoulos and Daniel Bergsma, *Editors*

No. 4 **Continuous Transcutaneous Blood Gas Monitoring,** A. Huch, R. Huch, and J. Lucey, *Editors*

No. 5 **Annual Review of Birth Defects, 1978,** Proceedings of the 1978 San Francisco Birth Defects Conference. Published in 3 volumes:
- 5A **Diagnostic Approaches to the Malformed Fetus, Abortus, Stillborn, and Deceased Newborn,** Mitchell S. Golbus and Bryan D. Hall, *Editors*
- 5B **Penetrance and Variability in Malformation Syndromes,** James J. O'Donnell and Bryan D. Hall, *Editors*
- 5C **Risks, Communication, and Decision Making in Genetic Counseling,** Charles J. Epstein, Cynthia J.R. Curry, Seymour Packman, Sanford Sherman, and Bryan D. Hall, *Editors*

No. 6 **Dermatoglyphics – Fifty Years Later,** Wladimir Wertelecki and Chris C. Plato, *Editors*

No. 7 **Newborn Behavioral Organization: Nursing Research and Implications,** Gene Cranston Anderson and Beverly Raff, *Editors*

No. 8 **Developmental Aspects of Craniofacial Dysmorphology,** Michael Melnick and Ronald Jorgenson, *Editors*

No. 9 **External Ear Malformations: Epidemiology, Genetics, and Natural History,** by Michael Melnick and Ntinos C. Myrianthopoulos